English for Pharmacy Writing
and Oral Communication

English for Pharmacy Writing and Oral Communication

Miriam Díaz-Gilbert

Assistant Director, Writing Center
Lecturer of English, Humanities Department
University of Sciences in Philadelphia
Philadelphia, PA

Wolters Kluwer | Lippincott Williams & Wilkins
Health

Philadelphia · Baltimore · New York · London
Buenos Aires · Hong Kong · Sydney · Tokyo

Acquisitions Editor: John Goucher
Managing Editor: Andrea M. Klingler
Marketing Manager: Christen D. Murphy
Creative Director: Doug Smock
Compositor: International Typesetting and Composition

351 West Camden Street   530 Walnut Street
Baltimore, MD 21201   Philadelphia, PA 19106

Printed in the United States of America.

9 8 7 6 5 4 3 2 1

DISCLAIMER

Care has been taken to confirm the accuracy of the information present and to describe generally accepted practices. However, the authors, editors, and publisher are not responsible for errors or omissions or for any consequences from application of the information in this book and make no warranty, expressed or implied, with respect to the currency, completeness, or accuracy of the contents of the publication. Application of this information in a particular situation remains the professional responsibility of the practitioner; the clinical treatments described and recommended may not be considered absolute and universal recommendations.

The authors, editors, and publisher have exerted every effort to ensure that drug selection and dosage set forth in this text are in accordance with the current recommendations and practice at the time of publication. However, in view of ongoing research, changes in government regulations, and the constant flow of information relating to drug therapy and drug reactions, the reader is urged to check the package insert for each drug for any change in indications and dosage and for added warnings and precautions. This is particularly important when the recommended agent is a new or infrequently employed drug.

Some drugs and medical devices presented in this publication have Food and Drug Administration (FDA) clearance for limited use in restricted research settings. It is the responsibility of the health care provider to ascertain the FDA status of each drug or device planned for use in their clinical practice.

To purchase additional copies of this book, call our customer service department at **(800) 638-3030** or fax orders to **(301) 223-2320**. International customers should call **(301) 223-2300**.

Visit Lippincott Williams & Wilkins on the Internet: http://www.lww.com. Lippincott Williams & Wilkins customer service representatives are available from 8:30 am to 6:00 pm, EST.

I dedicate this book to all of the pharmacy students, pharmacy technicians, and practicing pharmacists I have had the great pleasure of teaching and learning from, and to the future pharmacy professionals I will teach. They are the true inspiration for my writing this much-needed book. May they learn from it in good health. I also dedicate this book to my loving family for their everlasting support and love—my husband Jonathan, my daughter Jonna, and my son Sebastian. I love you!

Preface

English for Pharmacy Writing and Oral Communication is a language skills textbook that incorporates pharmacy and medical language and knowledge. The textbook is intended for pharmacy students, pharmacy technicians, and practicing pharmacists whose first or best language is not English. The book integrates vocabulary, pronunciation, listening, reading, and writing skills, along with idiomatic language. *English for Pharmacy Writing and Oral Communication* has been written with the following goals in mind: (i) to serve the English language needs of students and professionals studying and practicing pharmacy; (ii) to assist pharmacy faculty, who teach pharmacy, and pharmacy technician students, whose first or best language is not English, with their pharmacy language learning needs; (iii) to help pharmacy students, pharmacy technicians, and practicing pharmacists develop and gain communication confidence; and (iv) to help those for whom English is not their first or best language to master a solid foundation of pharmacy-related language dedicated to patient communication and care.

Organizational Philosophy

Effective and acceptable writing and oral communication skills are essential to success. In pharmacy, lack of good communication skills can lead to misspellings of words and drug names, medication errors, and much more. For pharmacy students, pharmacy technicians, and practicing pharmacists whose first or best language is not English, assessing patients, counseling patients, and documenting subjective information from patients who sometimes use idiomatic expressions can be challenging. Assessing, counseling, and documenting require a good command of spoken and written language and acceptable pronunciation and listening comprehension skills, as well as a solid knowledge of pharmacy-related language dedicated to patient communication and care.

 English for Pharmacy Writing and Oral Communication is written with the learner in mind. The language and learning activities are presented in a straightforward, meaningful, purposeful, and engaging manner. The textbook and accompanying audio files found on thePoint (thePoint.lww.com/diaz-gilbert) will help prepare students to enter their pharmacy education and the profession with the communication skills, knowledge, and confidence essential to function effectively in the pharmacy health care setting.

Chapter Organization

The design of each chapter provides students opportunities to acquire new medical and pharmacy-related language, to practice and reinforce new skills in an interactive and engaging manner, to retain these new language skills and knowledge, and to then reinforce them in subsequent chapters. Each chapter is dedicated to a body system and contains meaningful and purposeful medical and pharmacy-related language related to that body system.

 Chapters 1 through 12 are organized similarly. Each chapter begins with a Pre-Assessment section containing true/false and multiple choice questions to gauge the student's existing knowledge of language related to that body system, medical conditions, and general medical and pharmacy-related language. The Post-Assessment section at the end of each chapter contains true/false and multiple choice questions and listening comprehension dialogues followed by multiple choice questions to gauge the learner's thorough understanding of the chapter's content and his or her listening comprehension skills.

The first half of each chapter is devoted to the following written language skills and exercises:

Medical Vocabulary—In this section, students are presented with medical vocabulary related to the chapter body system.

Parts of Speech—In this section, students will learn, develop, enhance, and demonstrate their knowledge of the English parts of speech and word forms using sentences related to the chapter body system.

Typical Medical Conditions and Patient Complaints—In this section, students will learn, develop, enhance, and demonstrate their knowledge of the English parts of speech and word forms using sentences related to typical medical conditions and patient complaints related to the chapter body system.

Medical Vocabulary Comprehension—In this section, students will demonstrate their understanding and comprehension of the content presented in the Parts of Speech and Word Forms section and in the Typical Medical Conditions and Patient Complaints section by answering true/false multiple choice questions.

Writing Exercise—In this section, students will demonstrate their comprehension and their ability to write about designated medical conditions and diseases presented in the chapter.

These sections will help students to learn, read, recognize, and retain language found in written medical and pharmacy-related language in the context of the body system, medical conditions, and patient complaints. The student will also practice his or her reading comprehension, writing, and spelling skills by completing the various exercises.

The second half of each chapter is devoted to the following aural, oral, and pronunciation skills and exercises:

Listening and Pronunciation—In this section, students will listen to the audio files found on thePoint (thePoint.lww.com/diaz-gilbert) for correct pronunciation of the medical vocabulary presented in the Medical Vocabulary section and will practice the pronunciation of the provided terms.

Listening/Spelling—In this section, students will listen to dictated sentences in the audio files found on thePoint (thePoint.lww.com/diaz-gilbert) related to the chapter, and then write down what they hear. Students will integrate their listening and writing skills and practice and demonstrate their ability to write what they hear.

Pharmacist/Patient Dialogues—In this section, students will listen to authentic dialogues in the audio files found on thePoint (thePoint.lww.com/diaz-gilbert) typically found during pharmacist/patient communication in a pharmacy and other pharmacy-related health care settings. The dialogues integrate the content from the chapter with authentic patient medical conditions and disorders, prescriptions, side effects, and general patient counseling. Students will practice listening to authentic spoken communication between a pharmacist and patients and then demonstrate their comprehension skills by answering a series of multiple choice questions.

Idiomatic Expressions—In this section, students will learn idioms that contain body parts vocabulary. They will learn the meaning of the idioms and listen to mini-dialogues in the audio files found on thePoint (thePoint.lww.com/diaz-gilbert) that contain the idiom. The students will then demonstrate their comprehension through a short multiple choice exercise.

These activities will help students to learn, recognize, aurally and orally comprehend, write, and pronounce language commonly encountered in pharmacy and medical settings and in pharmacist/patient communication. Each chapter also contains a sidebar of English sounds that are difficult for speakers of other languages to pronounce.

Chapter 13 consists of a Pre-Assessment section containing true/false and multiple choice questions that gauge the student's knowledge of pharmacy documentation vocabulary, medical and pharmacy abbreviations, and pharmacy documentation forms. The Post-Assessment section contains true/false and multiple choice questions to gauge the learner's comprehension of that chapter's content. The chapter is devoted to the following written pharmacy documentation skills and exercises:

Pharmacy Documentation Vocabulary—In this section, students are presented with key vocabulary related to written pharmacy documentation.

Pharmacy Documentation Vocabulary and Abbreviations—In this section, students are presented with abbreviations related to medical and pharmacy documentation. The students will practice and demonstrate their ability to recognize pharmacy documentation language and abbreviations through fill-in-the-blank and multiple choice exercises.

Pharmacy and Medical Abbreviations Exercises—In this section, students will practice and demonstrate their ability to read written documentation in the form of short passages and provide abbreviations for designated vocabulary words from the passages.

Abbreviations Writing Exercises—In this section, students will put into practice their ability to comprehend abbreviations by rewriting abbreviated sentences into complete sentences.

Pharmacy Documentation Abbreviations Comprehension—In this section, students will demonstrate comprehension of written pharmacy documentation and abbreviations presented in the chapter by answering multiple choice and true/false questions.

Pharmacy Documentation and Standardized Patient Forms—In this section, students will be introduced to the SOAP note and the Patient History and Physical Database models of patient pharmacy documentation. Students will be introduced to a patient scenario and will practice completing a SOAP note and a Patient History and Physical Database to demonstrate their comprehension.

Pharmacy Documentation Forms Comprehension—In this section, students will demonstrate their understanding of the patient scenarios documentation and abbreviations in the patient scenario by answering true/false and multiple choice questions.

These sections will help students to read, recognize, and write patient pharmacy documentation and abbreviations, and to successfully complete a SOAP note and the Patient History and Physical Database. Students will practice and enhance their written pharmacy documentation skills.

Using the Textbook and the Website

English for Pharmacy Writing and Oral Communication and the accompanying website have been designed to meet, develop, and enhance the English language needs of pharmacy students and professionals whose first or best language is not English. It can be used as a supplement in a pharmacy communication class, as a textbook in ESL classes composed of pharmacy technician students and pharmacy students, and as a self-taught textbook for practicing pharmacy technicians and practicing pharmacists who cannot be in a classroom setting but who are able to use the textbook and website at their own pace and in the comfort of their home, the workplace, or school. The website can be accessed at thePoint.lww.com/diaz-gilbert.

For Instructors and Students

English for Pharmacy Writing and Oral Communication contains several appendices to further aid learning. The online Answer Key provides the answers to the exercises in each chapter (available at thePoint.lww.com/diaz-gilbert). Students and instructors can quickly check answers as soon as they complete an exercise and monitor their progress. Appendix A contains all the scripts from the pharmacist/patient dialogues and the mini-dialogues that are on the accompanying website. Students and instructors can quickly refer to the scripts for further practice or for clarification. Appendix B contains a sample Pharmacotherapy Patient Work-Up, which students and instructors will find a useful additional source of patient pharmacy documentation.

Acknowledgments

I would like to thank the reviewers of my book proposal and my manuscript. Their fabulous reviews, positive feedback, and support kept me energized as I wrote each chapter. I can't express my gratitude enough to my Managing Editor, Karen Ruppert. I could not have done it without her support and enthusiasm for each chapter. We laughed out loud a lot through our e-mail exchanges. I would also like to thank David Troy, Senior Acquisitions Editor, and Barrett Kroger, Acquisitions Editor, for their enthusiasm and support through the writing of the manuscript. A great big thanks to Andrea Klingler, Managing Editor, Michael Marino, Managing Editor-Ancillaries, Ed Schultes, Jr. and Freddie Patane from Media Services at Lippincott Williams & Wilkins, Michael Licisyn, and to voice over artists Michael Yurcaba, Deneane Richburg and Karen Ballerini for their enthusiastic participation in the success of my book. And to Rasika Mathur, for assisting me with "marathon" proofing.

Finally, I want to thank my student staff and tutoring staff in the writing center for their support, for being excited for me, for putting up with my kookiness, and for patiently listening to my dialogue ideas. They are Jenny, Melanie, Gayana, Sneha, Alice, Tonia, Jamie, Judi, Norma, Michelle, and Mary Ellen.

Reviewers

Rachel Abrishami, PharmD
USC/Ralphs Community Pharmacy Resident
University of Southern California
Compton, CA

Linda Albrecht, RPh, MBA
Instructor and Externship Coordinator
Richland College, UT Austin
Arlington, TX

Jennifer Borowski, PharmD
Assistant Professor
Long Island University and Bronx East
  Montefiore Medical Center
Bronx, NY

Tracy Call-Schmidt, MSN, FNP
Assistant Professor
University of Utah
Salt Lake City, UT

Shelley Chambers-Fox, PhD
Associate Professor
Washington State University
Pullman, WA

Patricia Darbishire, PharmD
Purdue University
Lafayette, IN

Beverly Hawkins, CPhT
Lab Instructor
AH/Pharm Tech
Chattanooga State Community College
Chattanooga, TN

Karl Hess, PharmD
Community Pharmacy Practice Resident
University of Southern California
Los Angles, CA

Scott Higgins, MA
Technology Education College
Columbus, OH

Doris C. Kalamut, RPh, BScPhm
Coordinator in Professional Practice
University of Toronto
Toronto, Ontario

Candace Smith, PharmD
Associate Clinical Professor
Clinical Pharmacy Practice Department
St. John's University
College of Pharmacy and Allied Health Professions
Queens, NY

Kristy J. Spetz, PharmD
Concord Pharmacy
Glen Mills, PA

Contents

Preface **vii**
Acknowledgments **xi**
Reviewers **xiii**

Chapter 1: Skin, Hair, and Nails 1

Chapter 2: Ears and Eyes 25

Chapter 3: Mouth and Nose 51

Chapter 4: Endocrine and Lymphatic System 77

Chapter 5: Chest, Lung, and Respiratory System 103

Chapter 6: Heart and Cardiovascular System 129

Chapter 7: The Abdomen and Gastrointestinal System 155

Chapter 8: The Musculoskeletal System 181

Chapter 9: Neurologic System and Mental Health 207

Chapter 10: The Urinary System 231

Chapter 11: Hepatic System 253

Chapter 12: Reproductive System 275

Chapter 13: Writing Pharmacy Documentation 301

Appendix A: Dialogues 333

Appendix B: Pharmacotherapy Workup Notes 393

Index 401

English for Pharmacy Writing and Oral Communication

Skin, Hair, and Nails | 1

True/False Questions

Indicate whether each sentence below is true (T) or false (F).

1. _____ A **scar** is a cut on the skin.
2. _____ **Dandruff** is dead skin that falls from a person's head.
3. _____ **Flaky** is an adjective form.
4. _____ Some individuals allergic to certain detergents can develop a very **itchy rash** on their hands.
5. _____ The adjective form of **blister** is blistery.
6. _____ Irritants such as solvents and cosmetics do not **trigger** contact dermatitis.
7. _____ **Prickly heat** can cause a skin rash.
8. _____ **Blisters** on the toes and feet, which may **ooze** a clear or bloody liquid, can be caused by wearing brand new shoes or shoes that are too tight.
9. _____ A **rough, scaly** patch of skin is very moist.
10. _____ The noun form of **itchy** is itch.
11. _____ **Brittle** nails are strong.
12. _____ **Athlete's foot** is a fungal infection that causes itching and burning between the toes.
13. _____ If **pus** is produced in an infected part of the body, the infected part is healing itself.
14. _____ If a person is allergic to penicillin, he or she can **break out in hives.**
15. _____ The word **scarred** is a past tense verb and adjective form.

Multiple Choice Questions

Choose the correct answer from a, b, and c.

1. _____ "It hurts a lot when I **bump the area**" means:
a. when I hit the area
b. when I massage the area
c. when I rub the area

2. _____ If you are **tearing your hair out** while sitting in a traffic jam on your way to the pharmacy, you are:
a. pulling your hair, one strand at a time
b. very angry and anxious
c. breaking off the split ends

3. _____ A **cluster of lesions** on the arm means:

a. many scabs

b. a few scars

c. a group of wounds

4. _____ He passed the exam **by the skin of his teeth** means:

a. he had a skin rash on the day of the exam

b. he is an expert and very experienced

c. he almost failed the exam

5. _____ If a patient complains of **flaky** skin on the head, the patient most likely has:

a. dandruff

b. alopecia

c. head lice

6. _____ A common skin condition in adolescents is:

a. acne

b. sunburn

c. impetigo

7. _____ A **keloid** is:

a. brittle

b. scar tissue

c. a laceration

8. _____ The verb and adjective from of **laceration:**

a. lacerated

b. lacerate

c. laceration

9. _____ A **zit** is another word for:

a. scab

b. wound

c. pimple

10. _____ The patient complained that her fingernail was **oozing pus.** This could indicate she has:

a. a brittle nail

b. a sharp nail

c. an ingrown nail

How did you do? Check your answers in the Answer Key online.

MEDICAL VOCABULARY

A good understanding of vocabulary words in pharmacy is very important for communication with professors, fellow students, patients, and coworkers. Knowledge and understanding of vocabulary leads to successful communication and success as a pharmacy student, as a pharmacy technician, and as a practicing pharmacist. You may already know many of the vocabulary words in this chapter, but for words that are unfamiliar, pay careful attention to them and make every effort to know their correct spelling, meaning, and pronunciation. It is a good idea to keep a list of new words and to look up these new words in a bilingual dictionary or dictionary in your first language. A good command of pharmacy-related vocabulary and good pronunciation of vocabulary will help to prevent embarrassing mistakes and increase effective verbal communication skills.

Skin Vocabulary

abscess	flaky	rupture
acne	gash	scabies
birthmark	hangnail	scabs
black nail	hives	scales
black toe	inflammation	scar
blister	irritation	scrape
boils	itch	scratch
break out	keloid	shingles
bruise	laceration	sore
bump	lesion	spider bite
chiggers	moist	superficial
clear up	mole	sweat
cracked	ooze	tick bite
crusty	patch	ulcers
cyst	pimple	wart
dermatitis	pins and needles	wound
diaper rash	prickly heat rash	wrinkles
dry	psoriasis	zit
eczema	pus	
excrete	pustules	

Hair Vocabulary

alopecia	fine	scalp
coarse	hair loss	silky
dandruff	head lice	
dry	oily	

Nail Vocabulary

black nail	cuticle	peeling nail
black toe	floating	splitting nail
brittle	fungal infection	
clubbing	ingrown nail	

PARTS OF SPEECH

A good understanding of parts of speech, such as verbs, nouns, adjectives, and adverbs, is important for successful communication when speaking or writing. It is equally important to know the various forms of words and to use them appropriately.

Word Forms

The table below lists the main forms of some terms that you will likely encounter in pharmacy practice. Review the table and then do the exercises that follow to assess your understanding.

Noun (n)	Infinitive/Verb (v) —Past Tense	Adjective (adj)	Adverb (adv)
a blister	to blister; blistered	blistery	
a boil	to boil; boiled	boiling; boiled	
brittleness		brittle	brittlely
a bruise	to bruise; bruised	bruised	
a bump	to bump; bumped	bumpy	
a crack	to crack; cracked	cracked; cracking	
a crust	to crust; crusted	crusty; crusting	
dryness	to dry; dried	dry; dried; drying	dryly
eczema		eczematous	
excretion	to excrete; excreted	excreted	
flakes; flakiness	to flake; flaked	flaky	flakily
inflammation	to inflame; inflamed	inflamed; inflammatory	
irritation; irritant	to irritate; irritated	irritable; irritated; irritating	irritably
itch; itchiness	to itch; itched	itchy; itching	
laceration	to lacerate; lacerated	lacerated	
moistness	to moisten; moistened	moist	moistly
oil; oiliness	to oil; oiled	oily; oiled	
ooze	to ooze; oozed	oozy	
a patch	to patch; patched	patchy; patched	
a pimple		pimply; pimpled	pimplier
psoriasis		psoriatic	
pus		pussy*	
a rupture	to rupture; ruptured	rupturing; ruptured	
a scab	to scab; scabbed	scabby; scabbed	
a scar	to scar; scarred	scarred; scarring	
a scrape	to scrap; scraped	scraped	
a sore		sore	sorely
sweat	to sweat; sweated	sweaty; sweating	sweatily
a swell	to swell; swelled	swollen; swelling; swelled	
an ulcer; an ulceration		ulcerated	
a wound	to wound; wounded	wounded; wounding	

*Caution: When *pussy* **is pronounced (p$\overline{oo}$ s$'\overline{e}$), the speaker is referring to a cat, as in** *pussy cat,* **or to a gentle person, or using it as a vulgar word to refer to a female sexual organ or to a male who is weak. However, when used in** *pussy sore,* **pussy is pronounced (p$\overset{\smile}{u}$ s$'\overline{e}$).**

Word Forms Exercise

Read the following sentences carefully. Then indicate the word form of the bolded word(s), choosing from v, n, adj, or adv.

1. Her lips are **cracked** as a result of the cold weather.

   cracked _____

2. The **rash** on her skin is very **itchy.**

   rash _____   itchy _____

3. Her scalp is **dry** but her hair is **oily.**

   dry _____   oily _____

4. She **dried** her skin completely before she applied the ointment.

   dried _____

5. The **scab** did not heal well and now the area is **scarred.**

   scab _____   scarred _____

6. It was not a superficial **wound,** but a deep **laceration.**

   wound _____   laceration _____

7. She **lacerated** her hand while opening the sharp lid of the cat food can.

   lacerated _____

8. The **wound** was filled with **pus.**

   wound _____   pus _____

9. Keep the sterile gauze on the **laceration** and be careful not to **wound** it again.

   laceration _____   wound _____

10. Her fingernails left big **scratch** marks on her **itchy** skin.

    scratch _____   itchy _____

11. The **boil** under her skin **ruptured.**

    boil _____   ruptured _____

12. The new body lotion she rubbed on her skin **irritated** her skin.

    irritated _____

13. If he doesn't get treatment for his acne, his face is going to become more **pimply.**

    pimply _____

14. He **scraped** his already **bruised** knees after he fell off his bike again.

    scraped _____   bruised _____

15. When she is speaking in front of an audience, she becomes very nervous and her hands become very **sweaty.**

    sweaty _____

How did you do? Check your answers against the Answer Key online.

Typical Medical Conditions and Patient Complaints

The sentences below contain vocabulary that describes and explains typical medical conditions, diseases, symptoms, and patient complaints that a pharmacist encounters. Read the sentences carefully. Then indicate the word form of the bolded word(s), choosing from v, n, adj, or adv. Look up words you do not know in your bilingual or first-language dictionary.

1. **Acne** is a skin condition that many adolescents and some adults experience, usually on the face. The acne, which is also called **pimples,** can consist of **white heads** or **black heads.** White heads are pimples that are white in color, and black heads are black in color.

   acne _____   pimples _____   white heads _____   black heads_____

2. After washing the dishes with a new liquid detergent, the woman's hands and wrists **broke out** in a very itchy rash. The pharmacist recommended an over-the-counter ointment, which stopped the **itchy rash.** Soon the woman stopped **scratching** her hands and wrists, and the rash **cleared up.**

   broke out _____   itchy_____   rash _____   scratching _____   cleared up_____

3. Some individuals develop a **keloid** after a **wound** or a surgical incision has healed. The keloid is a thick **scar tissue.**

   keloid _____   wound _____   scar tissue _____

4. Another word for **alopecia** is baldness, which is hair loss.

   alopecia _____

5. It is not uncommon for children to contract **head lice,** wingless insects that live in their hair or scalp, from other children.

   head lice _____

6. People with **dandruff** will experience **dry, itchy scalp.** Whether or not they **scratch** their head, **flakes** of dead skin can be seen on their hair and on their clothes, especially on their shoulders.

   dandruff _____   dry _____   itchy _____   scalp _____   scratch _____   flakes _____

7. **Brittle** nails break easily.

   brittle _____

8. A **scab** is mainly dry blood that forms over a cut or a **wound** on the skin. If it does not heal properly, the scab may **ooze pus** and become infected.

   scab _____   wound _____   ooze _____   pus _____

9. The young boy's knees became **inflamed** after he fell off his skateboard. Not only did he **scrape** his right elbow, he also got a deep bloody **gash,** a **wound,** on both knees that did not heal right away.

   inflamed _____   scrape _____   gash _____   wound _____

10. She **lacerated** her left index finger while slicing the tomato and tore off a piece of skin at the tip of the finger below the nail. What she thought was a **superficial wound** was actually a deep **wound** that required sutures.

    lacerated _____   superficial wound _____   wound _____

11. Some medications may cause the skin to **sweat.**

    sweat _____

12. He developed a **bump** on the right wrist after being hit with a baseball. Two days later, the bump turned a reddish black color and began to **ooze** liquid.

    bump _____   ooze _____

13. The red, **itchy patch** of **flaky** dry skin on her left forearm caused her to **scratch** so hard that soon it began to bleed.

    itchy _____   patch _____   flaky _____   scratch _____

14. The **scrape** on his knee healed nicely and did not form a **scab** or a **scar.**

    scrape _____   scab _____   scar _____

15. The **cyst** on her forehead **ruptured** and **oozed** bloody pus.

    cyst _____   ruptured _____   oozed _____

16. The **fungal infection** in his right toe caused **black toe,** and the nail eventually fell off.

fungal infection _____   black toe _____

17. Children with **head lice** will scratch their head because it itches.

head lice _____

18. A **wart** is a small **bump** on the foot or hand that is caused by a virus.

wart _____   bump _____

19. **Shingles** is a very painful **rash** caused by a virus.

shingles _____   rash _____

20. The skin of nervous people will sometimes **break out into hives** that are itchy and bumpy, as will the skin of some people who are allergic to cats.

break out into _____   hives _____

How did you do? Check your answers against the Answer Key online.

Medical Vocabulary Comprehension

Now that you have read sentences 1 through 20 describing language regarding skin, hair, and nails, assess your understanding by doing the exercises below.

Multiple Choice Questions

Choose the answer that correctly completes each sentence below.

1. _____ **Pimples** are:
a. lacerations on the skin
b. flakes of dead skin
c. acne, a skin condition that consists of black heads or white heads

2. _____ A **scab:**
a. is dry blood that forms on the skin
b. causes the skin to sweat
c. is a patch of flaky skin

3. _____ A **gash:**
a. is a superficial cut
b. oozes pus
c. is a deep wound

4. _____ People with **alopecia:**
a. have gray hair
b. are bald
c. have a full head of hair

5. _____ People with **dandruff** have:
a. a dry and flaky scalp
b. bumps on their head
c. brittle hair

6. _____ If a skin condition **clears up,** it means:
a. the pus is clear
b. it has healed
c. it is itchy

7. _____ A **ruptured cyst** is:

a. another word for scab

b. another word for laceration

c. a growth on the skin that has broken open or burst

8. _____ A **superficial wound** is:

a. a deep laceration

b. a bump

c. not deep

9. _____ A **scrape** on the skin is a:

a. cyst

b. scar

c. small mark on the skin caused by a rough surface

10. _____ An example of thick **scar tissue** is a:

a. keloid

b. laceration

c. pimple

11. _____ Small wingless insects on children's hair and scalp are:

a. hives

b. head lice

c. dandruff

12. _____ A **wart** is a:

a. white head

b. pimple

c. bump on the skin caused by a virus

13. _____ **Shingles** is a:

a. painful rash on the skin caused by a virus

b. skin condition caused by prickly heat

c. scrape that hasn't cleared up

14. _____ White heads and black heads are examples of:

a. alopecia

b. head lice

c. acne

15. _____ **Sweaty** skin is:

a. dry

b. moist

c. flaky

True/False Questions

Indicate whether each sentence below is true (T) or false (F).

1. _____ If a patient complains that pus is oozing from his skin, it means that the skin is dry.

2. _____ If a patient complains that she needs an over-the-counter treatment for acne, it means that the patient needs treatment for baldness.

3. _____ If the pharmacist tells a patient that the medicine may make the skin itch, it means the patient's skin will sweat.

4. _____ A scrape on the skin is a much more serious injury than a gash.

5. _____ If fingernails are brittle, they are strong and healthy.

6. _____ If you are allergic to cats, you might break out in hives.

7. _____ The word "itchy" is a noun.

8. _____ The word "wound" is both a verb and a noun.

9. _____ If a lesion is oozing blood, it means the lesion has formed into a scab.

10. _____ A scrape on the skin is a gash.

How did you do? Check your answers against the Answer Key online.

Writing Exercise

An important part of communication is the ability to write about what you read, to write correctly, and to spell correctly. In the exercises below, write your understanding of the meaning of the bolded words.

1. Describe in writing what a **laceration,** a superficial **wound,** a **gash,** and a **scrape** are.

_____

_____

_____

_____

2. Describe in writing what a **scab,** a **scar,** and a **keloid** are.

_____

_____

_____

_____

3. Describe in writing what **acne,** a **pimple,** a **black head,** and a **white head** are.

_____

_____

_____

_____

4. Describe in writing what **baldness, dandruff,** and **head lice** are.

_____

_____

_____

_____

5. Describe in writing what **athlete's foot** and **ingrown nail** are.

_____

_____

_____

_____

Check what you have written with acceptable answers that appear in the Answer Key online.

LISTENING AND PRONUNCIATION

The ability to listen and understand what is being said and heard, and the ability to pronounce words clearly, is extremely important. A word misheard and a word mispronounced will lead to poor communication and can seriously put both the pharmacist and patient in danger. Therefore, it is very important that one hear clearly what another person has said, and that one speak clearly with correct pronunciation.

Listen carefully to the pharmacy-related words presented in the audio files found in Chapter 1 on thePoint (thePoint.lww.com/diaz-gilbert), and then pronounce them as accurately as you can. Listen and then repeat. You will listen to each word once and then you will repeat it. You will do this twice for each word. Listening and pronunciation practice will increase your listening and speaking confidence. Many languages do not produce or emphasize certain sounds produced and emphasized in English, so pay careful attention to the pronunciation of each word.

Pronunciation Exercise

Listen to the audio files found in Chapter 1 on thePoint (thePoint.lww.com/diaz-gilbert). Listen and repeat the words. Then say the words aloud for additional practice.

1. abscess — ăb′sĕs
2. acne — ăk′nē
3. alopecia — ăl′ə-pē′shə
4. birthmark — bûrth′märk′
5. black nail — blăk nāl
6. black toe — blăk tō
7. blister — blĩs′t ə r
8. boil — boil
9. breakout — brāk out
10. brittle — brĩt′l
11. bruise — brōōz
12. bump — bŭmp
13. chiggers — chĭg′ərz
14. clear up — klîr ŭp
15. coarse — kôrs
16. cracked — krăkt
17. crusty — krŭs′tē
18. cuticule — kyōō′tĭ-kəl
19. cyst — sĭst
20. dandruff — dăn′drəf
21. dermatitis — dûr′mə-tī′tĭs
22. diaper rash — dī′ə-pər răsh
23. dry — drī
24. eczema — ĕk′sə-mə
25. excrete — ĭk-skrēt′
26. fine — fīn
27. flaky — flā′kē
28. fungal infection — fŭng′gəl ĭn-fĕk′shən
29. gash — găsh
30. hair loss — hâr lôs
31. head lice — hĕd līs
32. hives — hīvz
33. inflammation — ĭn′flə-mā′shən
34. ingrown nail — ĭn′grōn′ nāl
35. irritation — ĭr′ĭ-tā′shən
36. itch — ĭch

37. keloid	kē′loid
38. laceration	lăs′ə-rā′shən
39. lesion	lē′zhən
40. moist	moist
41. mole	mōl
42. oily	oi′lē
43. ooze	ōoz
44. patch	păch
45. peeling	pē′lĭng
46. pimple	pĭm′pəl
47. pins and needles	pĭns ənd nēd′ls
48. prickly heat	prĭk′lē hēt
49. psoriasis	sə-rī′ə-sĭs
50. pus	pŭs
51. rash	răsh
52. rupture	rŭp′chə
53. scab	skăb
54. scabies	skā′bēz
55. scales	skālz
56. scar	skär
57. scrape	skrāp
58. scratch	skrăch
59. shingles	shĭng′gəlz
60. silk	sĭlk
61. sore	sôr
62. sunscreen	sŭn′skrēn′
63. superficial	sōo′pər-fĭsh′əl
64. sweat	swĕt
65. swollen	swō′lən
66. tick bite	tĭk bīt
67. ulcer	ŭl′sər
68. wart	wôrt
69. wound	wōond
70. wrinkles	rĭng′kəls
71. zit	zĭt

Which words are easy to pronounce? Which are difficult to pronounce? Use the space below to write in the words that you find difficult to pronounce. These are words you should practice saying often.

_____

_____

_____

_____

_____

_____

_____

Listen to the audio files found in Chapter 1 on thePoint (thePoint.lww.com/diaz-gilbert) as many times as you need to increase your pronunciation ability of the difficult words. Pronounce these words with a friend or a colleague who speaks English.

English Sounds That Are Difficult for Speakers of Other Languages to Pronounce

Spanish

In Spanish, there is no English "v" sound, but the "v" consonant in Spanish is pronounced like the English "b." The vowel "i" is pronounced like a long "e." Pay careful attention to the "v" sound in English when pronouncing words that begin with "v." Also pay careful attention to English words that begin with "s;" do not use the Spanish "es" sound when pronouncing English words that begin with "s."

For example, in English,

vane is not pronounced bane
scratch is not pronounced escratch
scar is not pronounced escar
itch is not pronounced eetch

Vietnamese

In Vietnamese, the "t" consonant is pronounced "s," but in English the "t" is pronounced "t" and "s" is pronounced "s." Be careful with English words that begin with "t." In Vietnamese, the "b" consonant is pronounced "p," but in English "p" is pronounced "p" and "b" is pronounced "b."

In Vietnamese, words do not end in "b," "ch," "f," "d," "j," "l," "p," "r," "s," "sh," "v," and "z." In English, words end in these letters. Pay special attention to pronouncing these English sounds. In Vietnamese, there is no "dzh" or "zh" sound, so English words like "judge" (dzh) and "rupture" (zh) will be hard for Vietnamese speakers to pronounce.

For example, in English,

bump is not pronounced pum
gash is not pronounced gah
dandruff is not pronounced dandruh
rash is not pronounced rah

Gujarati

In Gujarati, "v" is pronounced "w," "f" is pronounced "p," "p" is pronounced "f," and "z" is pronounced "j." Short "i" is pronounced long "e," "x" is pronounced "ch," and "th" is pronounced "s." In English, "v" is pronounced "v," "f" is pronounced "f," "z" is pronounced "z" or "s," "j" is pronounced "j," and "x" is pronounced "x." Pay careful attention when pronouncing these sounds.

For example, in English,

wart is not pronounced vart
fungal is not pronounced pungal
bump is not pronounced bumf
tick is not pronounced teek
path is not pronounced pass
zit is not pronounced jit

Korean

In Korean, the "v" consonant is pronounced "b" and the "f" consonant is pronounced "p." In English, the "v" is pronounced "v," the "f" is pronounced "f," and the "p" is pronounced "p." Pay special attention when pronouncing these sounds.

(continued)

For example, in English,

fungal is not pronounced pungal
vane is not pronounced bane

Chinese

In Chinese, the "r" consonant is pronounced "l" or "w," and "b," "d," "g," and "ng" are not pronounced at all. Pay careful attention to English words that begin with "r" because the "r" is not pronounced "l" or "w," and "b," "d," "g," and "ng" are pronounced in English.

For example, in English,

rash is not pronounced lash
keloid is not pronounced keloi
peeling is not pronounced peelin
scab is not pronounced sca

Russian

The "w" consonant is pronounced like a "v" and the "v" sounds like a "w." Pay careful attention to the English "th." It is not pronounced "s."

For example, in English,

wart is not pronounced vart
vein is not pronounced wein
thank is not pronounced sank
thought is not pronounced sought

DICTATION

Listening/Spelling Exercise: Word and Word Pairs

Listen to the words or word pairs on the audio files found in Chapter 1 on thePoint (thePoint.lww.com/diaz-gilbert), and then write them down on the lines below.

1. _____
2. _____
3. _____
4. _____
5. _____
6. _____
7. _____
8. _____
9. _____
10. _____
11. _____
12. _____
13. _____
14. _____
15. _____

Listening/Spelling Exercise: Sentences

Listen to the sentences on the audio files found in Chapter 1 on thePoint (thePoint.lww.com/diaz-gilbert), and then write them down on the lines below.

1. _____
   _____
2. _____
   _____
3. _____
   _____
4. _____
   _____
5. _____
   _____
6. _____
   _____
7. _____
   _____
8. _____
   _____
9. _____
   _____
10. _____
    _____

Now, check your sentences against the correct answers in the Answer Key online. If there are any new words that you do not know or that you spelled incorrectly, make a list of those words and study them for meaning and spelling.

PHARMACIST/PATIENT DIALOGUES

The ability to orally communicate effectively with your professors, colleagues, and especially with patients is very important. As a pharmacist, you will be counseling patients; patients will come to you for advice. They will have questions about a condition and symptoms they may experience and will ask you to help treat the condition. Therefore, it is extremely important that you understand what they are saying and that you respond to them and their questions appropriately. Your patients will speak differently. For example, some may speak very quickly, others too low, and yet others may speak angrily. To help you improve your listening skills, listen to the following dialogues, or short conversations, between a pharmacist and a patient and between a pharmacy technician and a patient.

 Listening and Comprehension Exercises
Dialogue #1

Listen to Dialogue #1, stop, listen again and take notes. Listen to the dialogue as many times as you need or until you feel you have written sufficient notes and feel confident. You can use your notes to answer the multiple choice questions at the end of the dialogue.

Notes _____
_____
_____
_____
_____

Answer the questions below by selecting the answer that correctly completes each sentence.

1. _____ What is the patient's complaint?
a. she can't swallow tablets
b. she is allergic to jellyfish
c. she has bumps on her body from the waist down

2. _____ Which part of the body does the patient claim has bumps?
a. from the waist down
b. her arms only
c. her entire body

3. _____ Before recommending treatment, what does the pharmacist ask the patient?
a. how long she had been scratching
b. if she is allergic to any medication
c. how long she was swimming in the ocean

4. _____ What over-the-counter medicine does the pharmacist recommend?
a. betadine in liquid form only
b. Benadryl in liquid form only and a shot of hydrocortisone
c. Benadryl in liquid form because the patient can't swallow tablets, and hydrocortisone cream

5. _____ The pharmacist tells the patient:
a. to call her doctor if the rash and itching continue
b. that she can continue to swim in the ocean as long as she takes the medication
c. that her skin will become very dry

Check your answers in the Answer Key online. How did you do? Are there new words you do not know? Take the time now to look them up in your bilingual or first-language dictionary.

Dialogue #2

Listen to Dialogue #2, stop, listen again and take notes. Listen to the dialogue as many times as you need or until you feel you have written sufficient notes and feel confident. You can use your notes to answer the multiple choice questions at the end of the dialogue.

Notes _____

_____

_____

_____

_____

Answer the questions below by selecting the answer that correctly completes each sentence.

1. _____ The patient is complaining that:
a. he has an ingrown nail on his big left toe
b. his left toe has a laceration
c. his right toe is oozy and blistery

2. _____ The patient is wearing open-toe sandals because:
a. it is summertime
b. his right toe is sensitive to the touch
c. he has foot odor

3. _____ The pharmacist tells the patient that:

a. he has an infected toe caused by wearing tight shoes with no socks

b. his toe is peeling

c. he has a fungal infection caused by the moist environment of a wet sneaker and wet socks rubbing against his toe

4. _____ The patient is allergic to:

a. sulfa only

b. sulfa and iodine

c. iodine only

5. _____ The pharmacist tells the patient to find:

a. fungicide in aisle 5

b. Lidocaine in aisle 3

c. Lamisil in aisle 3

6. _____ The patient's right toenail will:

a. never grow back

b. grow back in 1 week

c. grow back in a few months

7. _____ The pharmacist suggests that the patient:

a. continue to run in wet socks

b. see a podiatrist or a primary care doctor if the toe does not get better

c. run races in open-toe shoes

Check your answers in the Answer Key online. How did you do? Are there new words you do not know? Take the time now to look them up in your bilingual or first-language dictionary.

Dialogue #3

Listen to Dialogue #3, stop, listen again and take notes. Listen to the dialogue as many times as you need or until you feel you have written sufficient notes and feel confident. You can use your notes to answer the multiple choice questions at the end of the dialogue.

Notes _____

_____

_____

_____

_____

Answer the questions below by selecting the answer that correctly completes each sentence.

1. _____ The child's mother is concerned because her daughter:

a. has dandruff

b. has an itchy scalp

c. is not happy in day camp

2. _____ Her daughter is:

a. 16 months old

b. 6 years old

c. 6 weeks old

3. _____ The pharmacist tells the mother that:

a. head lice taste like sesame seeds

b. head lice look like sesame seeds

c. sesame seed is another name for head louse

4. _____ The pharmacist recommends that the mother:

a. purchase a louse comb and Nix, a medicated anti-lice treatment

b. wash only her daughter's hair and the pillowcases

c. remove the head lice with her fingers

5. _____ Nix is:

a. a type of head lice

b. a cream rinse applied to the hair after shampooing to remove head lice

c. an antibiotic

6. _____ The pharmacist tells the mother that she and her husband should also treat their hair with Nix because head lice are:

a. contagious

b. not contagious

c. infectious

7. _____ The mother thinks her daughter may have picked up head lice:

a. on vacation

b. in day care

c. in day camp

Check your answers in the Answer Key online. How did you do? Are there new words you do not know? Take the time now to look them up in your bilingual or first-language dictionary.

IDIOMATIC EXPRESSIONS

Idioms and idiomatic expressions are made up of a group of words that have a different meaning from the original meaning of each individual word. Native speakers of the English language use such expressions comfortably and naturally. However, individuals who are new speakers of English or who have studied English for many years may still not be able to use idioms and idiomatic expressions as comfortably or naturally as native speakers. As pharmacy students, pharmacy technicians, and practicing pharmacists, you will hear many different idiomatic expressions. Some of you will understand and know how to use these expressions correctly. At times, however, you may not understand what your professors, colleagues, and patients are saying. This of course can lead to miscommunication, embarrassment, and possibly dangerous mistakes.

To help you improve your knowledge of idioms and idiomatic expressions, carefully read the following idiomatic expressions that contain the body words of skin, hair, and nail.

Idiomatic Expressions using "Skin"

1. **by the skin of my teeth** means that the person succeeded in doing something but almost failed.

    For example: I passed my pharmacy exam **by the skin of my teeth.**

2. **to be thick skinned** means that the person does not get easily upset.

    For example: Because I'm **thick skinned,** almost failing the exam did not upset me.

3. **to get under my skin** means that someone annoys or upsets others by the way that they behave.

    For example: People who behave like they know it all really **get under my skin.**

4. *to make my skin crawl* means that a person has made others uncomfortable, upset, or afraid.

For example: Sometimes patients who are very impatient and who demand their prescriptions immediately *make my skin crawl*.

5. *to be skin deep* is used to mean that something that is seen as important is not really important because it only appears that way.

For example: Beauty is only *skin deep*.

Idiomatic Expressions using "Hair"

1. *to get in my hair* means that someone is annoying or bothering me.

For example: I try not to let the sick patients at the pharmacy *get in my hair* during the cold season.

2. *to let my hair down* means that I am behaving in a relaxed manner.

For example: I'm usually a very serious and professional person, but sometimes I *let my hair down* after work and go dancing with my friends.

3. *to tear my hair out* means to become very anxious or worried.

For example: I began to *tear my hair out* after I was told that I needed to fill 25 prescriptions in 1 hour.

4. *to keep your hair on* means to stay calm.

For example: *Keep your hair on!* Don't let the stress of the job upset you.

5. *make your hair stand on end* means to be frightened and shocked.

For example: My professor's rude behavior in class sometimes makes the students' *hair stand on end*.

Idiomatic Expressions using "Nail"

1. *to be hard as nails* or *tough as nails* means one is strong and determined.

For example: My boss is *tough as nails.*

2. to be *nail biting* means the situation makes you nervous because you are waiting for something important to happen.

For example: Waiting to hear whether I had gotten into pharmacy school was a real *nail biting* experience because there were only 10 seats for more than 100 applicants.

Mini Dialogues Listening Exercise

How much did you understand? Listen to the following mini dialogues on the audio files found in Chapter 1 on thePoint (thePoint.lww.com/diaz-gilbert), read the questions below, and then choose the correct answer.

 Mini Dialogue #1

1. _____ *Let your hair down* means:

a. to wear one's hair long

b. to relax

c. to fill the prescriptions quickly

Mini Dialogue #2

2. _____ ***Hair stand on end*** means:

a. to remain calm

b. to have no tender feelings

c. to be frightened and shocked

 Mini Dialogue #3

3. _____ ***Getting under my skin*** means:

a. the new pharmacist gets easily upset

b. to annoy others with one's behavior

c. to stay calm

 Mini Dialogue #4

4. _____ ***Get in my hair*** means:

a. to bother and annoy

b. to be worried and anxious

c. to say or do the right thing

 Mini Dialogue #5

5. _____ ***Tearing my hair out*** means:

a. to worry and to be anxious

b. to relax

c. to not worry

 Mini Dialogue #6

6. _____ ***Tough as nails*** means:

a. brittle

b. strong and determined

c. to be mean

How did you do? Check your answers against the Answer Key online.

POST-ASSESSMENT

True/False Questions

Indicate whether each sentence below is true (T) or false (F).

1. _____ The idiom **pulling my hair out** means the individual has head lice.

2. _____ The noun form of **to inflame** is inflammatory.

3. _____ Another word for pimple is keloid.

4. _____ The adjective form of the word **scratch** is scratchy.

5. _____ If a person **gets under your skin,** the person annoys you by the way he or she behaves.

6. _____ Another word for head lice is dandruff.

7. _____ A bloody toe blister is an example of a white head.

8. _____ The past tense and adjective forms of **scrape** is scraped.

9. _____ Acne is a form of dry skin.

10. _____ A laceration is a superficial wound.

11. _____ If a person is **thick skinned,** it means he or she has a big bump on the skin.

12. _____ If a patient complains that his foot is burning and itching, he most likely has an infected ingrown toenail.

13. _____ A keloid is a swollen scab.

14. _____ Head lice are insects that bite the skin.

15. _____ A person with alopecia has head lice.

Multiple Choice Questions

Choose the correct answer from a, b, and c.

1. _____ The adjective form of **scratch** is:

a. scratched

b. scratchy

c. scratched and scratchy

2. _____ If a person has **athlete's foot,** the person:

a. is a fast runner

b. plays many sports

c. has a fungal infection

3. _____ If a person is **tearing his or her hair out,** the person:

a. is balding

b. is worried and anxious

c. has alopecia

4. _____ A child with head lice:

a. needs to scratch his or her head

b. needs to remove the head lice with his or her fingers

c. needs to have his or her hair combed with a louse comb and treated with anti-lice treatment

5. _____ In the sentence, "I have a bruised bump on my head," the word **bruised** is:

a. a past tense verb

b. an adjective

c. a noun

6. _____ The adjective form of **sweat** is:

a. sweaty, sweating, and sweatily

b. sweaty and sweating

c. sweating and sweated

7. _____ Scratch marks are:

a. produced on the skin from scratching too much

b. caused by a jellyfish sting

c. caused by a laceration

8. _____ A person who is **tough as nails:**

a. has healthy nails

b. has brittle nails

c. is strong and determined

9. _____ Dried blood that is formed on the skin after a cut or wound is healed is called:

a. a laceration

b. a scab

c. a scrape

10. _____ In the sentence, "The girl complained of an itchy sensation on her arm," the word **itchy** is:

a. an adjective

b. a verb

c. a noun

11. _____ The word **wound** is:

a. both a verb and a noun

b. a verb only

c. a noun only

12. _____ A superficial wound is:

a. a deep gash

b. a deep laceration

c. not deep

13. _____ An oozy blister can contain:

a. pus

b. lice

c. scabs

14. _____ The word **swell** is:

a. a noun, a verb, and an adjective

b. a noun only

c. an adjective

15. _____ In the sentence, "Because the scab on the skin did not heal properly, the area is scarred," the word **scarred** is used as:

a. an adjective

b. a past tense verb

c. a noun

Listening and Comprehension Exercises

Dialogue #1

Listen to Dialogue #1, stop, listen again and take notes. Listen to the dialogue as many times as you need or until you feel you have written sufficient notes and feel confident. You can use your notes to answer the multiple choice questions at the end of the dialogue.

Notes_____

_____

_____

_____

_____

Answer the questions below by selecting the answer that correctly completes each sentence.

1. _____ The patient tells the pharmacist her arm:

a. has itchy bumps

b. has a deep gash

c. is painful and itchy

2. _____ The patient asks the pharmacist for:

a. a cream to reduce the swelling and itchiness

b. Tylenol

c. an antibiotic

3. _____ The pharmacist asks the patient if she:

a. has been bitten by an insect

b. went camping on Labor Day

c. has called her doctor

4. _____ The pharmacist tells the patient she has:

a. impetigo

b. inflammation

c. itchiness

5. _____ The pharmacist recommends the patient contact the doctor for an antibiotic:

a. today

b. in 1 week

c. in 1 day

Dialogue #2

Listen to Dialogue #2, stop, listen again and take notes. Listen to the dialogue as many times as you need or until you feel you have written sufficient notes and feel confident. You can use your notes to answer the multiple choice questions at the end of the dialogue.

Notes _____

_____

_____

_____

_____

Answer the questions below by selecting the answer that correctly completes each sentence.

1. _____ The patient complains that his feet are:

a. oozing pus

b. burning and itching

c. dry

2. _____ When the patient says that he is tearing his hair out, he means that:

a. he is bald

b. his hair is dry

c. he is anxious and worried

3. _____ Characteristics of athlete's foot are:

a. blistering skin

b. dry and itchy skin

c. scaliness, in combination with burning and itching

4. _____ The pharmacist recommends:

a. a cream to help stop the burning and itchiness on his foot

b. an antibiotic to stop the burning and itchiness on his foot

c. a pill he can take

5. _____ The pharmacist instructed the patient to:

a. wash and completely dry his feet, even between the toes, before applying Lamisil

b. apply the cream with the feet still wet

c. wash and completely dry his feet, even between the toes, before applying Lamisil and to change his socks daily

 Dialogue #3

Listen to Dialogue #3, stop, listen again and take notes. Listen to the dialogue as many times as you need or until you feel you have written sufficient notes and feel confident. You can use your notes to answer the multiple choice questions at the end of the dialogue.

Notes _____

_____

_____

_____

_____

Answer the questions below by selecting the answer that correctly completes each sentence.

1. _____ The patient's bad habit is:

a. splitting her nails

b. biting her nails

c. painting her nails

2. _____ The patient complains that her finger is:

a. red, swollen, and painful

b. lacerated

c. breaking out in hives

3. _____ The patient noticed that her finger discharged:

a. a white head

b. a rash

c. yellow pus

4. _____ The patient's finger is:

a. red only

b. red, inflamed, painful, and discharging pus

c. discharging pus only

5. _____ The pharmacist recommends that she soak her finger in:

a. table salt

b. Epsom salts

c. iodized salt

6. _____ The pharmacist also recommends the patient apply:

a. peroxide and Neosporin

b. peroxide only

c. Neosporin only

How did you do on the Post-Assessment in Chapter 1? Check your answers in the Answer Key online.

Ears and Eyes | 2

PRE-ASSESSMENT

True/False Questions

Indicate whether each sentence below is true (T) or false (F).

1. _____ A person with **conjunctivitis** has swollen eyes.
2. _____ A **cataract** can make lamplight or sunlight seem too bright or glaring.
3. _____ Children with an **ear infection** will sometimes tug on their ears.
4. _____ One way to reduce **ear wax** is to put drops of baby oil in the ear.
5. _____ The adjective form of **infection** is infected.
6. _____ A **foreign body** in the eye can cause it to become irritated, red, and painful.
7. _____ A **stye** is a bumpy, red, itchy infection in the middle ear.
8. _____ Infants with an **ear infection** will experience inconsolable crying.
9. _____ A **cataract** is a yellow discharge from the eye.
10. _____ The noun form of **itchy** is itch.
11. _____ **Pink eye** is another term for conjunctivitis.
12. _____ A person should never use a warm compress over the ear to relieve an **earache.**
13. _____ **Glaucoma** can lead to blindness.
14. _____ A **droopy eye** is swollen and itchy.
15. _____ The word **swell** is a noun and verb form.

Multiple Choice Questions

Choose the correct answer from a, b, and c.

1. _____ "My ear feels like it's clogged up" means:
a. the ear is infected
b. the ear is closed
c. the ear feels tight

2. _____ If you are **all ears** while listening to the professor's lecture, you are:
a. putting your hands over your ears during the lecture
b. very interested in the lecture and paying attention
c. you can't hear the lecture

3. _____ **Ear popping** is caused by:
a. pressure in the ear
b. wax in the ear
c. a broken eardrum

4. _____ If you can't see **eye to eye** with another person, it means:

a. you have weak vision

b. the other person is blind

c. you can't agree with the person

5. _____ If a patient complains of **blurred vision,** the patient should be tested for:

a. glaucoma

b. dry eye

c. conjunctivitis

6. _____ A common ear condition in infants is:

a. swimmer's ear

b. middle ear infection

c. fungal infection

7. _____ If a person has **tunnel vision,** he or she:

a. can only see things that are straight ahead

b. can only see in the dark

c. can only see around them

8. _____ The word **discharge** is:

a. a verb

b. a verb and a noun

c. a noun

9. _____ **Pink eye** is another term for:

a. crusty eyes

b. a stye

c. conjunctivitis

10. _____ The patient complained that she had a yellow, green, and watery **discharge** from her eye. This could indicate she has:

a. a droopy eye

b. an eye infection

c. an eyelash in her eye

How did you do? Check your answers in the Answer Key online.

MEDICAL VOCABULARY

A good understanding of vocabulary words in pharmacy is very important for communication with professors, fellow students, patients, and coworkers. Knowledge and understanding of vocabulary leads to successful communication and success as a pharmacy student, as a pharmacy technician, and as a practicing pharmacist. You may already know many of the vocabulary words in this chapter, but for words that are unfamiliar, pay careful attention to them and make every effort to know their correct spelling, meaning, and pronunciation. It is a good idea to keep a list of new words and to look up these new words in a bilingual dictionary or dictionary in your first language. A good command of pharmacy-related vocabulary and good pronunciation of vocabulary will help to prevent embarrassing mistakes and increase effective verbal communication skills.

Ear Vocabulary

airplane ear	cauliflower ear	dizziness
buzzing	deafness	drainage

ear lobe	middle ear infection	tinnitus
ear plug	perforated eardrum	tugging
fluid	pressure	vertigo
foreign body	ringing	wax
hearing loss	swimmer's ear	

Eye Vocabulary

astigmatism	dry eye	lazy eye
blinking	eyeball	macular degeneration
bloodshot	eyelid	nearsightedness
blurred	eye herpes	night vision
bulging eye	eye pressure	optic nerve
cataract	eye strain	peripheral vision
clogged	farsightedness	photophobia
conjunctivitis	floaters	pink eye
contact lens	focus	pupils
cornea	fuzzy vision	retina
cross-eyed	glare	secrete
crusty eyelid	glaucoma	squinting
distorted vision	grittiness	tears
double vision	halos	twitching
droopy eyelid	jaundice	watery

PARTS OF SPEECH

A good understanding of parts of speech, such as verbs, nouns, adjectives, and adverbs, is important for successful communication when speaking or writing. It is equally important to know the various forms of words and to use them appropriately.

Word Forms

The table below lists the main forms of some terms that you will likely encounter in pharmacy practice. Review the table and then do the exercises that follow to assess your understanding.

Noun (n)	Infinitive/Verb (v) —Past Tense	Adjective (adj)	Adverb (adv)
a blink	to blink; blinked	blinking	
a blur	to blur; blurred	blurred; blurry	
a bulge; bulginess	to bulge; bulged	bulged; bulging; bulgy	
a clog	to clog; clogged	clogged	
distortion	to distort; distorted	distorted; distorting	
deafness		deaf; deafening	
dizziness		dizzy; dizzier	dizzily; dizzyingly

(*continued*)

Noun (n)	Infinitive/Verb (v) —Past Tense	Adjective (adj)	Adverb (adv)
drainage	to drain; drained	drained; draining; drainable	
droop	to droop; drooped	droopy; drooping	droopingly
focus	to focus; focused	focused	
fluid; fluidity	to flow; flowed	flowing	flowingly
fuzziness; fuzz		fuzzy	fuzzily
glare	to glare; glared	glaring	glaringly
grit; grittiness	to grit; gritted	gritty	grittily
jaundice		jaundiced	
lump	to lump; lumped	lumpy	
presbyopia		presbyopic	
pressure	to pressure; pressured	pressured	
ring	to ring; rang	ringing	
squint; squinter	to squint; squinted	squinting	
tear;* tearfulness	to tear; teared	tearing; teary; tearful; tearless	tearfully
tug	to tug; tugged	tugging	tuggingly
twitch	to twitch; twitched	twitching	twitchily
wax	to wax; waxed	waxing; waxy	

*Caution: The pronunciation of this form of tear is (tîr) and not (târ); tore is the past tense of (târ).

Word Forms Exercise

Read the following sentences carefully. Then indicate the word form of the bolded word(s), choosing from v, n, adj, or adv.

1. The foreign body in his eye caused him to **blink.**

   blink _____

2. The doctor told her that **tugging** and pulling on her earlobe might be a sign of swimmer's ear.

   tugging _____

3. Because her eyes are sensitive to light, she **squints** a lot when she's outdoors on a sunny day.

   squints _____

4. A buildup of **fluid** or **wax** in the ear can cause hearing problems.

   fluid _____   wax _____

5. **Jaundice** is a yellowish discoloration of the whites of the eyes.

   jaundice _____

6. Some of the symptoms experienced by people with **airplane ear** are **hearing loss** and **ringing** in the ear.

   airplane ear _____   hearing loss _____   ringing _____

7. She accidentally **perforated** her **eardrum** after inserting a Q-tip in her ear to remove the **wax** from her ear.

   perforated _____   eardrum _____   wax _____

8. Dandruff and bacteria can cause inflammation of the **eyelid** and cause the eye to **tear** and the eyelids to become **crusty.**

   eyelid _____   tear _____   crusty _____

9. A sudden loud noise, explosion, or too much pressure from **fluid** in the ear can cause the eardrum to **rupture.**

   fluid _____   rupture _____

10. A **cataract** can cause a person's vision to **blur** and make him or her sensitive to sunlight and **glare.**

    cataract _____   blur _____   glare _____

11. The **stye** on her left eyelid was **itchy** and **bumpy** and looked like a **pimple.**

    stye _____   itchy _____   bumpy _____   pimple _____

12. **Foreign objects** in your ear, such as a cotton swab or a bobby pin, can cause an eardrum to **rupture;** and foreign objects in your eye, such as sand or dust particles, can cause the eye to become **infected.**

    foreign objects _____   rupture _____   infected _____

13. **Floaters,** which look like clouds and spots, are dark or gray spots that we see with our vision and that move as we move our eyes.

    floaters _____

14. During night driving, a person with **cataracts** will see **halos** and **glare.**

    cataracts _____   halos _____   glare _____

15. It is not unusual for the eyes of people in their 40s to have **presbyopia** or the inability to **focus** on reading materials or close objects.

    presbyopia _____   focus _____

How did you do? Check your answers against the Answer Key online.

Typical Medical Conditions and Patient Complaints

The sentences below contain vocabulary that describes and explains typical medical conditions, diseases, symptoms, and patient complaints that a pharmacist encounters. Read the sentences carefully. Then indicate the word form of the bolded word(s), choosing from v, n, adj, or adv. Look up words you do not know in your bilingual or first-language dictionary.

1. Children with **lazy eye** may have permanent eye problems if they do not get treatment.

   lazy eye _____

2. The patient complained he was experiencing tinnitus, some **hearing loss,** and **vertigo.**

   hearing loss _____   vertigo _____

3. After the mother picked up her child, who was crying inconsolably and **tugging** at her right ear, the mother noticed the child had a fever. She knew right away that her child had an **ear infection** and called the doctor.

   tugging _____   ear infection _____

4. If you experience **itching, hearing loss,** redness, **swelling, pressure,** or **fluid** in your ear, you should see your doctor.

   itching _____   hearing loss _____   swelling _____   pressure _____   fluid _____

5. Applying a warm compress to **inflamed** eyelids can help reduce the **inflammation** and help loosen the **crust** in the eye.

   inflamed _____   inflammation _____   crust _____

6. It is not uncommon for children to experience **fluid** and **wax** buildup in their ears.

   fluid _____   wax _____

7. People with **conjunctivitis** should avoid spreading it to others and re-infecting themselves by washing their hands often and by avoiding contact with their eyes such as rubbing and touching.

   conjunctivitis _____

8. **Pressure** in your ear as a result of a hit to the ear, a loud noise, or traveling in an airplane can easily **rupture** your eardrum.

   pressure _____   rupture _____

9. The eyes of people with **dry eye,** which is caused by a lack of **tears,** can appear **swollen** and feel **gritty.**

   dry eye _____   tears _____   swollen _____   gritty _____

10. One way to prevent **swimmer's ear** is to place drops of half alcohol and half white vinegar solution in your ear.

    swimmer's ear _____

11. People with eye herpes, which is a viral infection that can cause **scarring** and **inflammation** of the cornea, will experience **tearing** and **swelling** around the eye.

    scarring _____   inflammation _____   tearing _____   swelling _____

12. If you are experiencing **drainage** from your ear, see a doctor as soon as you can.

    drainage _____

13. If a person has a **bloodshot** eye, the whites of the eye are red.

    bloodshot _____

14. People who are **farsighted** have difficulty seeing objects that are close but can see objects that are far away or at a distance without difficulty.

    farsighted _____

15. To prevent **airplane ear,** people should swallow and yawn frequently and wear **ear plugs.**

    airplane ear _____   ear plugs _____

16. Working too long in front of the computer can cause **eye strain** and fatigue.

    eye strain _____

17. A **stye** is an infection near the eyelash and forms into a red **lump** filled with **pus** that will eventually burst.

    stye _____   lump _____   pus _____

18. It is not uncommon for people who are feeling faint, who have had too much alcohol, or who have had a head injury to have **double vision.**

    double vision _____

19. Swimmer's ear is caused by a fungus and will cause the ear to **itch,** the skin inside the ear canal to **flake,** and pus to **discharge** from the ear.

    itch _____   flake _____   discharge _____

20. You should be tested for **tinnitus** if you hear **ringing, buzzing,** or **hissing** sounds.

    tinnitus _____   ringing _____   buzzing _____   hissing _____

How did you do? Check your answers against the Answer Key online.

Medical Vocabulary Comprehension

Now that you have read sentences 1 through 20 describing language regarding ears and eyes, assess your understanding by doing the exercises below.

Multiple Choice Questions

Choose the answer that correctly completes each sentence below.

1. _____ **Styes** are:
a. a kind of ear infection
b. an infected lump on the eyelid
c. floaters

2. _____ Swallowing and yawning often during a plane ride will help to prevent:
a. swimmer's ear
b. ear wax
c. a ruptured ear drum

3. _____ To prevent airplane ear during a plane ride, a person should:
a. cover their ears with their hands
b. yawn and swallow frequently
c. not wear ear plugs

4. _____ In children, symptoms of an **ear infection** include:
a. tugging at the ear and crying inconsolably
b. airplane ear
c. ringing and buzzing sounds

5. _____ People experiencing **itchiness, fluid, pressure,** or **swelling** in their ear should:
a. insert a Q-tip in the ear
b. chew gum
c. see a doctor

6. _____ Another term for **pink eye** is:
a. lazy eye
b. droopy eye
c. conjunctivitis

7. _____ A **ruptured eardrum** can be caused by:
a. fungus in the ear
b. a loud noise, a foreign object, or pressure
c. wax buildup

8. _____ To help remove the **crust** from an inflamed eyelid, you should:
a. wash the eyelid with water
b. put an ice pack on the eyelid
c. put a warm compress on the eyelid

9. _____ A person who is **farsighted** sees:
a. halos
b. floaters
c. objects that are far away without difficulty

10. _____ **Dry eye** is caused by:

a. crying

b. the inability to produce tears

c. grittiness

11. _____ A person who is feeling faint or who has had too much alcohol may experience:

a. droopy eye

b. hearing loss

c. double vision

12. _____ A yellowish discoloration of the eyes is:

a. mucus

b. jaundice

c. dry crust

13. _____ Working in front of a computer for a long time can:

a. make you cross-eyed

b. cause eye strain and fatigue

c. cause macular degeneration

14. _____ **Presbyopia** is:

a. the ability to focus on close objects

b. tunnel vision

c. the inability to focus on close objects

15. _____ **Swimmer's ear** is caused by:

a. a fungus

b. an inner ear infection

c. a rupture

True/False Questions

Indicate whether each sentence below is true (T) or false (F).

1. _____ If a patient complains that his eyelid is irritated and is secreting pus that gets crusty, it means that he has dry eye.

2. _____ If a patient complains that she can see objects close up, the patient probably has tunnel vision.

3. _____ Swimmer's ear is caused by rupturing the eardrum with a Q-tip.

4. _____ If you have glaucoma, you will not see halos or have night vision problems.

5. _____ A droopy eye is a symptom of middle ear infection in children.

6. _____ A stye is a pus-filled lump inside the ear.

7. _____ The word "gritty" is an adjective.

8. _____ The word "tear" is both a verb and a noun.

9. _____ If you hear whistling, hissing, and ringing in your ears, it means you are tone deaf.

10. _____ Allergies can trigger conjunctivitis.

How did you do? Check your answers against the Answer Key online.

Writing Exercise

An important part of communication is the ability to write about what you read, to write correctly, and to spell correctly. In the exercises below, write your understanding of the meaning of the bolded words.

1. Describe in writing what a **cataract** and a **stye** are.

_____

_____

_____

_____

2. Describe in writing what a **ruptured eardrum, airplane ear,** and **swimmer's ear** are.

_____

_____

_____

_____

3. Describe in writing what **nearsightedness, farsightedness, photophobia,** and **tunnel vision** are.

_____

_____

_____

_____

4. Describe in writing what **pink eye** and **dry eye** are.

_____

_____

_____

_____

Check what you have written with acceptable answers that appear in the Answer Key online.

LISTENING AND PRONUNCIATION

The ability to listen and understand what is being said and heard, and the ability to pronounce words clearly, is extremely important. A word misheard and a word mispronounced will lead to poor communication and can seriously put both the pharmacist and patient in danger. Therefore, it is very important that one hear clearly what another person has said, and that one speak clearly with correct pronunciation.

Listen carefully to the pharmacy-related words in the audio files found in Chapter 2 on thePoint (thePoint.lww.com/diaz-gilbert), and then pronounce them as accurately as you can. Listen and then repeat. You will listen to each word once and then you will repeat it. You will do this twice for each word. Listening and pronunciation practice will increase your listening and speaking confidence. Many languages do not produce or emphasize certain sounds produced and emphasized in English, so pay careful attention to the pronunciation of each word.

 Pronunciation Exercise

Listen to the audio files found in Chapter 2 on thePoint (thePoint.lww.com/diaz-gilbert) and repeat the words. Then say the words aloud for additional practice.

1. airplane ear   âr′plā̄n′ îr
2. astigmatism   ə-stĭg′mə-tĭz′əm
3. blinking   blĭngk ŋ
4. bloodshot   blŭd′shŏt′
5. blur   blûr
6. bulging eye   bŭljŋ ī

7. buzzing   bŭzɳ

8. cataract   kăt′ə-răkt′

9. cauliflower ear   kô′lī-flou′ər îr

10. clog   klôg

11. conjunctivitis   kən-jŭngk′tə-vī′tĭs

12. contact lens   kŏn′tăkt′ lĕnz

13. cornea   kôr′nē-ə

14. cross-eyed   krôs īd

15. crusty eyelid   krŭs′tē ī′lĭd′

16. deaf   def

17. distorted   dĭ-stôrt ĭd

18. dizzy   dĭz′ē

19. double vision   dŭb′əl vĭzh′ən

20. drain   drān

21. dry eye   drī ī

22. earache   îr′āk′

23. ear lobe   îr′ lōb′

24. eyeball   ī′bôl′

25. eye herpes   ī hûr′pēz

26. eye pressure   ī prĕsh′ər

27. eye strain   ī strān

28. farsighted   fär′sī′tĭd

29. floaters   flō′tərs

30. fluid   flōō′ĭd

31. focus   fō′kəs

32. foreign body   fôr′ĭn bŏd′ē

33. fuzzy   fŭz′ē

34. glare   glâr

35. glaucoma   glou-kō′mə

36. gritty   grĭt′ē

37. halos   hā′lōs

38. hearing loss   hîr′ĭng lôs

39. jaundice   jôn′dĭs

40. lazy eye   lā′zē ī

41. macular degeneration   măkyōō lär dĭ-jĕn′ə-rā′shən

42. middle ear infection   mĭd′l îr ĭn-fĕk′shən

43. nearsighted   nîr′sī′tĭd

44. night vision   nīt vĭzh′ən

45. optic nerve   ŏp′tĭk nûrv

46. perforated eardrum   pûr′fə-rā′tĭd îr′drŭm

47. peripheral vision   pə-rĭf′ər-əl vĭzh′ən

48. photophobia   fō′tə-fō′bē-ə

49. pink eye   pĭngk ī

50. presbyopia   prĕz′bē-ō′pē-ə

51. pupil   pyōō′pəl

52. retina   rĕt′n-ə

53. ringing   rĭng ɳ

54. secrete   sĭ-krēt′

55. squint   skwĭnt

56. swimmer's ear   swĭmərz îr

57. tear   tîr

58. tinnitus   tĭ-nī′təs

59. tug   tŭg
60. twitch   twĭch
61. vertigo   vûr′tĭ-gō′
62. wax   wăks

Which words are easy to pronounce? Which are difficult to pronounce? Use the space below to write in the words that you find difficult to pronounce. These are words you should practice saying often.

_____

_____

_____

_____

_____

_____

_____

_____

Listen to the audio files found in Chapter 2 on thePoint (thePoint.lww.com/diaz-gilbert) as many times as you need to increase your pronunciation ability of the difficult words. Pronounce these words with a friend or a colleague who speaks English.

English Sounds That Are Difficult for Speakers of Other Languages to Pronounce

Spanish

In Spanish, there is no English "v" sound, but the "v" consonant in Spanish is pronounced like the English "b." The vowel "i" is pronounced like a long "e." Pay careful attention to the "v" sound in English when pronouncing words that begin with "v." Also pay careful attention to English words that begin with "s;" do not use the Spanish "es" sound when pronouncing English words that begin with "s."

For example, in English,

vertigo is not pronounced berteego
swimmer's ear is not pronounced esweemmer's ear
squint is not pronounced esqueent
secrete is not pronounced esecrete

Vietnamese

In Vietnamese, the "t" consonant is pronounced "s," but in English the "t" is pronounced "t" and "s" is pronounced "s." Be careful with English words that begin with "t." In Vietnamese, the "b" consonant is pronounced "p," but in English "p" is pronounced "p" and "b" is pronounced "b."

In Vietnamese, words do not end in "b," "ch," "f," "d," "j," "l," "p," "r," "s," "sh," "v," and "z." In English, words end in these letters. Pay special attention to pronouncing these English sounds. In Vietnamese, there is no "dzh" or "zh" sound, so English words like "judge" (dzh) and rupture (zh) will be hard for Vietnamese speakers to pronounce.

For example, in English,

buzzing is not pronounced puzzing
twitch is not pronounced twih
nearsighted is not pronounced nearsigh
pressure is not pronounced prehso

(continued)

Gujarati

In Gujarati, "v" is pronounced "w," "f" is pronounced "p," "p" is pronounced "f," and "z" is pronounced "j." Short "i" is pronounced long "e," "x" is pronounced "ch," and "th" is pronounced "s." In English, "v" is pronounced "v," "f" is pronounced "f," "z" is pronounced "z" or "s," "j" is pronounced "j," and "x" is pronounced "x." Pay careful attention when pronouncing these sounds.

For example, in English,

wax is not pronounced vax
farsighted is not pronounced parsighted

Korean

In Korean, the "v" consonant is pronounced "b" and the "f" consonant is pronounced "p." In English, the "v" is pronounced "v," the "f" is pronounced "f," and the "p" is pronounced "p." Pay special attention when pronouncing these sounds.

For example, in English,

focus is not pronounced pocus
vertigo is not pronounced bertigo

Chinese

In Chinese, the "r" consonant is pronounced "l" or "w," and "b," "d," "g," and "ng" are not pronounced at all. Pay careful attention to English words that begin with "r" because the "r" is not pronounced "l" or "w," and "b," "d," "g," and "ng" are pronounced in English.

For example, in English,

eyelid is not pronounced eyelih
bloodshot is not pronounced bluhshah

Russian

The "w" consonant is pronounced like a "v" and the "v" sounds like a "w." Pay careful attention to the English "th." It is not pronounced "s."

For example, in English,

wax is not pronounced vax
vertigo is not pronounced wertigo

DICTATION

 ### Listening/Spelling Exercise: Word and Word Pairs

Listen to the words or word pairs on the audio files found in Chapter 2 on thePoint (thePoint.lww.com/diaz-gilbert) and then write them down on the lines below.

1. _____
2. _____
3. _____
4. _____
5. _____
6. _____
7. _____

8. _____

9. _____

10. _____

11. _____

12. _____

13. _____

14. _____

15. _____

Listening/Spelling Exercise: Sentences

Listen to the sentences on the audio files found in Chapter 2 on thePoint (thePoint.lww.com/diaz-gilbert) and then write them down on the lines below.

1. _____
_____

2. _____
_____

3. _____
_____

4. _____
_____

5. _____
_____

6. _____
_____

7. _____
_____

8. _____
_____

9. _____
_____

10. _____
_____

Now, check your sentences against the correct answers in the Answer Key online. If there are any new words that you do not know or that you spelled incorrectly, make a list of those words and study them for meaning and spelling.

PHARMACIST/PATIENT DIALOGUES

The ability to orally communicate effectively with your professors, colleagues, and especially with patients is very important. As a pharmacist, you will be counseling patients; patients will come to you for advice. They will have questions about a condition and symptoms they may experience and will ask you to help treat the condition. Therefore, it is extremely important that you understand what they are saying and that you respond to them and their questions appropriately. Your patients will speak differently. For example, some may speak very quickly, others too low, and yet others may speak angrily. To help you improve your listening skills, listen to the following dialogues, or short conversations, between a pharmacist and a patient and between a pharmacy technician and a patient.

Listening and Comprehension Exercises

Dialogue #1

Listen to Dialogue #1, stop, listen again and take notes. Listen to the dialogue as many times as you need or until you feel you have written sufficient notes and feel confident. You can use your notes to answer the multiple choice questions at the end of the dialogue.

Notes _____

_____

_____

_____

_____

Answer the questions below by selecting the answer that correctly completes each sentence.

1. _____ What is the patient's complaint?
a. She can't wear contact lenses
b. She woke up with her left eye crusted and shut tight
c. She woke up with her right eye crusted and shut tight

2. _____ Throughout the day the patient's eye:
a. got worse
b. got better
c. stayed the same

3. _____ The patient's eye is:
a. itchy
b. itchy, swollen, and really red
c. gritty

4. _____ What condition does the patient have?
a. a stye
b. crusty eye syndrome
c. conjunctivitis

5. _____ The patient has a prescription for:
a. tobramycin tablets
b. tobramycin ointment
c. tobramycin solution

6. _____ The pharmacist tells the patient to use:
a. 4 eyedrops once a day
b. 1 eyedrop every 4 hours
c. 4 eyedrops every hour

Check your answers in the Answer Key online. How did you do? Are there new words you do not know? Take the time now to look them up in your bilingual or first-language dictionary.

Dialogue #2

Listen to Dialogue #2, stop, listen again and take notes. Listen to the dialogue as many times as you need or until you feel you have written sufficient notes and feel confident. You can use your notes to answer the multiple choice questions at the end of the dialogue.

Notes _____

_____

_____

_____

_____

Answer the questions below by selecting the answer that correctly completes each sentence.

1. _____ The patient's mother is complaining that her daughter:

a. has an earache

b. has an ear infection and is crying non-stop

c. is crying non-stop

2. _____ The doctor prescribed:

a. penicillin

b. baby oil eardrops

c. an antibiotic

3. _____ The antibiotic is:

a. astigmatism

b. amoxicillin

c. Augmentin

4. _____ The patient is:

a. almost 3 years old

b. 3 months old

c. 36 months old

5. _____ The pharmacist recommends that the patient's mother buy a:

a. measuring spoon

b. dose-measuring spoon

c. regular spoon

6. _____ The pharmacist tells the patient's mother to call the doctor immediately if her daughter:

a. has some diarrhea

b. gets a rash, starts itching, or starts wheezing

c. stops crying

7. _____ The pharmacist tells the patient's mother to:

a. keep the medicine in the refrigerator

b. make sure her daughter takes the entire medicine even if she starts to feel better

c. both a and b

Check your answers in the Answer Key online. How did you do? Are there new words you do not know? Take the time now to look them up in your bilingual or first-language dictionary.

Dialogue #3

Listen to Dialogue #3, stop, listen again and take notes. Listen to the dialogue as many times as you need or until you feel you have written sufficient notes and feel confident. You can use your notes to answer the multiple choice questions at the end of the dialogue.

Notes _____

_____

_____

_____

_____

Answer the questions below by selecting the answer that correctly completes each sentence.

1. _____ The patient tells the pharmacist that the eye doctor gave him a prescription to treat his:

a. glaucoma

b. hematoma

c. high blood pressure

2. _____ The name of the prescription is:

a. Isopto Cetamide

b. Isopto Carpine

c. Isopto Tears

3. _____ The pharmacist explains that the medication will help:

a. increase pressure in the eyes and decrease vision problems

b. reduce pressure in the eyes and help to prevent vision problems

c. decrease pressure in the eyes but not increase vision

4. _____ The patient:

a. lives at the same address and is allergic to Visine

b. lives at the same address, has the same insurance, and has no allergies

c. lives at the same address and has no insurance

5. _____ The pharmacist instructs the patient that after squirting the drops in his eyes, the patient should:

a. try to wink

b. try not to blink

c. try to shut his eyes tight

6. _____ The patient's name is:

a. Al Mangini and he is 60 years old

b. Aldo Mancine and he is 44 years old

c. Aldo Mancini and he is 62 years old

7. _____ The patient's birth date is:

a. April 15, 1945

b. April 4, 1944

c. April 5, 1944

8. _____ Common side effects of the medication include:

a. watery discharge

b. irritation, burning, and stinging

c. swelling and stinging

9. _____ The correct spelling of the eyes drops is:

a. I-S-O-T-O-P-E   C-A-R-B-O-N

b. I-S-O-T-O-P   C-A-R-P-I-N

c. I-S-O-P-T-O   C-A-R-P-I-N-E

10. _____ The following information is on the prescription label:
  a. the pharmacist's name, the pharmacy phone number, and number of times patient will need to use the eyedrops
  b. the pharmacy phone number and the number of times the patient will need to use the eyedrops
  c. the side effects only

Check your answers in the Answer Key online. How did you do? Are there new words you do not know? Take the time now to look them up in your bilingual or first-language dictionary.

IDIOMATIC EXPRESSIONS

Idioms and idiomatic expressions are made up of a group of words that have a different meaning from the original meaning of each individual word. Native speakers of the English language use such expressions comfortably and naturally. However, individuals who are new speakers of English or who have studied English for many years may still not be able to use idioms and idiomatic expressions as comfortably or naturally as native speakers. As pharmacy students, pharmacy technicians, and practicing pharmacists, you will hear many different idiomatic expressions. Some of you will understand and know how to use these expressions correctly. At times, however, you may not understand what your professors, colleagues, and patients are saying. This of course can lead to miscommunication, embarrassment, and possibly dangerous mistakes.

To help you improve your knowledge of idioms and idiomatic expressions, carefully read the following idiomatic expressions that contain the body words of eye and ear.

Idiomatic Expressions using "Eye"

1. ***keep an eye out*** for something means that the person should look for, watch, find, or notice something.

   For example: You need to ***keep an eye out*** for any allergic reactions to the medication.

2. ***to have eyes in the back of one's head*** means that the person knows everything that is happening around him or her even with the back turned.

   For example: Mothers with children usually have ***eyes in the back of their head*** when their children are playing outdoors.

3. ***to have eyes like a hawk*** means that the person can notice every small detail so it would be difficult to deceive that person.

   For example: My boss has ***eyes like a hawk,*** so I try not to eat while I'm dispensing medicines to patients.

4. ***to have a good eye*** for something means that a person has the ability to notice and recognize something of good quality, something that is valuable, etc.

   For example: The pharmacy technician who pays attention to every detail ***has a good eye*** for recognizing fake prescriptions.

5. ***to have your eyes glued*** to something means you are watching something with all your attention, or you are not able to move because you are frightened of something.

   For example: Everyone in the office had their ***eyes glued*** to the TV news report about the pharmacist who went to jail for stealing prescription medicines.

6. ***to be hit between the eyes*** means the person has received surprising and shocking news.

   For example: She was really ***hit between the eyes*** when she did not receive the promotion to pharmacy regional manager.

Idiomatic Expressions using "Ear"

1. ***to lend an ear*** means to listen sympathetically to someone.

   For example: It important to ***lend an ear*** to patients who are medically ill when they speak to you.

2. *to turn a deaf ear* means that the person is ignoring and pretending not to hear what the other person is saying.

For example: It's not always a good idea to ***turn a deaf ear*** to patient complaints that you feel are not serious.

3. *to be wet/green behind the ears* means to be new at your job or to have little experience.

For example: Because I was still ***wet/green behind the ears,*** I made several nonfatal mistakes switching the patient labels on the prescription bottles.

4. *to be up to your ears* in something means that you are very busy.

For example: Because she was ***up to her ears*** in work, she called another pharmacist to help her fill the prescriptions.

5. *to bend someone's ear* means to talk to someone for a long time about your problems or concerns.

For example: Some patients will ***bend their pharmacist's ear*** about their health problems.

6. *to smile/grin from ear to ear* means to be very happy.

For example: She ***smiled from ear to ear*** for a week after learning she had passed the pharmacy licensing exam.

Mini Dialogues Listening Exercise

How much did you understand? Listen to the following mini dialogues in the audio files found in Chapter 2 on thePoint (thePoint.lww.com/diaz-gilbert), read the questions below, and then choose the correct answer.

Mini Dialogue #1

1. _____ *Smiling from ear to ear* means:

a. the person has been hired by three pharmacies

b. the person took the licensing exam three times before she passed

c. the person is very happy

Mini Dialogue #2

2. _____ *My eyes were glued* means:

a. I sat close to the TV because I could not see

b. I watched the soccer game with all my attention

c. I was frightened and shocked

Mini Dialogue #3

3. _____ *Up to his ears* means:

a. the new head pharmacist can talk for a long time

b. the new head pharmacist is very busy with work

c. the new pharmacist is in shock

Mini Dialogue #4

4. _____ *Bend your ear* means:

a. to pay careful attention to someone's problems

b. to damage your ear

c. to talk a very long time to someone else about one's problems

Mini Dialogue #5

5. _____ ***Green behind the ears*** means:

a. to worry and to be anxious

b. to be happy

c. to be new at your job and have little experience

 Mini Dialogue #6

6. _____ ***To have eyes like a hawk*** means:

a. the boss is strong and determined

b. the boss has poor vision

c. the boss can't be easily deceived because he notices every detail

 Mini Dialogue #7

7. _____ ***To have eyes in the back of your head*** means:

a. to be able to see what's going on when our backs are turned

b. to look directly at people

c. to be unable to see

How did you do? Check your answers against the Answer Key online.

POST-ASSESSMENT

True/False Questions

Indicate whether each sentence below is true (T) or false (F).

1. _____ The idiom **to bend someone's ear** means the individual is breaking someone's ear.
2. _____ The noun form of **deaf** is deafness.
3. _____ An infected eyelid causes lazy eye.
4. _____ The adjective form of **lump** is lumpy.
5. _____ If a person's **eyes are glued to something,** it means he or she has crusty eyes.
6. _____ Another word for squinting is blinking.
7. _____ Floaters are dark spots that cause tunnel vision.
8. _____ The past tense and adjective form of **tug** is tugged.
9. _____ A stye is a one kind of ear infection.
10. _____ A halo is a ringing sound in the ear.
11. _____ If a person is **up to his or her ears in work,** it means he or she is not busy.
12. _____ Jaundice is a yellowish discoloration of ear wax.
13. _____ Photophobia means sensitivity to sound.
14. _____ People with presbyopia have no difficulty seeing close objects or reading print.
15. _____ Working on the computer for a long time helps to reduce eye strain.

Multiple Choice Questions

Choose the correct answer from a, b, and c.

1. _____ The adjective form of **swell** is:

a. swollen and swelled

b. swelled

c. swell

2. _____ If a person has airplane ear, the person:

a. is an airline pilot

b. flies many planes

c. has ear pressure

3. _____ If a person is **all ears,** the person is:

a. deaf in both ears

b. worried and anxious

c. paying attention

4. _____ A child with a middle ear infection:

a. will wear ear plugs

b. will tug at the ear and cry inconsolably

c. needs to have the wax in the ear removed

5. _____ In the sentence, "If you are experiencing drainage from your ear, see a doctor," the word **drainage** is:

a. a past tense verb

b. an adjective

c. a noun

6. _____ The adjective form of **bulge** is:

a. bulgy

b. bulged only

c. bulged, bulging, and bulgy

7. _____ Cataracts cause:

a. farsightedness

b. blurred vision

c. tunnel vision

8. _____ A person who has **eyes like a hawk:**

a. has perfect vision

b. is difficult to deceive because he or she notices every small detail

c. is strong and determined

9. _____ Dry eye is caused by:

a. contact lenses

b. the inability to produce tears

c. styes

10. _____ In the sentence, "The girl complained of an itchy bump on her eye," the word **bump** is:

a. an adjective

b. a verb

c. a noun

11. _____ The word **perforated** is:

a. both a verb and a noun

b. a verb and an adjective

c. a verb only

12. _____ A crusty eyelid is caused by:

a. having your eyes glued to something

b. dry eye

c. discharge from the eye that will dry

13. _____ If your ears are clogged, you will:

a. hear perfectly

b. have difficulty hearing

c. hear hissing sounds

14. _____ The word **focused** is:

a. a verb only

b. an adjective only

c. a verb and an adjective

15. _____ In the sentence, "The child tugged at her ear," **tugged** is:

a. an adjective

b. a verb

c. a noun

Listening and Comprehension Exercises

Dialogue #1

Listen to Dialogue #1, stop, listen again and take notes. Listen to the dialogue as many times as you need or until you feel you have written sufficient notes and feel confident. You can use your notes to answer the multiple choice questions at the end of the dialogue.

Notes _____

_____

_____

_____

_____

Answer the questions below by selecting the answer that correctly completes each sentence.

1. _____ The patient has a prescription for:

a. a topical antibiotic

b. an antibiotic

c. an antihistamine

2. _____ The patient tells the pharmacist he:

a. is a fast swimmer

b. has swimmer's ear

c. can only swim above his ears

3. _____ The pharmacist tells the patient the prescription is for:

a. cortisol

b. cortisone

c. Cortisporin

4. _____ The patient probably got the ear infection:

a. swimming in a pool

b. swimming in Cooper River

c. swimming in a pool and in Cooper River

5. _____ The patient tells the pharmacist he has:

a. never had swimmer's ear before

b. had swimmer's ear a couple of times

c. had swimmer's ear only one time before

6. _____ The patient tells the pharmacist that he:

a. usually puts diluted vinegar in his ear and takes Tylenol for pain when he has swimmer's ear

b. never puts diluted vinegar in his ear when he has swimmer's ear

c. has only taken Tylenol when he has swimmer's ear

7. _____ The pharmacist tells the patient that the antibiotic will:

a. stop the growth of bacteria only

b. reduce the swelling and inflammation only

c. stop and reduce the growth of bacteria and reduce the swelling and inflammation

8. _____ The doctor prescribed the patient to put drops in his ear:

a. three to four times a week

b. thirty-four times a day

c. three to four times a day

9. _____ The pharmacist told the patient he should start feeling better in:

a. 35 days

b. 3 to 5 days

c. 3 to 5 weeks

10. _____ The side effects of the antibiotic could include:

a. a plugged ear

b. a ruptured ear

c. hearing loss

11. _____ The patient told the pharmacist he will:

a. read the directions and instructions in the package and run a marathon in 1 week

b. read the directions and instructions in the package and run a triathlon in 1 month

c. read the directions and instructions in the package and run a biathlon in about 1 month

12. _____ The patient's name is:

a. Michael E. Frank and his birth date is February 2, 1960

b. Michael P. Frances and his birth date is February 2, 1960

c. Michael P. Francis and his birth date is February 2, 1960

Dialogue #2

Listen to Dialogue #2, stop, listen again and take notes. Listen to the dialogue as many times as you need or until you feel you have written sufficient notes and feel confident. You can use your notes to answer the multiple choice questions at the end of the dialogue.

Notes _____

_____

_____

_____

_____

Answer the questions below by selecting the answer that correctly completes each sentence.

1. _____ The patient has just had:

a. hip surgery

b. cataract surgery

c. foot surgery

2. _____ The pharmacist on duty is:

a. Miss Newman

b. Dr. Newmark

c. Mr. Newmark

3. _____ The patient's prescription is for:

a. conjunctivitis

b. inflammation

c. a laceration

4. _____ The name of the drug is:

a. Levitra

b. Lotemax

c. Lamisil

5. _____ The patient's name is:

a. Edeline Burn

b. Ethel Burns

c. Ethel Byrnes

6. _____ The patient's birth date is:

a. December 14, 1928

b. December 4, 1938

c. December 4, 1948

7. _____ The patient is allergic to:

a. penicillin and is taking other medications

b. ampicillin and is taking other medications

c. penicillin and is not taking other medications

8. _____ Upon putting the eyedrops in the eye, the patient may experience:

a. dry eye

b. burning and stinging

c. crusty eye

9. _____ The patient should call the doctor immediately if she:

a. goes for her 2-mile walk

b. experiences dizziness, a rash, itching, and difficulty breathing

c. gets itchy while she walks

10. _____ The pharmacist is glad the patient has:

a. a good sense of humor

b. no sense of humor

c. a bad sense of humor

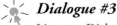

Dialogue #3

Listen to Dialogue #3, stop, listen again and take notes. Listen to the dialogue as many times as you need or until you feel you have written sufficient notes and feel confident. You can use your notes to answer the multiple choice questions at the end of the dialogue.

Notes _____
_____
_____
_____
_____

Answer the questions below by selecting the answer that correctly completes each sentence.

1. _____ The patient has a ruptured eardrum as a result of:
a. swimming
b. a brawl
c. inserting a Q-tip in his ear

2. _____ The patient tells the pharmacist that the emergency room doctor told him he has:
a. a plugged ear
b. a ruptured eardrum
c. airplane ear

3. _____ The patient went to the emergency room:
a. immediately after the brawl
b. a week after the brawl
c. a couple of days after the brawl

4. _____ The prescription is for:
a. hydrocortisone
b. Cortisporin Otic
c. cortisone

5. _____ The patient's name is:
a. Tom Mill
b. Thomas Milner
c. Thomas Miller

6. _____ The patient's birth date is:
a. November 6, 1980
b. November 16, 1980
c. November 16, 1986

7. _____ The patient's home address is:
a. 17 Oak Bluff Road in Middle Berry, Connecticut
b. 7 Oak Bluff Road in Middlebury, Connecticut
c. 17 Oak Bluff Road in Middlebury, Connecticut

8. _____ The pharmacist told the patient:
a. to use a shower cap when showering and to blow his nose gently if he needs to
b. that it is not necessary to wear a shower cap
c. that it is not necessary to blow his nose gently

9. _____ The patient:
a. has insurance and a credit card
b. has no credit card
c. has no insurance, but has a credit card

10. _____ The patient said "Yikes!" to express:

    a. his shock at the cost of the prescription

    b. how happy he was he had his credit card

    c. he will try to not get in another brawl in the future

How did you do on the Post-Assessment in Chapter 2? Check your answers in the Answer Key online.

Mouth and Nose | 3

True/False Questions

Indicate whether each sentence below is true (T) or false (F).

1. _____ A person who has **halitosis** should use mouthwash regularly.
2. _____ Drinking water regularly can help to reduce **dry mouth.**
3. _____ The slang term for **rhinoplasty** is nose job.
4. _____ Allergies or a cold can cause a person to experience **postnasal drip.**
5. _____ The adjective form of **infection** is infected.
6. _____ A **canker sore** is a small but painful ulcer in the mouth, which can make eating and talking unpleasant.
7. _____ If a child's **runny nose** is not wiped as needed, the **mucous discharge** will become dry and crusted.
8. _____ A **cold sore** appears on the lip and can look red and crusted.
9. _____ Colds, allergies, nose picking, dryness, and cocaine use can cause a **nosebleed.**
10. _____ Whitish patches on the tongue and the back of the mouth can be a sign of **thrush.**
11. _____ Saline nose drops, a humidifier, or a vaporizer can help alleviate **nasal dryness.**
12. _____ If you are experiencing pain and pressure in your face, a headache, and a **congested** and **stuffy** nose that is discharging a thick yellow-green **mucus,** you might have **sinusitis.**
13. _____ **Chapped lips** are soft and healthy.
14. _____ A **deviated septum** can block one or both **nostrils** and cause **nasal congestion.**
15. _____ The word **swell** is a noun and verb form.

Multiple Choice Questions

Choose the correct answer from a, b, and c.

1. _____ "My nose is **stuffy**" means:
   a. the nose is infected
   b. the nose is bleeding
   c. the nose is congested

2. _____ "I **paid through the nose** for my medicine" means:
   a. I bought nose drops for my congested nose
   b. the medicine is very expensive
   c. the medicine is inexpensive

51

3. _____ A **canker sore** is:

a. a benign mouth ulcer

b. a blister on the lip

c. a malignant ulcer

4. _____ A person who **shoots his or her mouth off:**

a. accidentally shoots their mouth with a gun

b. talks too much about matters they shouldn't talk about

c. is protesting

5. _____ If the patient complains of **hay fever,** the patient will experience:

a. a low-grade fever

b. itchy eyes with a clear discharge and sneezing

c. fever blisters

6. _____ A common mouth condition in infants is:

a. oral thrush

b. sinusitis

c. hay fever

7. _____ If a person has **fever blisters,** he or she:

a. need to only apply Blistex on them

b. should get treatment, because fever blisters are contagious

c. should cover the nose when he or she sneezes

8. _____ The word **congested** is:

a. a verb

b. an adjective and a verb

c. an adverb

9. _____ **Stuffy nose** is another term for:

a. bloody nose

b. nasal congestion

c. nasal passages

10. _____ A person who **snores:**

a. may temporarily stop breathing during sleep

b. is a sound sleeper

c. has too much mucus in the nose

How did you do? Check your answers in the Answer Key online.

MEDICAL VOCABULARY

A good understanding of vocabulary words in pharmacy is very important for communication with professors, fellow students, patients, and coworkers. Knowledge and understanding of vocabulary leads to successful communication and success as a pharmacy student, as a pharmacy technician, and as a practicing pharmacist. You may already know many of the vocabulary words in this chapter, but for words that are unfamiliar, pay careful attention to them and make every effort to know their correct spelling, meaning, and pronunciation. It is a good idea to keep a list of new words and to look up these new words in a bilingual dictionary or dictionary in your first language. A good command of pharmacy-related vocabulary and good pronunciation of vocabulary will help to prevent embarrassing mistakes and increase effective verbal communication skills.

Nose Vocabulary

adenoids
antihistamine
blocked nose
boogers
clogged nose
cloudy discharge
congestion
coughing
decongestant
deviated septum
dry cough

halitosis
hay fever
mucus
nasal congestion
nasal discharge
nosebleed
nose job
nostril
pick the nose
pollen
postnasal drip

ragweed
rhinoplasty
roof of the mouth
runny nose
sinus infection
sinus passages
sneezing
snoring
tonsils

Mouth Vocabulary

canker sore
chapped lips
cheek
chipped tooth
cold sore
cracked lips
dentures
drool
dry mouth
fever blister
gag reflex
gargle

gingivitis
gums
hairy tongue
halitosis
hoarse voice
itchy throat
mouth sore
oral herpes
oral thrush
palate
phlegm
plaque

saliva
scratchy throat
spit
sputum
taste buds
sore throat
strep throat
swallow
teething
tingle
tooth
yeast infection

PARTS OF SPEECH

A good understanding of parts of speech, such as verbs, nouns, adjectives, and adverbs, is important for successful communication when speaking or writing. It is equally important to know the various forms of words and to use them appropriately.

Word Forms

The table below lists the main forms of some terms that you will likely encounter in pharmacy practice. Review the table and then do the exercises that follow to assess your understanding.

Noun (n)	Infinitive/Verb (v) —Past Tense	Adjective (adj)	Adverb (adv)
an allergen; an allergy		allergic	
a bleed	to bleed; bled	bleeding; bloody	
a block	to block; blocked	blocked; blockage	
a blow	to blow; blew	blowing	
a cloud; cloudiness	to cloud; clouded	clouded; cloudy; clouding	
congestion	to congest; congested	congested; congestive	
contagion		contagious	contagiously
a cough; coughing	to cough; coughed	coughing	
a crack	to crack; cracked	cracked; cracking	
a drip	to drip; dripped	dripping	

(continued)

Noun (n)	Infinitive/Verb (v) —Past Tense	Adjective (adj)	Adverb (adv)
a drool	to drool; drooled	drooling	
drowsiness		drowsy	
excessiveness		excessive	excessively
a gag	to gag; gagged	gagging	
a gargle	to gargle; gargled	gargling	
hoarseness		hoarse	hoarsely
mucus		mucous; mucousy; mucousal	
a recurrence	to recur; recurred	recurrent	
a relief	to relieve; relieved	relieved; relieving	
a sneeze	to sneeze; sneezed	sneezing	
stuffiness	to stuff; stuffed	stuffed	
snore	to snore; snored	snoring	
a spit	to spit; spitted		
sufferer; suffering	to suffer; suffered	suffering	
a swallow	to swallow; swallowed	swallowing	
tenderness	to tender; tendered	tender	tenderly
a tingle	to tingle; tingled	tingling	
a tooth	to teethe	teething	
water	to water; watered	watered; watering; watery	

Word Forms Exercise

Read the following sentences carefully. Then indicate the word form of the bolded word(s), choosing from v, n, adj, or adv.

1. One way to relieve a **stuffy nose,** which is caused by **swollen** membranes, is to use a **nasal** spray.

   stuffy nose _____   swollen _____   nasal _____

2. A **canker sore** is a red **bump** in the mouth that **ulcerates.**

   canker sore _____   bump ____   ulcerates _____

3. Because infants and small children do not know how to **blow** their noses, a **nasal** aspirator can be used to remove the **mucus** that **clogs** their **nostrils.**

   blow _____   nasal _____   mucus _____   clogs _____   nostrils _____

4. If you have a **mouth sore,** it's a good idea to **gargle** with cool water to help relieve the **irritation** in your mouth.

   mouth sore _____   gargle _____   irritation _____

5. People **allergic** to pollen, dust, and dander will experience a **stuffy** nose and **swollen, watering** eyes.

   allergic _____   stuffy _____   swollen _____   watering _____

6. Some people will experience the **irritating, tingling** sensation of a **canker sore** if they have bitten their tongue or cheek.

   irritating _____   tingling _____   canker sore _____

7. Over-the-counter **antihistamines** can help reduce the amount of **mucus** produced if you have a **runny nose,** but they may also make you **drowsy.**

   antihistamines _____   mucus _____   runny nose _____   drowsy _____

8. Though **coughing** helps us to **clear** our throats, you should see a doctor if you have **excessive** coughing.

   coughing _____   clear _____   excessive _____

9. If you feel pain and **scratchiness** in your throat and have difficulty **swallowing,** you probably have a **sore** throat.

   scratchiness _____   swallowing _____   sore _____

10. Hay fever **sufferers** may experience thick or discolored **drainage** from their **inflamed sinuses.**

    sufferers _____   drainage _____   inflamed _____   sinuses _____

11. Another word for **mucus** and **sputum** is **phlegm.**

    mucus _____   sputum _____   phlegm _____

12. The slang word for **mucus** is **boogers,** and is used more by children than adults.

    mucus _____   boogers _____

13. To **diagnose strep throat,** a throat culture test is needed.

    diagnose _____   strep throat _____

14. **Postnasal drip** is another word for the **mucus** that runs down the back of the throat.

    postnasal drip _____   mucus _____

15. To get some **relief** from a **painful** mouth sore, you should **gargle** with **cool** water.

    relief _____   painful _____   gargle _____   cool _____

How did you do? Check your answers against the Answer Key online.

Typical Medical Conditions and Patient Complaints

The sentences below contain vocabulary that describes and explains typical medical conditions, diseases, symptoms, and patient complaints that a pharmacist encounters. Read the sentences carefully. Then indicate the word form of the bolded word(s), choosing from v, n, adj, or adv. Look up words you do not know in your bilingual or first-language dictionary.

1. Children with **runny noses** can be treated with over-the-counter **decongestants** and a cool mist vaporizer.

   runny noses _____   decongestants_____

2. The patient complained that when he **blew** his nose, the **nasal discharge** was thick, **cloudy** and yellow-green in color.

   blew _____   nasal discharge _____   cloudy_____

3. If you **suffer** from a **sinus infection,** the **tenderness** you feel around your eyes and cheekbones will feel worse if you bend your head forward.

   suffer _____   sinus infection _____   tenderness _____

4. If you experience **itching** eyes, a **watery discharge** from your nose, and **sneezing,** you might have hay fever.

   itching _____   watery _____   discharge _____   sneezing _____

5. **Allergens,** such as dander and pollen, can cause a person's nose to **run, itch, swell,** and produce **mucus.**

   allergens _____   run _____   itch _____   swell _____   mucus _____

6. A person with **oral thrush,** which is caused by a **fungus,** will have yellow and white spots on the mouth and tongue.

   oral thrush _____   fungus _____

7. Toddlers who are **teething** will be cranky, **irritable,** and will cry and **drool** a lot.

   teething _____   irritable _____   drool _____

8. **Nosebleeds** can be caused by dry **nasal passages** and by rubbing and picking at a **blocked** or **itching** nose.

   nosebleeds _____   nasal passages _____   blocked _____   itching _____

9. A person with a **deviated septum** can suffer from **sinus infections** and **snoring,** and have difficulty breathing.

   deviated septum _____   sinus infections _____   snoring _____

10. Lozenges, mouthwashes, and mints can temporarily **relieve halitosis,** commonly known as bad **breath.**

    relieve _____   halitosis _____   breath _____

11. **Fever blisters,** or cold sores, are painful **fluid-filled blisters** found on the lips, **gums,** and roof of the mouth.

    fever blisters _____   fluid-filled _____   blisters _____   gums _____

12. **Sputum,** which is **coughed** up with saliva, is another word for **phlegm** and **mucus.**

    sputum _____   coughed _____   phlegm _____   mucus_____

13. It's not uncommon to lose one's **taste buds,** and for food to taste differently when one has a **cold** or a **stuffy nose.**

    taste buds _____   cold _____   stuffy nose _____

14. An **inflammation** of the throat can cause a sore throat, **scratchiness** in the throat, and difficulty **swallowing.**

    inflammation _____   scratchiness_____   swallowing _____

15. The patient complained that the **coughing** episodes were becoming more frequent and that she was **spitting** up **bloody,** green-yellow **phlegm.**

    coughing _____   spitting _____   bloody _____   phlegm _____

16. **Bruising** and **swelling** will occur around the eyes after rhinoplasty, commonly referred to as a nose surgery or a nose job.

    bruising _____   swelling _____

17. Even though canker sores are not **contagious,** it's a good idea not to kiss another person if you have one because the person can **infect** your canker sore.

    contagious _____   infect _____

18. If your gums are red, **sore, swollen,** and **bleed** easily, you should see your dentist.

    sore ____   swollen ____   bleed _____

19. To treat **chapped** lips, which can become red, **sore,** and **peel,** apply an over-the-counter antibiotic ointment to **prevent** an **infection.**

    chapped _____   sore ____   peel ____   prevent ____   infection ____

20. **Dry mouth** can be caused by certain health conditions, medications, smoking, **snoring,** and the inability to **produce saliva.**

    dry mouth _____   snoring _____   produce _____   saliva _____

How did you do? Check your answers against the Answer Key online.

Medical Vocabulary Comprehension

Now that you have read sentences 1 through 20 describing language regarding the nose and mouth, assess your understanding by doing the exercises below.

Multiple Choice Questions

Choose the answer that correctly completes each sentence below.

1. _____ **Nose spray** relieves:
a. a nosebleed
b. a stuffy nose
c. thrush

2. _____ **Teething** in toddlers can cause:
a. bite marks
b. drooling
c. fever blisters

3. _____ **Fever blisters** are:
a. painful fluid-filled blisters
b. blood-filled blisters
c. pus-filled blisters

4. _____ In children, a **nasal aspirator** can be used to:
a. prevent coughing
b. stop a runny nose
c. remove mucus

5. _____ A red bump that ulcerates in the mouth is:
a. a canker sore
b. fungus
c. sputum

6. _____ Another term for **phlegm** is:
a. sputum
b. cough
c. postnasal drip

7. _____ A **stuffy nose** can cause:
a. fungus in the nasal passage
b. teething
c. a loss of taste buds

8. _____ To help relieve the irritation of a **canker sore,** you should:
a. apply a warm compress
b. gargle with cool water
c. pick it

9. _____ **Postnasal drip** is another term for:
a. blowing your nose
b. allergens that produce mucus
c. the mucus that runs down the back of the throat

10. _____ Another term for **halitosis** is:
a. bad breath
b. halos
c. grittiness

11. _____ One way to relieve a stuffy nose is to:
a. blow your nose hard
b. use a nasal spray
c. pick your nose

12. _____ **Antihistamines** can:
a. make a person drowsy
b. cause a runny nose
c. cause mouth sores

13. _____ **Oral thrush** is caused by:
a. halitosis
b. fungus
c. pollen

14. _____ Another term for **palate** is:
a. tongue
b. roof of mouth
c. gums

15. _____ **Dry nasal passages** can cause:
a. a nosebleed
b. sputum
c. phlegm

True/False Questions

Indicate whether each sentence below is true (T) or false (F).

1. _____ If a patient complains that tenderness around the eyes and checks gets worse when bending the head forward, the patient may be suffering from a sinus infection.
2. _____ If a patient complains of pain and scratchiness in the throat, and is having difficulty swallowing, the patient probably has postnasal drip.
3. _____ People allergic to dander, pollen, and dust will not experience a stuffy nose or swollen and watering eyes.
4. _____ Because coughing helps us to clear our throats, if you have excessive coughing you should not see a doctor.
5. _____ Teething may cause some children to be irritable and to drool.
6. _____ Halitosis can be temporarily relieved by lozenges only.
7. _____ The word "drowsiness" is an adjective.
8. _____ The word "relieved" is both a verb and an adjective.
9. _____ Whitish patches on the tongue and back of the mouth can be a sign of thrush.
10. _____ Allergies or a cold can trigger postnasal drip.

How did you do? Check your answers against the Answer Key online.

Writing Exercise

An important part of communication is the ability to write about what you read, to write correctly, and to spell correctly. In the exercises below, write your understanding of the meaning of the bolded words.

1. Describe in writing what a **runny nose**, a **stuffy nose**, and a **nosebleed** are.

_____

_____

_____

_____

2. Describe in writing what a **canker sore** and a **fever blister** are.

_____

_____

_____

_____

3. Describe in writing what **a sore throat** and **strep throat** are.

_____

_____

_____

_____

4. Describe in writing what **phlegm, sputum,** and **mucus** are.

_____

_____

_____

_____

Check what you have written with acceptable answers that appear in the Answer Key online.

LISTENING AND PRONUNCIATION

The ability to listen and understand what is being said and heard, and the ability to pronounce words clearly, is extremely important. A word misheard and a word mispronounced will lead to poor communication and can seriously put both the pharmacist and patient in danger. Therefore, it is very important that one hear clearly what another person has said, and that one speak clearly with correct pronunciation.

Listen carefully to the pharmacy-related words presented in the audio files found in Chapter 3 on thePoint (thePoint.lww.com/diaz-gilbert), and then pronounce them as accurately as you can. Listen and then repeat. You will listen to each word once and then you will repeat it. You will do this twice for each word. Listening and pronunciation practice will increase your listening and speaking confidence. Many languages do not produce or emphasize certain sounds produced and emphasized in English, so pay careful attention to the pronunciation of each word.

Pronunciation Exercise

Listen to the audio files found in Chapter 3 on thePoint (thePoint.lww.com/diaz-gilbert) and repeat the words. Then say the words aloud for additional practice.

1. adenoids	ăd′n-oidz
2. antihistamine	ăn′tē-hĭs′tə-mēn
3. blocked nose	blŏkt nōz
4. booger	bo͞og′ər
5. chapped lips	chăpt lĭps
6. cheek	chēk

7.	chipped tooth	chĭp to͞oth
8.	clogged nose	klôgd nōz
9.	cloudy discharge	klou'dē dĭs-chärj
10.	cold sore	kōld sōr
11.	congestion	kon-jes'chŭn
12.	coughing	kôfŋ
13.	cracked lips	krăkt lĭpz
14.	decongestant	dē'kən-jĕs'tənt
15.	dentures	dĕn'chərs
16.	deviated septum	dē'vē-āt' sĕp'təm
17.	drool	dro͞ol
18.	dry cough	drī kôf
19.	dry mouth	drī mouth
20.	fever blister	fē'vər blĭs'tər
21.	gag reflex	găg rē'flĕks
22.	gargle	gär'gəl
23.	gingivitis	jĭn'jə-vī'tĭs
24.	gums	gumz
25.	hairy tongue	hâr'ē tŭng
26.	halitosis	hăl'ĭ-tō'sĭs
27.	hay fever	hā fē'vər
28.	hoarse voice	hōrs vois
29.	itchy throat	ĭch'ē thrōt
30.	mouth sore	mouth sōr
31.	mucus	myo͞o'kəs
32.	nasal discharge	nā'zəl dĭs-chärj'
33.	nosebleed	nōz blēd
34.	nose job	nōz jŏb
35.	nostril	nŏs'trəl
36.	oral herpes	ôr'əl hûr'pēz
37.	oral thrush	ôr'əl, ōr' thrŭsh
38.	palate	păl'ĭt
39.	phlegm	flĕm
40.	pick the nose	pĭk thə nŏz
41.	plaque	plăk
42.	pollen	pŏl'ən
43.	postnasal drip	pōst nā'zəl drĭp
44.	ragweed	răg'wēd'
45.	rhinoplasty	rī'nō-plăs'tē
46.	runny nose	rŭn'ē nōz
47.	saliva	sə-lī'və
48.	scratchy throat	skrăch'ē thrōt
49.	sinus infection	sī'nəs ĭn-fĕk'shən
50.	sinus passages	sī'nəs păs'ĭjs
51.	sneezing	snēzŋ
52.	snoring	snôrŋ
53.	sore throat	sôr thrōt
54.	spit	spĭt
55.	sputum	spyo͞o'təm
56.	strep throat	strĕp thrōt

57. taste buds	t$\bar{a}$st b$\breve{u}$ds
58. tingle	t$\breve{i}$ng′gϑl
59. tonsils	t$\breve{o}$n′sϑls
60. tooth	t$\overline{oo}$th

Which words are easy to pronounce? Which are difficult to pronounce? Use the space below to write in the words that you find difficult to pronounce. These are words you should practice saying often.

_____

_____

_____

_____

_____

_____

_____

Listen to the audio files found in Chapter 3 on thePoint (thePoint.lww.com/diaz-gilbert) as many times as you need to increase your pronunciation ability of the difficult words. Pronounce these words with a friend or a colleague who speaks English.

English Sounds That Are Difficult for Speakers of Other Languages to Pronounce

Spanish

In Spanish, there is no English "v" sound, but the "v" consonant in Spanish is pronounced like the English "b." The vowel "i" is pronounced like a long "e." Pay careful attention to the "v" sound in English when pronouncing words that begin with "v." Also pay careful attention to English words that begin with "s;" do not use the Spanish "es" sound when pronouncing English words that begin with "s."

For example, in English,

stuffy nose is not pronounced estuffy nose
sneezing is not pronounced esneezeen

Vietnamese

In Vietnamese, the "t" consonant is pronounced "s," but in English the "t" is pronounced "t" and "s" is pronounced "s." Be careful with English words that begin with "t." In Vietnamese, the "b" consonant is pronounced "p," but in English "p" is pronounced "p" and "b" is pronounced "b."

In Vietnamese, words do not end in "b," "ch," "f," "d," "j," "l," "p," "r," "s," "sh," "v," and "z." In English, words end in these letters. Pay special attention to pronouncing these English sounds. In Vietnamese, there is no "dzh" or "zh" sound, so English words like "judge" (dzh) and rupture (zh) will be hard for Vietnamese speakers to pronounce.

For example, in English,

blocked nose is not pronounced plo no
cracked lips is not pronounced crah lih
postnasal drip is not pronounced ponayso drih
discharge is not pronounced dihshar

(continued)

Gujarati

In Gujarati, "v" is pronounced "w," "f" is pronounced "p," "p" is pronounced "f," and "z" is pronounced "j." Short "i" is pronounced long "e," "x" is pronounced "ch," and "th" is pronounced "s." In English, "v" is pronounced "v," "f" is pronounced "f," "z" is pronounced "z" or "s," "j" is pronounced "j," and "x" is pronounced "x." Pay careful attention when pronouncing these sounds.

For example, in English,

fever blister is not pronounced pever bleester
deviated septum is not pronounced dewiated seftum
postnasal drip is not pronounced fostnasal dreef

Korean

In Korean, the "v" consonant is pronounced "b" and the "f" consonant is pronounced "p." In English, the "v" is pronounced "v," the "f" is pronounced "f," and the "p" is pronounced "p." Pay special attention when pronouncing these sounds.

For example, in English,

fever is not pronounced pever

Chinese

In Chinese, the "r" consonant is pronounced "l" or "w," and "b," "d," "g," and "ng" are not pronounced at all. Pay careful attention to English words that begin with "r" because the "r" is not pronounced "l" or "w," and "b," "d," "g," and "ng" are pronounced in English.

For example, in English,

runny nose is not pronounced lunny nose

Russian

The "w" consonant is pronounced like a "v" and the "v" sounds like a "w." Pay careful attention to the English "th." It is not pronounced "s."

For example, in English,

throat is not pronounced sroat

DICTATION

 ### Listening/Spelling Exercise: Word and Word Pairs

Listen to the words or word pairs on the audio files found in Chapter 3 on thePoint (thePoint.lww.com/diaz-gilbert) and then write them down on the lines below.

1. _____
2. _____
3. _____
4. _____
5. _____
6. _____
7. _____
8. _____

9. _____

10. _____

11. _____

12. _____

13. _____

14. _____

15. _____

 ## Listening/Spelling Exercise: Sentences

Listen to the sentences on the audio files found in Chapter 3 on thePoint (thePoint.lww.com/diaz-gilbert) and then write them down on the lines below.

1. _____
   _____

2. _____
   _____

3. _____
   _____

4. _____
   _____

5. _____
   _____

6. _____
   _____

7. _____
   _____

8. _____
   _____

9. _____
   _____

10. _____
    _____

Now, check your sentences against the correct answers in the Answer Key online. If there are any new words that you do not know or that you spelled incorrectly, make a list of those words and study them for meaning and spelling.

PHARMACIST/PATIENT DIALOGUES

The ability to orally communicate effectively with your professors, colleagues, and especially with patients is very important. As a pharmacist, you will be counseling patients; patients will come to you for advice. They will have questions about a condition and symptoms they may experience and will ask you to help treat the condition. Therefore, it is extremely important that you understand what they are saying and that you respond to them and their questions appropriately. Your patients will speak differently. For example, some may speak very quickly, others too low, and yet others may speak angrily. To help you improve your listening skills, listen to the following dialogues, or short conversations, between a pharmacist and a patient and between a pharmacy technician and a patient.

Listening and Comprehension Exercises

Dialogue #1

Listen to Dialogue #1, stop, listen again and take notes. Listen to the dialogue as many times as you need or until you feel you have written sufficient notes and feel confident. You can use your notes to answer the multiple choice questions at the end of the dialogue.

Notes _____

_____

_____

_____

_____

Answer the questions below by selecting the answer that correctly completes each sentence.

1. _____ What is the patient's complaint?
a. She has a runny nose
b. She has nasal blockage
c. She has a nosebleed

2. _____ The doctor prescribed
a. a nasal pump
b. a nasal aspirator
c. Nasonex

3. _____ The pharmacist demonstrates to the patient how to
a. spray her nose
b. prime the pump
c. blow her nose

4. _____ The patient's name is
a. Debbie Allen
b. Debra Allen
c. Deborah Allan

5. _____ The pharmacist tells the patient
a. it can take up to 2 days to get relief
b. it can take up to 2 weeks to get relief
c. it's OK to skip a day

6. _____ The side effects of Nasonex are
a. headache
b. headache, sore throat, nosebleeds, and coughing
c. headache and coughing

Check your answers in the Answer Key online. How did you do? Are there new words you do not know? Take the time now to look them up in your bilingual or first-language dictionary.

Dialogue #2

Listen to Dialogue #2, stop, listen again and take notes. Listen to the dialogue as many times as you need or until you feel you have written sufficient notes and feel confident. You can use your notes to answer the multiple choice questions at the end of the dialogue.

Notes _____
_____
_____
_____
_____

Answer the questions below by selecting the answer that correctly completes each sentence.

1. _____ The patient is getting a prescription for:
a. Valium
b. Vicodin
c. Valtrex

2. _____ The patient complained of a:
a. tingling, itching, burning sensation in her mouth
b. core sore on both lips
c. tingling, itching, burning sensation in her lower lip

3. _____ The patient's name is:
a. Rebekah Low
b. Rebecca Lowe
c. Rebekah Lowe

4. _____ Valtrex is:
a. a 12-day ointment treatment
b. a caplet taken every 12 hours
c. a caplet taken once and then 12 hours later

5. _____ The pharmacist tells the patient:
a. not to kiss others, even though the cold sore is not contagious
b. not to kiss others or touch the cold sore with her hands
c. that the cold sore is contagious but she can touch the sore with her hands

6. _____ Valtrex has:
a. no side effects
b. side effects such as headache, dizziness, nausea, and a sore throat.
c. side effects such as drowsiness and inconsolable crying

7. _____ The patient said the doctor told her:
a. she will not have a recurrence
b. she may have a recurrence
c. she will definitely have a recurrence

Check your answers in the Answer Key online. How did you do? Are there new words you do not know? Take the time now to look them up in your bilingual or first-language dictionary.

Dialogue #3

Listen to Dialogue #3, stop, listen again and take notes. Listen to the dialogue as many times as you need or until you feel you have written sufficient notes and feel confident. You can use your notes to answer the multiple choice questions at the end of the dialogue.

Notes _____

_____

_____

_____

_____

_____

Answer the questions below by selecting the answer that correctly completes each sentence.

1. _____ The child's mother is complaining that her:

a. 6-month-old son is teething

b. 6-month-old daughter has infected gums

c. 6-month-old daughter is teething and drooling

2. _____ To relieve her daughter's teething pain, the mother has:

a. fed her daughter bananas

b. rubbed her daughter's gums, given her a frozen washcloth, and massaged her daughter's gums with a frozen banana

c. cleaned her daughter's gums with a frozen washcloth

3. _____ The pharmacist asks the mother if she has given her child:

a. Children's Tylenol

b. Zilactin Baby

c. Tylenol Baby

4. _____ The pharmacist recommends that the mother:

a. purchase prescription Zilactin

b. purchase non-prescription Zilactin Baby

c. purchase a grape gel

5. _____ Zilactin Baby is:

a. a grape-flavored medicated gel

b. a medicated ointment to rub on the gums

c. an antibiotic

6. _____ The pharmacist tells the mother to keep her eye on the following side effects:

a. vomiting

b. a rash and hives

c. diarrhea

7. _____ The pharmacist instructs the mother to apply Zilactin Baby on her daughter's gums:

a. with her fingertip or a cotton swab no more than four times a day

b. with a cotton swab only for 4 days only

c. with her fingertip only no more than twice a day

Check your answers in the Answer Key online. How did you do? Are there new words you do not know? Take the time now to look them up in your bilingual or first-language dictionary.

IDIOMATIC EXPRESSIONS

Idioms and idiomatic expressions are made up of a group of words that have a different meaning from the original meaning of each individual word. Native speakers of the English language use such expressions comfortably and naturally. However, individuals who are new speakers of English or who have studied English for many years may still not be able to use idioms and idiomatic expressions as comfortably or naturally as native speakers. As pharmacy students, pharmacy technicians, and practicing pharmacists, you will hear many different idiomatic expressions. Some of you will understand and know how to use these expressions correctly. At times, however, you may not understand what your professors, colleagues, and patients are saying. This of course can lead to miscommunication, embarrassment, and possibly dangerous mistakes.

To help you improve your knowledge of idioms and idiomatic expressions, carefully read the following idiomatic expressions that contain the body words of nose, mouth, lips, and tongue.

Idiomatic Expressions using "Nose"

1. ***to be hard-nosed*** means that the person is strong, stubborn, and determined to get want he or she wants.

   For example: Because he is such a ***hard-nosed*** negotiator, he got the ten percent salary increase he wanted.

2. ***to keep your nose clean*** means to stay out of trouble.

   For example: If you don't want to get fired, come to work on time, do your work, and ***keep your nose clean.***

3. ***to keep your nose to the grindstone*** means to keep very busy and work very hard.

   For example: She was warned by her supervisor to ***keep her nose to the grindstone,*** and to fill as many prescriptions as possible during her shift.

4. ***to stick or poke your nose into something*** means that a person gets involved in private matters that do not concern him or her.

   For example: The new pharmacist and the supervisor do not get along because the supervisor likes ***to poke her nose into*** the new pharmacist's private life.

5. ***to nose around*** means to look for information, to explore, and to inquire.

   For example: From time to time, the regional manager of the pharmacy likes to ***nose around*** the pharmacy to see how the pharmacists and pharmacy technicians are doing their jobs.

6. ***no skin off one's nose*** is used to show that the person is not interested in or concerned about a matter.

   For example: It's ***no skin off my nose*** if I don't get hired by this pharmacy because I have another job offer.

7. ***under one's nose*** means that what a person is looking for is in his or her sight.

   For example: The pharmacy technician was about to panic when she realized the prescription she thought she had misplaced was right ***under her nose.***

Idiomatic Expressions using "Mouth"

1. ***to bad mouth*** means to say bad things about someone.

   For example: The student was so angry he failed the exam that he started ***to bad mouth*** the professor.

2. ***to foam at the mouth*** means to be very angry.

   For example: After the patient was given the wrong antibiotic prescription for the second time, the patient's mother was ***foaming at the mouth.***

3. ***to make one's mouth water*** means food looks and smells good and makes you want to eat it.

   For example: Certain foods, such as Chinese food and freshly baked chocolate chip cookies, ***make my mouth water.***

4. ***to melt in your mouth*** means that the food you are eating is very delicious and so tender that it doesn't need to be chewed.

   For example: Even people with high cholesterol can't stop themselves from eating delicious roast pork, which just ***melts in their mouth.***

5. *to take someone's words out of his or her mouth* means that you say what another person is thinking and say it before he or she says it.

For example: The pharmacist *took the words right out of the pharmacy technician's mouth* when he announced she could leave early.

Idiomatic Expressions using "Lips"

1. *to keep a stiff upper lip* means to be brave and strong in a difficult situation.

For example: The patient managed to *keep a stiff upper lip* after the doctor told her she was having a recurrence of her fever blisters on her lip.

2. *lips are sealed* means a person knows a secret and will not tell others.

For example: *My lips are sealed;* I cannot tell you who has been promoted to regional manager.

Idiomatic Expressions using "Tongue"

1. *a slip of the tongue* means a person has said something in error or had not planned to say something.

For example: The pharmacy technician made a *slip of the tongue* when she told the patient her prescription for Predisol, instead of Prednisone, would be ready for pickup in one hour.

2. *hold your tongue* means to be silent and not speak.

For example: You're very angry right now; don't say anything you'll regret so *hold your tongue.*

Mini Dialogues Listening Exercise

How much did you understand? Listen to the following mini dialogues in the audio files found in Chapter 3 on thePoint (thePoint.lww.com/diaz-gilbert), read the questions below, and then choose the correct answer.

 Mini Dialogue #1

1. _____ *Keep my nose to the grindstone* means:

a. her nose was hit by a stone

b. she can relax

c. she has to work very hard

 Mini Dialogue #2

2. _____ *Foaming at the mouth* means:

a. to have a mouth infection

b. to have no tender feelings

c. to be very angry

 Mini Dialogue #3

3. _____ *Poking her nose* means:

a. the new pharmacist is a private person

b. the new pharmacist gets involved in matters that don't concern her

c. she likes to blow her nose in front of other people

Mini Dialogue #4

4. _____ ***No skin off my nose*** means:

a. some skin came off the nose

b. to be worried and anxious

c. not to be concerned about the matter

 Mini Dialogue #5

5. _____ ***Melts in your mouth*** means:

a. to be hot

b. to burn the mouth

c. it's delicious and doesn't need to be chewed

 Mini Dialogue #6

6. _____ ***To bad mouth*** means:

a. to have bad breath

b. to say nice things about someone

c. to say bad things about someone

 Mini Dialogue #7

7. _____ ***Keep your nose clean*** means:

a. to remove mucus from one's nose

b. to blow one's nose

c. to stay out of trouble

How did you do? Check your answers against the Answer Key online.

POST-ASSESSMENT

True/False Questions

Indicate whether each sentence below is true (T) or false (F).

1. _____ The idiom **to be hard-nosed** means the individual cannot blow his or her nose.

2. _____ The adjective form of the word **recurrence** is recurrent.

3. _____ Another word for rhinoplasty is nose job.

4. _____ The adjective form of the word **dry** is dryness.

5. _____ If a person **noses around,** the person is spreading their cold.

6. _____ Another word for cold sore is fever blister.

7. _____ A canker sore is an example of a mouth sore.

8. _____ Bulge and bulginess are both noun forms.

9. _____ Phlegm is a kind of allergen.

10. _____ Another word for roof of the mouth is palate.

11. _____ If food **makes a person's mouth water,** it means they are producing excessive saliva.

12. _____ If a person's **lips are sealed,** the lips are cracked and dry.

13. _____ A nosebleed can be caused by picking the nose.

14. _____ The slang word for **mucus** is boogers.

15. _____ A person who has a cold sore on the lip will feel a cold, sweaty sensation.

Multiple Choice Questions

Choose the correct answer from a, b, and c.

1. _____ The adverb form of **excessive** is:

a. excessively

b. excessiveness

c. excessive

2. _____ If a person has **halitosis,** the person has:

a. a sinus infection

b. bad breath

c. speaks badly of others

3. _____ If a person is **foaming at the mouth,** the person is:

a. vomiting

b. making bubbles with saliva

c. very angry

4. _____ A child who is teething:

a. will tug at the ear

b. will cry and drool a lot

c. needs head lice removed with a fine-tooth comb

5. _____ In the sentence, "Mints can temporarily relieve halitosis," the word **relieve** is:

a. a noun

b. a verb

c. an adjective

6. _____ The adjective form of **stuff** is:

a. stuffed

b. stuffy

c. stuffed and stuffy

7. _____ Excessive mucus can produce:

a. a runny nose

b. a stuffy nose

c. a bloody nose

8. _____ A person who is **hard-nosed:**

a. is stubborn and determined

b. cannot smell

c. is always getting in trouble

9. _____ Pollen, dander, and dust can cause:

a. thrush

b. a canker sore

c. hay fever

10. _____ In the sentence, "The woman complained of a tingling sensation on her lip," the word **tingling** is:

a. an adjective

b. a verb

c. a noun

11. _____ The word **wound** is:

a. both a verb and noun

b. a verb only

c. a noun only

12. _____ The part of the mouth that hurts when a child is teething is:

a. the tongue

b. the gums

c. the roof of the mouth

13. _____ A fever blister is:

a. contagious

b. not contagious

c. the same as a canker sore

14. _____ The noun form of **allergic** is:

a. allergy only

b. allergen only

c. both allergy and allergen

15. _____ In the sentence, "Chapped lips can be treated with over-the-counter antibiotic ointment," the word **chapped** is:

a. an adjective

b. a past tense verb

c. a noun

Listening and Comprehension Exercises

Dialogue #1

Listen to Dialogue #1, stop, listen again and take notes. Listen to the dialogue as many times as you need or until you feel you have written sufficient notes and feel confident. You can use your notes to answer the multiple choice questions at the end of the dialogue.

Notes _____

_____

_____

_____

_____

Answer the questions below by selecting the answer that correctly completes each sentence.

1. _____ The patient's mother tells the pharmacist she needs a prescription filled for:

a. her baby girl

b. herself

c. her baby boy

2. _____ The patient's mother does not know the name of the prescription or how to pronounce it:

a. because she can't read

b. because she forgot her glasses

c. because she can't understand the doctor's handwriting

3. _____ The pharmacist tells the patient's mother the prescription is for:

a. Nasonex

b. Nystatin Suspension

c. Neosporin

4. _____ The patient's name is:

a. Sabastian Hofmen

b. Sebastian Hoffman

c. Sebastian Hofman

5. _____ The patient is:

a. 45 months old

b. 45 days old

c. 4 days old

6. _____ The patient was born on:

a. June 6, 2002

b. June 2, 2006

c. June 6, 2006

7. _____ The patient's address is:

a. 7 Treelane Rd

b. 77 Tree Rd

c. 77 Tree Lane

8. _____ The pharmacist instructs the patient's mother to:

a. squirt the liquid drops of Nystatin in her mouth four times a day

b. squirt drops of Nystatin in her son's cheek using a dropper once a day

c. squirt drops of Nystatin in her son's cheek four times a day using a dropper

9. _____ The pharmacist instructs the patient's mother to:

a. sterilize the bottles and nipples, and to keep an eye out for side effects such as vomiting and diarrhea

b. sterilize the bottles and nipples only

c. watch out for side effects only

Dialogue #2

Listen to Dialogue #2, stop, listen again and take notes. Listen to the dialogue as many times as you need or until you feel you have written sufficient notes and feel confident. You can use your notes to answer the multiple choice questions at the end of the dialogue.

Notes _____

_____

_____

_____

_____

Answer the questions below by selecting the answer that correctly completes each sentence.

1. _____ The patient wants to speak to:

a. Sam the pharmacy technician

b. Sam the pharmacist

c. the technician on duty

2. _____ The patient's full name is:

a. Jennie Braun

b. Jennifer Browne

c. Jenny Browne

3. _____ The patient also calls herself:

a. Jenne

b. Jenny

c. Jennie

4. _____ The patient's date of birth is:

a. October 10, 1980

b. October 6, 1980

c. June 10, 1980

5. _____ The patient is complaining about:

a. her canker sores

b. her doctor

c. her fever blisters

6. _____ The patient tells the pharmacist that:

a. Orabase helped heal her canker sores

b. Orabase did not help heal her canker sores

c. she wants to buy more Orabase

7. _____ The doctor gave her a prescription for:

a. Diflucan

b. Debacterol

c. Duclolax

8. _____ Debacterol is:

a. a cream

b. a liquid

c. an ointment

9. _____ The pharmacist tells the patient that after applying the Debacterol, she:

a. will feel a tingling sensation and be pain-free

b. will feel a stinging sensation and be pain-free

c. will feel a numbing sensation and get no relief

10. _____ The patient's insurance plan is:

a. Life and Health Insurance

b. Healthy Life Insurance

c. Health and Life Plan

Dialogue #3

Listen to Dialogue #3, stop, listen again and take notes. Listen to the dialogue as many times as you need or until you feel you have written sufficient notes and feel confident. You can use your notes to answer the multiple choice questions at the end of the dialogue.

Notes _____

_____

_____

Answer the questions below by selecting the answer that correctly completes each sentence.

1. _____ What medical condition does the patient have?
a. phlebitis
b. arthritis
c. sinusitis

2. _____ The patient has just left:
a. her home
b. her doctor's office
c. her office

3. _____ The patient thinks the name of the prescription begins with the letter:
a. A
b. M
c. L

4. _____ The prescription was phoned in to the pharmacy by the:
a. doctor
b. patient
c. nurse

5. _____ The doctor's name is:
a. Rob Dixon
b. Robert Dixson
c. Robert Dixon

6. _____ The prescription is for:
a. Ampicillin
b. Amoxicillin
c. Augmentin

7. _____ The patient asks the pharmacist if she can:
a. take the medication with food and if it will make her feel different and sick
b. take the medication with a full glass of water and if there are side effects
c. break open the capsules and mix it in a full glass of water

8. _____ The pharmacist instructs the patient to get immediate medical attention if:
a. she experiences diarrhea and hairy tongue
b. she experiences hives, swelling, closing of her throat, and difficulty breathing
c. she experiences thrush

9. _____ The pharmacist also instructed the patient to:
a. read the side effects on the computer printout
b. call her doctor if she has any concerns
c. both a and b

10. _____ The name of the patient's insurance is:
a. Good Health Insurance
b. Best Health Insurance
c. Total Health Insurance

11. _____ The patient's name is:

a. Melinda Costanza

b. Melissa Costello

c. Melissa Constanza

12. _____ The patient's home number is:

a. 555-1710

b. 505-0172

c. 555-0171

13. _____ The pharmacy is located in a:

a. mall

b. supermarket

c. discount store

How did you do on the Post-Assessment in Chapter 3? Check your answers in the Answer Key online.

Endocrine and Lymphatic System | 4

True/False Questions

Indicate whether each sentence below is true (T) or false (F).

1. _____ Bleeding and bruising is a common symptom of **leukemia.**
2. _____ **Thyroid** hormones are produced by the lymph glands.
3. _____ **Lymph nodes** are filled with red blood cells.
4. _____ **Hypothyroidism** is the term used to refer to lower-than-normal production of thyroid hormone.
5. _____ The adjective form of **lethargy** is lethargic.
6. _____ A person with hypothyroidism will suffer from cold **intolerance.**
7. _____ Another word for trachea is **windpipe.**
8. _____ A person with leukemia will suffer swelling in the abdomen as a result of an **enlarged spleen.**
9. _____ Non-Hodgkin's **lymphoma** is a type of cancer that begins in the thyroid.
10. _____ The noun form of **agitated** is agitation.
11. _____ **Protruding eyes** are deep-set eyes.
12. _____ Signs of **diabetes** are lack of thirst and urination.
13. _____ If a person experiences **constipation,** cold intolerance, and fatigue, he or she should be tested for **hyperthyroidism.**
14. _____ **Hypoglycemia** refers to above normal levels of **glucose** in the blood.
15. _____ The word **delirium** is the adjective form of **delirious,** which is the noun form.

Multiple Choice Questions

Choose the correct answer from a, b, and c.

1. _____ An **overactive** thyroid:
a. does not produce enough thyroid hormones
b. produces too much thyroid hormone
c. produces too little thyroid hormone

2. _____ The front of the neck that sticks out a little bit and moves when we swallow is the:
a. trachea
b. Adam's apple
c. windpipe

3. _____ Clusters of **lymph nodes** are found in the:
a. groin
b. groin, armpits, neck, chest, and abdomen
c. armpits

4. _____ A person with **Graves disease** will experience:
a. heat intolerance
b. cold intolerance
c. the inability to sweat

5. _____ People who experience frequent urinating and increased thirst should be tested for:
a. enlargement of the lymph nodes
b. bacterial infection
c. diabetes

6. _____ The enlargement of the thyroid gland is called:
a. a cyst
b. an Adam's apple
c. a goiter

7. _____ A **thyroid nodule:**
a. is a fluid-filled cyst
b. is scar tissue
c. regulates metabolism

8. _____ The adjective and verb form of **breath** is:
a. breathe
b. breathing
c. breathed

9. _____ The term used to refer to cancers in the lymphatic system is:
a. carcinoma
b. melanoma
c. lymphoma

10. _____ Gangrene can develop in people suffering from:
a. colds
b. diabetes
c. fluid-filled cysts

How did you do? Check your answers against the Answer Key online.

MEDICAL VOCABULARY

A good understanding of vocabulary words in pharmacy is very important for communication with professors, fellow students, patients, and coworkers. Knowledge and understanding of vocabulary leads to successful communication and success as a pharmacy student, as a pharmacy technician, and as a practicing pharmacist. You may already know many of the vocabulary words in this chapter, but for words that are unfamiliar, pay careful attention to them and make every effort to know their correct spelling, meaning, and pronunciation. It is a good idea to keep a list of new words and to look up these new words in a bilingual dictionary or dictionary in your first language. A good command of pharmacy-related vocabulary and good pronunciation of vocabulary will help to prevent embarrassing mistakes and increase effective verbal communication skills.

Endocrine System Vocabulary

ache
Adam's apple
Addison's disease
agitation
appetite
benign
bowel movement
cold intolerance
constipation
coordination
Cushing's disease
delirium
diabetes
drowsy
enlarged
exhaustion
gangrene
gland

glucose
goiter
Graves disease
Hashimoto's disease
heat intolerance
hormone
hypoglycemia
hyperthyroidism
hypothyroidism
indigestion
insulin
lethargy
malignant
mask
metabolism
mood swings
muscle cramps
nausea

nervousness
nodule
overactive
overproduction
pituitary gland
protruding
puffy
regulate
stiffness
swallow
tender
thirst
tremble
underactive
underproduction
urination
water retention
windpipe

Blood Disorders and Lymphatic System Vocabulary

abdomen
anemia
armpit
blood
bone marrow
enlarged spleen
fatigue

groin
Hodgkin's lymphoma
immune system
lightheaded
lymph node
malaise
measles

mononucleosis
mumps
non-Hodgkin's lymphoma
numbness
pallor
relapse
underarm

PARTS OF SPEECH

A good understanding of parts of speech, such as verbs, nouns, adjectives, and adverbs, is important for successful communication when speaking or writing. It is equally important to know the various forms of words and to use them appropriately.

Word Forms

The table below lists the main forms of some terms that you will likely encounter in pharmacy practice. Review the table and then do the exercises that follow to assess your understanding.

Noun (n)	Infinitive/Verb (v) —Past Tense	Adjective (adj)	Adverb (adv)
abdomen		abdominal	abdominally
an ache	to ache; ached	achy; aching	
agitation	to agitate; agitated	agitated; agitating	
blood		bloody; bloodied	
constipation		constipated	
coordination	to coordinate; coordinated	coordinated	
delirium		delirious	deliriously
diabetes; a diabetic		diabetic	
drowsiness		drowsy	drowsily

(continued)

Noun (n)	Infinitive/Verb (v) —Past Tense	Adjective (adj)	Adverb (adv)
enlargement	to enlarge; enlarged	enlarged; enlarging	
exhaustion	to exhaust; exhausted	exhausted; exhausting	
fatigue	to fatigue; fatigued	fatigued; fatiguing	
gangrene		gangrened	gangrenous
hormone		hormonal	hormonally
hypoglycemia; hyperglycemic		hypoglycemic	
hyperthyroidism		hyperthyroid	
hypothyroidism		hypothyroid	
incontinence		incontinent	
insomnia; insomniac		insomniac	
intolerance		intolerant; intolerable	
lethargy		lethargic	
lightheadedness		lightheaded	
mask	to mask	masked; masking	
metabolism	to metabolize	metabolized; metabolizing	
nausea; nauseation	nauseate; nauseated	nauseous; nauseating	
nervousness		nervous	nervously
numbness	to numb; numbed	numbed; numbing	
overactivity		overactive	
pallor; paleness		pale; pallid	
protrusion	to protrude; protruded	protruding	
puffiness; puff	to puff; puffed	puffy	puffily
regulation	to regulate	regulated; regulating	
relapse	to relapse; relapsed	relapsing	
retention; retentiveness	to retain; retained	retentive	retentively
stiffness	to stiff; stiffed	stiff; stiffing	stiffly
a swallow	to swallow; swallow	swallowed	
tenderness		tender	tenderly
thirst		thirsty	
thyroid; thyroiditis			
tolerance	to tolerate; tolerated	tolerant; tolerable	
a tremble; tremor; trembler	to tremble; trembled	trembled; trembling; trembly	tremblingly
urination; urine	to urinate; urinated; urinating		

Word Forms Exercise

Read the following sentences carefully. Then indicate the word form of the bolded word(s), choosing from v, n, adj, or adv.

1. Early signs of hypothyroidism are **puffiness** around the face, constant **fatigue,** and **constipation.**

    puffiness _____   fatigue _____   constipation _____

2. **Paleness, bruising,** and **fatigue** may be signs of leukemia.

    paleness _____   bruising _____   fatigue _____

3. Because she complained of **weight loss** despite an increased **appetite,** frequent **diarrhea,** and feeling **nervous,** her doctor tested her for possible thyroid conditions.

    weight loss _____   appetite _____   diarrhea _____   nervous _____

4. The lymphatic system helps to fight **infection** and disease.

    infection _____

5. **Painless swelling** in the lymph nodes in the groin, armpit, or neck and **recurrent** fevers should not be ignored.

    painless _____   swelling _____   recurrent _____

6. People with type I **diabetes** are not able to **produce insulin,** whereas people with type II diabetes **resist** insulin and are not able to use it properly.

    diabetes _____   produce _____   insulin _____   resist _____

7. After complaining to her doctor that she was experiencing **insomnia, tremors** of her hands, weight loss, and that her eyes were **protruding,** she was given a series of thyroid tests and **diagnosed** with Graves disease.

    insomnia_____   tremors _____   protruding _____   diagnosed _____

8. Some symptoms of hypothyroidism include, but are not limited to, **cold intolerance,** body **aches, coarse** hair, and decreased **concentration.**

    cold intolerance _____   aches _____   coarse_____   concentration _____

9. A person experiencing **involuntary** loss of **urine** or **stool,** and experiencing **mental** confusion and **drowsiness,** should seek medical attention immediately.

    involuntary _____   urine _____   stool _____   mental _____   drowsiness _____

10. Graves disease is a **form** of hyperthyroidism that causes the patient to **overproduce** thyroid hormone and to have **protruding** eyes.

    form_____   overproduce_____   protruding _____

11. A **goiter,** which is an **enlargement** of the thyroid gland, can be reduced in size with thyroid **hormone.**

    goiter _____   enlargement _____   hormone _____

12. Symptoms of non-Hodgkin's lymphoma may include **swelling** in the armpits, groin, and neck, **night sweats,** weight loss, itchy skin, and **recurrent** fevers.

    swelling _____   night sweats _____   recurrent _____

13. A common thyroid **disorder** is Hashimoto's disease, which is caused by **inflammation** of the thyroid **gland** and can lead to an **underactive** thyroid, **stiffness,** and problems with concentration.

    disorder_____   inflammation_____   gland_____   underactive_____   stiffness_____

14. Some symptoms of leukemia include fatigue resulting from **anemia,** and **bruises,** a **rash,** and **swollen** lymph nodes.

    anemia _____   bruises _____   rash _____   swollen _____

15. **Diabetics** should exercise to help them control their blood **glucose,** weight, and blood **pressure.**

    diabetics _____   glucose _____   pressure _____

How did you do? Check your answers against the Answer Key online.

Typical Medical Conditions and Patient Complaints

The sentences below contain vocabulary that describes and explains typical medical conditions, diseases, symptoms, and patient complaints that a pharmacist encounters. Read the sentences carefully. Then indicate the word form of the bolded word(s), choosing from v, n, adj, or adv. Look up words you do not know in your bilingual or first-language dictionary.

1. People with type II **diabetes** are not able to properly use their sugar, which is called **glucose.**

   diabetes _____   glucose _____

2. Radioactive iodine **therapy** is one way to **treat thyroid cancer.**

   therapy _____   treat _____   thyroid _____   cancer _____

3. Some individuals suffering with either Hodgkin's lymphoma, a cancer of the **lymphatic** system, or non-Hodgkin's **lymphoma,** a cancer of the lymphatic system, may experience soaking night **sweats** and **severely itchy** skin.

   lymphatic _____   lymphoma ___   sweats _____   severely _____   itchy _____

4. Another word for **trachea** is **windpipe.**

   trachea _____   windpipe _____

5. **Insulin** is a **hormone** that helps the body to use **glucose,** the main source of fuel in the body.

   insulin ____   hormone _____   glucose ____

6. Leukemia is not a single disease but a number of **related blood** cancers that begin in the **bone marrow.**

   related _____   blood _____   bone marrow ____

7. **Cold intolerance** and excessive **sleepiness** are experienced by some individuals with hypothyroidism, but some individuals with hyperthyroidism are not able to **tolerate** heat and experience **excessive sweating** and weight gain.

   cold intolerance ___   sleepiness ___   tolerate ____   excessive ___   sweating ___

8. Patients suffering from diseases of the lymph and blood will **exhibit** many of the same symptoms, such as fatigue, **numbness, paleness, night sweats,** and **incontinence.**

   exhibit ____   numbness ___   paleness ___   night sweats ___   incontinence ___

9. The **bone marrow** of a person with leukemia will **produce abnormal** white blood cells.

   bone marrow ____   produce ____   abnormal _____

10. Because people with type II diabetes are not able to have **normal levels** of sugar, other **complications** such as kidney, heart, and eye disease can **occur.**

    normal ____   levels ____   complications _____   occur _____

11. Type I diabetes is an **autoimmune disease** in which the pancreas is not able to **produce** insulin.

    autoimmune disease _____   produce _____

12. People with diabetes need to be watchful of **slow-healing sores,** which can **typically** be found on their feet.

    slow-healing _____   sores____   typically ____

13. Thyroid hormones will help people with hypothyroidism **restore** their **metabolism.**

    restore _____   metabolism ____

14. A thyroid **nodule** is an **abnormal** growth that forms a **lump** in the thyroid gland, which is located below the **Adam's apple** in the front of the neck.

    nodule ____   abnormal ____   lump ____   Adam's apple ____

15. Depending on the **stage** and **grade** of the disease, non-Hodgkin's lymphoma may be treated with radiation, chemotherapy, a **combination** of both, and stem cell transplantation.

    stage _____   grade _____   combination _____

16. People with non-Hodgkin's lymphoma may experience a wide range of symptoms, including **swollen** lymph nodes, weight loss, **swelling** in the **abdomen,** night sweats, and trouble breathing.

    swollen _____   swelling _____   abdomen _____

17. After her daughter had experienced **unexplained** fevers, night **sweats,** weight loss, and **abdominal discomfort,** a series of blood tests **confirmed** the daughter had leukemia.

    unexplained _____   sweats _____   abdominal _____   discomfort _____   confirmed _____

18. Diabetes can lead to **hyperglycemia,** which can lead to blindness, kidney **failure,** and foot **ulcers.**

    hyperglycemia _____   failure _____   ulcers _____

19. If a person is feeling **lightheaded,** he or she is feeling a bit **dizzy** and is not able to think clearly or move **steadily.**

    lightheaded _____   dizzy _____   steadily _____

20. Some **medical** conditions and diseases can cause a person to **experience delirium** and confusion.

    medical _____   experience _____   delirium _____

How did you do? Check your answers against the Answer Key online.

Medical Vocabulary Comprehension

Now that you have read sentences 1 through 20 describing language regarding the endocrine and lymphatic systems, assess your understanding by doing the exercises below.

Multiple Choice Questions

Choose the answer that correctly completes each sentence below.

1. _____ **Hypothyroidism** symptoms include:
a. sweaty skin and constipation
b. constipation, weight gain, and fatigue
c. an enlarged spleen

2. _____ The **Adam's apple** is located:
a. in the thyroid gland
b. in the lymph node
c. in front of the neck

3. _____ An enlarged spleen and malaise might be experienced by a person who may have:
a. Hashimoto's disease
b. leukemia
c. a deep wound

4. _____ People with **type I diabetes:**
a. can make their own insulin
b. have protruding eyes
c. cannot make their own insulin

5. _____ Another word for **windpipe** is:
a. tonsils
b. esophagus
c. trachea

6. _____ Radioactive iodine therapy is treatment for:
a. lymphoma
b. Graves disease
c. thyroid cancer

7. _____ Slow-healing sores can be found in patients suffering from:
a. diabetes
b. lymphoma
c. leukemia

8. _____ If you are unable to tolerate heat and experience excessive sweating, you should be tested for:
a. hypothyroidism
b. hyperthyroidism
c. a blood disease

9. _____ **Hyperglycemia** is caused by diabetes and can lead to:
a. ulcers
b. ulcers, blindness, and kidney failure
c. a skin rash

10. _____ A **goiter** is an enlargement of:
a. a lymph node
b. the thyroid gland
c. the abdomen

11. _____ Puffiness around the face and constipation are symptoms of:
a. hives
b. hyperthyroidism
c. hypothyroidism

12. _____ Signs of leukemia include:
a. itchy, flaky skin
b. irritability and agitation
c. paleness, bruising, and fatigue

13. _____ Frequent urination and unquenchable thirst may be signs of:
a. incontinence
b. diabetes
c. ulcers

14. _____ Hashimoto's disease is:
a. a disorder of the lymph nodes
b. inflammation of the thyroid gland and can lead to an underactive thyroid
c. a kind of leukemia

15. _____ A person who is feeling lightheaded is:
a. wide awake
b. delirious
c. feeling dizzy and unsteady

True/False Questions

Indicate whether each sentence below is true (T) or false (F).

1. _____ A patient diagnosed with hypothyroidism may require life-long treatment with hormones.
2. _____ A person diagnosed with Graves disease may have protruding eyes.
3. _____ If the patient complains that he is constipated, it means he cannot urinate.
4. _____ A diabetic with a sore on the foot should not be concerned because the sore will heal quickly.
5. _____ If a patient complains of abdominal discomfort, frequent fevers, and fatigue, she should be tested for Hashimoto's disease.
6. _____ "Incontinence" is the adjective form and "incontinent" is the noun form.
7. _____ The word "intolerable" is a noun form.
8. _____ The word "diabetic" is both an adjective and a noun.
9. _____ A person with an underactive thyroid may experience stiffness.
10. _____ People with type II diabetes have normal sugar levels.

How did you do? Check your answers against the Answer Key online.

Writing Exercise

An important part of communication is the ability to write about what you read, to write correctly, and to spell correctly. In the exercises below, write your understanding of the meaning of the bolded words.

1. Describe in writing what **hypothyroidism** and **hyperthyroidism** are.

_____

_____

_____

_____

2. Describe in writing what **type I diabetes** and **type II diabetes** are.

_____

_____

_____

_____

3. Describe in writing what **Hodgkin's lymphoma** and **non-Hodgkin's lymphoma** are.

_____

_____

_____

_____

4. Describe in writing what **Hashimoto's disease** and **Graves disease** are.

_____

_____

_____

_____

Check what you have written with acceptable answers that appear in the Answer Key online.

LISTENING AND PRONUNCIATION

The ability to listen and understand what is being said and heard, and the ability to pronounce words clearly, is extremely important. A word misheard and a word mispronounced will lead to poor communication and can seriously put both the pharmacist and patient in danger. Therefore, it is very important that one hear clearly what another person has said, and that one speak clearly with correct pronunciation.

Listen carefully to the pharmacy-related words presented in the audio files found in Chapter 4 on thePoint (thePoint.lww.com/diaz-gilbert), and then pronounce them as accurately as you can. Listen and then repeat. You will listen to each word once and then you will repeat it. You will do this twice for each word. Listening and pronunciation practice will increase your listening and speaking confidence. Many languages do not produce or emphasize certain sounds produced and emphasized in English, so pay careful attention to the pronunciation of each word.

 ### Pronunciation Exercise

Listen to the audio files found in Chapter 4 on thePoint (thePoint.lww.com/diaz-gilbert) and repeat the words. Then say the words aloud for additional practice.

1. abdomen ăb-dōˈmən
2. ache āk
3. Addison's disease ădˈĭ-sənz dĭ-zēzˈ
4. agitation ăjˈĭ-tāˈshən
5. anemia ə-nēˈmē-ə
6. appetite ăpˈĭ-tītˈ
7. armpit ärmˈpĭtˈ
8. benign bĭ-nīnˈ
9. blood blŭd
10. bone marrow bōn mărˈō
11. bowel movement bouˈəl mōōvˈmənt
12. cold intolerance kōld ĭn-tŏlˈər-əns
13. constipation kŏnˈstə-pāˈshən
14. coordination kō-ôrˈdn-āˈshən
15. Cushing's disease kōōshˈĭngz dĭ-zēzˈ
16. delirium dĭ-lîrˈē-əm
17. diabetes dīˈə-bēˈtĭs
18. drowsy drouˈzē
19. enlargement ĕn-lärjˈmənt
20. exhaustion ĭg-zôsˈchən
21. fatigue fə-tēgˈ
22. gangrene găngˈgrēn
23. gland glănd
24. glucose glōōˈkōsˈ
25. goiter goiˈtər
26. Graves disease gräˈvāz dĭ-zēzˈ
27. groin groin
28. Hashimoto's disease häˈshē-mōˈtōzˈ dĭ-zēz
29. Hodgkin's lymphoma ˈhŏjˈkĭnz lĭm-fōˈmə
30. heat intolerance hēt ĭn-tŏlˈər-əns
31. hormone hôrˈmōnˈ
32. hyperthyroidism hīˈpər-thīˈroi-dĭzˈəm
33. hypoglycemia hīˈpō-glīˈ-sēˈmĭk
34. hypothyroidism hīˈpō-thīˈroi-dĭzˈəm
35. immune system ĭ-myōōnˈ sĭsˈtəm
36. incontinence ĭn-kŏnˈtə-nəns
37. indigestion ĭnˈdĭ-jĕsˈchən

38. insomnia	ĭn-sŏm′nə
39. insulin	ĭn′sə-lĭn
40. lethargy	lĕth′ər-jē
41. lightheaded	līt′hĕd′ĭd
42. lymph node	lĭmf nōd
43. malaise	mă-lāz
44. malignant	mə-lĭg′nənt
45. mask	măsk
46. measles	mē′zəlz
47. metabolism	mĭ-tăb′ə-lĭz′əm
48. mononucleosis	mŏn-′onoo′klē-ō′sĭs
49. mood swings	mood swĭngs
50. mumps	mŭmps
51. muscle cramp	mŭs′əl krămp
52. nausea	nô′zē-ə
53. nervous	nûr′vəs
54. nodule	nŏj′ool
55. non-Hodgkin's lymphoma	nŏn′hŏj′kĭnz lĭm-fō′mə
56. numb	nŭm
57. overactive	ō′vər-ăk′tĭv
58. overproduction	ō′vər prə-dŭk′shən
59. pallor	păl′ər
60. pituitary gland	pĭ-too′ĭ-tĕr′ē glănd
61. protruding	prō-trood′ng
62. puffy	pŭf′ē
63. regulate	rĕg′yə-lāt′
64. relapse	rĭ-lăps′
65. stiff	stĭf
66. swallow	swŏl′ō
67. tender	tĕn′dər
68. thirst	thûrst
69. tremble	trĕm′bəl
70. underactive	ŭn′dər ăk′tĭv
71. underarm	ŭn′dər ärm′
72. underproduction	ŭn′dər prō dŭk′shən
73. unquenchable	ŭn-kwĕn′chə-bəl
74. urinate	yoor′ə-nāt′
75. water retention	wô′tər rĭ-tĕn′shən
76. windpipe	wĭnd′pīp′

Which words are easy to pronounce? Which are difficult to pronounce? Use the space below to write in the words that you find difficult to pronounce. These are words you should practice saying often.

_____

_____

_____

_____

_____

Listen to the audio files found in Chapter 4 on thePoint (thePoint.lww.com/diaz-gilbert) as many times as you need to increase your pronunciation ability of the difficult words. Pronounce these words with a friend or a colleague who speaks English.

English Sounds That Are Difficult for Speakers of Other Languages to Pronounce

Spanish

In Spanish, there is no English "v" sound, but the "v" consonant in Spanish is pronounced like the English "b." The vowel "i" is pronounced like a long "e." Pay careful attention to the "v" sound in English when pronouncing words that begin with "v." Also pay careful attention to English words that begin with "s;" do not use the Spanish "es" sound when pronouncing English words that begin with "s."

For example, in English,

stiff is not pronounced esteef
insulin is not pronounced eensuleen

Vietnamese

In Vietnamese, the "t" consonant is pronounced "s," but in English the "t" is pronounced "t" and "s" is pronounced "s." Be careful with English words that begin with "t." In Vietnamese, the "b" consonant is pronounced "p," but in English "p" is pronounced "p" and "b" is pronounced "b."

In Vietnamese, words do not end in "b," "ch," "f," "d," "j," "l," "p," "r," "s," "sh," "v," and "z." In English, words end in these letters. Pay special attention to pronouncing these English sounds. In Vietnamese, there is no "dzh" or "zh" sound, so English words like "judge" (dzh) and "rupture" (zh) will be hard for Vietnamese speakers to pronounce.

For example, in English,

blood is not pronounced plud
armpit is not pronounced ahmpih
malaise is not pronounced malai

Gujarati

In Gujarati, "v" is pronounced "w," "f" is pronounced "p," "p" is pronounced "f," and "z" is pronounced "j." Short "i" is pronounced long "e," "x" is pronounced "ch," and "th" is pronounced "s." In English, "v" is pronounced "v," "f" is pronounced "f," "z" is pronounced "z" or "s," "j" is pronounced "j," and "x" is pronounced "x." Pay careful attention when pronouncing these sounds.

For example, in English,

puffy is not pronounced fuffy
fatigue is not pronounced patigue
mumps is not pronounced mumfs
stiff is not pronounced steef
lethargy is not pronounced lesargy

Korean

In Korean, the "v" consonant is pronounced "b" and the "f" consonant is pronounced "p." In English, the "v" is pronounced "v," the "f" is pronounced "f," and the "p" is pronounced "p." Pay special attention when pronouncing these sounds.

For example, in English,

fatigue is not pronounced patigue
windpipe is not pronounced vinpipe

(continued)

Chinese

In Chinese, the "r" consonant is pronounced "l" or "w," and "b," "d," "g," and "ng" are not pronounced at all. Pay careful attention to English words that begin with "r" because the "r" is not pronounced "l" or "w," and "b," "d," "g," and "ng" are pronounced in English.

For example, in English,

gland is not pronounced glan
protruding is not pronounced plotludin

Russian

The "w" consonant is pronounced like a "v" and the "v" sounds like a "w." Pay careful attention to the English "th." It is not pronounced "s."

For example, in English,

windpipe is not pronounced vinpipe
thirst is not pronounced sirst

DICTATION

Listening/Spelling Exercise: Word and Word Pairs

Listen to the words or word pairs on the audio files found in Chapter 4 on thePoint (thePoint.lww.com/diaz-gilbert) and then write them down on the lines below.

1. _____
2. _____
3. _____
4. _____
5. _____
6. _____
7. _____
8. _____
9. _____
10. _____
11. _____
12. _____
13. _____
14. _____
15. _____

Listening/Spelling Exercise: Sentences

Listen to the sentences on the audio files found in Chapter 4 on thePoint (thePoint.lww.com/diaz-gilbert) and then write them down on the lines below.

1. _____
_____
2. _____
_____

3. _____

_____

4. _____

_____

5. _____

_____

6. _____

_____

7. _____

_____

8. _____

_____

9. _____

_____

10. _____

_____

Now, check your sentences against the correct answers in the Answer Key online. If there are any new words that you do not know or that you spelled incorrectly, make a list of those words and study them for meaning and spelling.

PHARMACIST/PATIENT DIALOGUES

The ability to orally communicate effectively with your professors, colleagues, and especially with patients is very important. As a pharmacist, you will be counseling patients; patients will come to you for advice. They will have questions about a condition and symptoms they may experience and will ask you to help treat the condition. Therefore, it is extremely important that you understand what they are saying and that you respond to them and their questions appropriately. Your patients will speak differently. For example, some may speak very quickly, others too low, and yet others may speak angrily. To help you improve your listening skills, listen to the following dialogues, or short conversations, between a pharmacist and a patient and between a pharmacy technician and a patient.

Listening and Comprehension Exercises
Dialogue #1

Listen to Dialogue #1, stop, listen again and take notes. Listen to the dialogue as many times as you need or until you feel you have written sufficient notes and feel confident. You can use your notes to answer the multiple choice questions at the end of the dialogue.

Notes _____

_____

_____

_____

_____

Answer the questions below by selecting the answer that correctly completes each sentence.

1. _____ Why is the patient in the pharmacy?

a. to pick up a prescription

b. to get a prescription filled

c. to pay for her prescription

To help you improve your knowledge of idioms and idiomatic expressions, carefully read the following idiomatic expressions that contain the word "blood."

Idiomatic Expressions using "Blood"

1. ***to make one's blood boil*** means to be very angry.

    For example: Patients who say they have insurance, but do not have their insurance cards with them, sometimes ***make my blood boil,*** especially when we are really busy.

2. ***to make one's blood run cold*** means to be frightened or scared.

    For example: Scary movies such as "The Exorcist" and "Friday the 13th" ***make my blood run cold.***

3. ***to be after one's blood*** means a person hates or wants to harm another person.

    For example: The pharmacist, who was arrested for stealing drugs from cancer patients, is now under police protection because many patients are ***after his blood.***

4. ***to run in one's blood*** means that a person's characteristic is passed down by family tradition.

    For example: The parents and their two adult children are pharmacists; it ***runs in their blood.***

5. ***to get blood from a stone*** means it is difficult to get something, such as money, from a person.

    For example: I will never lend her money again; the first time I lent her money it was like ***getting blood from a stone*** before she repaid me.

6. ***blood is thicker than water*** means that family relationships are more important than relationships with other people.

    For example: Even though family members often fight with each other, they will always come to the defense of their family members because ***blood is thicker than water.***

Mini Dialogues Listening Exercise

How much did you understand? Listen to the following mini dialogues in the audio files found in Chapter 4 on thePoint (thePoint.lww.com/diaz-gilbert), read the questions below, and then choose the correct answer.

 ## *Mini Dialogue #1*

1. _____ Don't let them ***make your blood boil*** means:

a. don't let them yell at you

b. don't let them make you angry

c. don't let them get angry

 ## *Mini Dialogue #2*

2. _____ ***Make my blood run cold*** means:

a. to stay calm

b. to feel cold

c. to make me frightened and scared

 ## *Mini Dialogue #3*

3. _____ ***Run in your blood*** means:

a. the blood disease is hereditary

b. it's part of family tradition

c. family relationships are very important

Mini Dialogue #4

4. _____ *Getting blood from a stone* means:

a. to bleed because she was hit by a stone

b. her sister will pay her with pennies

c. she will have a difficult time getting the money back from her sister

 Mini Dialogue #5

5. _____ *Blood is thicker than water* means:

a. relationships with other people are important

b. relationships with relatives are not important

c. relationships with relatives are more important than relationships with other people

How did you do? Check your answers against the Answer Key online.

POST-ASSESSMENT

True/False Questions

Indicate whether each sentence below is true (T) or false (F).

1. _____ The idiom **makes my blood boil** means the individual's blood is very hot.

2. _____ The noun form of **delirium** is delirious.

3. _____ Another word for windpipe is Adam's apple.

4. _____ **Diabetic** is both a noun and adjective form.

5. _____ If a person's **blood runs cold,** the person is scared and frightened.

6. _____ Another word for trachea is windpipe.

7. _____ Paleness, bruising, and fatigue are signs of diabetes.

8. _____ The adjective form of **constipation** is constipated.

9. _____ Hypothyroidism is one type of thyroid disease.

10. _____ A goiter is a reduced thyroid gland.

11. _____ If a person believes **blood is thicker than water,** she believes relationships with friends are more important than relationships with relatives.

12. _____ If a patient complains his eyes are protruding and that he is experiencing sleepless nights and tremors, he should be tested for Graves disease.

13. _____ People with type II diabetes are able to use sugar properly.

14. _____ People with diabetes need to be watchful of fast-healing sores.

15. _____ If a person is feeling lightheaded, he or she barely has a headache.

Multiple Choice Questions

Choose the correct answer from a, b, and c.

1. _____ The adjective form of **tremble** is:

a. trembled

b. trembling

c. trembled, trembling, trembly

Answer the questions below by selecting the answer that correctly completes each sentence.

1. _____ The customer is picking up a prescription for:
a. his wife
b. himself
c. his wife and himself

2. _____ The patient's name is:
a. Christine Gramm
b. Christina Gram
c. Christina Graham

3. _____ The prescription is for:
a. Aricept
b. Aranesp
c. Arimidex

4. _____ The medication is used:
a. in chemotherapy
b. to treat cancer
c. to treat anemia caused by chemotherapy

5. _____ The patient's doctor's name is:
a. Ahmed Patel
b. Amid Patel
c. Amit Patel

6. _____ The patient's birth date is:
a. February 12, 1955
b. February 12, 1905
c. February 12, 1912

7. _____ The patient's husband is:
a. an asthmatic
b. a diabetic
c. anemic

8. _____ Side effects of the medication include:
a. headache, body aches, and diarrhea
b. dry mouth
c. irritability

9. _____ The pharmacist tells the customer that the doctor should be called if she experiences:
a. swelling, redness, and weakness in the arms and legs
b. weakness in the arms
c. swelling in the arms and legs

10. _____ The patient's insurance:
a. has changed and has a co-pay
b. is the same and has no co-pay
c. has changed and has no co-pay

How did you do on the Post-Assessment in Chapter 4? Check your answers in the Answer Key online.

Chest, Lung, and Respiratory System | 5

PRE-ASSESSMENT

True/False Questions

Indicate whether each sentence below is true (T) or false (F).

1. _____ **Asthma** is a chronic heart condition.
2. _____ **Bronchitis** is a respiratory infection that causes a hacking cough and produces phlegm.
3. _____ **Inhalation** and **inhaler** are noun forms.
4. _____ Some individuals with **pneumonia** will experience a cold, a fever, **shaking chills,** and cough with sputum production.
5. _____ The adjective form of **perspiring** is perspiration.
6. _____ **Tuberculosis** cannot be treated successfully with antibiotics.
7. _____ The most common cause of **emphysema** is cigarette smoking.
8. _____ People with chronic obstructive pulmonary disease (COPD) experience **wheezing** and **shortness of breath.**
9. _____ **Pneumothorax** refers to a collapsed lung.
10. _____ The adjective form of **asthma** is asthmatic.
11. _____ A person with **bronchitis** may experience fatigue, shortness of breath, and itchiness.
12. _____ The most common forms of **COPD** are asthma and tuberculosis.
13. _____ **Pleurisy** is a blood clot in the lung, and a **pulmonary embolism** is fluid in the lung.
14. _____ Allergens such as pet dander, dust mites, molds, and pollen can trigger **asthma.**
15. _____ The word **wheeze** is a noun and an adjective.

Multiple Choice Questions

Choose the correct answer from a, b, and c.

1. _____ "She was **shouting at the top of her lungs**" means:
   a. she was speaking very loudly
   b. the top of her lungs are in a lot of pain
   c. her lungs had collapsed

2. _____ **"To get something off your chest"** means:
   a. to remove the heavy pressure on your chest
   b. to let someone know that something has been annoying or bothering you for a long time
   c. to be very angry and anxious

3. _____ Another word for pertussis is:

a. hacking cough

b. persistent cough

c. whooping cough

4. _____ If someone is experiencing shallow breathing, they are:

a. breathing heavily

b. wheezing

c. breathing in small amounts of air

5. _____ If a patient complains of **shortness of breath,** wheezing, and fatigue, he or she might have:

a. pleurisy

b. bronchitis

c. tuberculosis

6. _____ **Emphysema** is a common problem in:

a. children with cystic fibrosis

b. asthmatics

c. smokers

7. _____ **Dyspnea** is another word for:

a. wheezing

b. shortness of breath

c. puffs

8. _____ The word **tightness** is:

a. a noun

b. a verb

c. an adjective

9. _____ A **hacking cough** is:

a. a loud, repeated, painful cough

b. a dry cough

c. a cough that produces a lot of phlegm

10. _____ The patient complained that she was having shaking chills, a high fever, some chest pain, and that she was coughing with sputum. This could indicate she has:

a. a collapsed lung

b. pneumonia

c. bronchitis

How did you do? Check your answers in the Answer Key online.

MEDICAL VOCABULARY

A good understanding of vocabulary words in pharmacy is very important for communication with professors, fellow students, patients, and coworkers. Knowledge and understanding of vocabulary leads to successful communication and success as a pharmacy student, as a pharmacy technician, and as a practicing pharmacist. You may already know many of the vocabulary words in this chapter, but for words that are unfamiliar, pay careful attention to them and make every effort to know their correct spelling, meaning, and pronunciation. It is a good idea to keep a list of new words and to look up these new words in a bilingual dictionary or dictionary in your first language. A good command of pharmacy-related vocabulary and good pronunciation of vocabulary will help to prevent embarrassing mistakes and increase effective verbal communication skills.

Chest, Lung, and Respiratory System Vocabulary

acute	diphtheria	pertussis
airway	dyspnea	pleurisy
asthma	edema	puffs
blood-streaked	episodic	pulmonary embolism
blood-tinged	exertion	rapid breathing
bluish color	exhale	shaking chills
bronchitis	expectorate	shallow breathing
chills	febrile	sharp pain
chronic obstructive	frothy	shivering
pulmonary disease	hacking cough	shortness of breath
(COPD)	influenza	spit
clammy	inhale	tightness
collapsed lung	knife-like pain	walking pneumonia
crackles	labored breathing	wheezing
creaking	nasal flaring	whooping cough
croup	persistent cough	
cystic fibrosis	perspiration	

PARTS OF SPEECH

A good understanding of parts of speech, such as verbs, nouns, adjectives, and adverbs, is important for successful communication when speaking or writing. It is equally important to know the various forms of words and to use them appropriately.

Word Forms

The table below lists the main forms of some terms that you will likely encounter in pharmacy practice. Review the table and then do the exercises that follow to assess your understanding.

Noun (n)	Infinitive/Verb (v) —Past Tense	Adjective (adj)	Adverb (adv)
acuteness		acute	acutely
asthma; asthmatic		asthma; asthmatic	asthmatically
bronchitis; bronchodilator		bronchial; bronchitic; bronchiolar	bronchially
chills	to chill; chilled	chilled; chilly; chilling	
chronicity		chronic	chronically
collapse; collapsibility;	to collapse; collapsed	collapsed; collapsible; collapsable	
creak	to creak; creaked	creaking; creaky	creakingly
croup		croupous; croupy	
diphtheria		diphtheric; diphtheritic; diphtherial	
dyspnea		dyspneic	
edema		edematous	
embolism		embolismic	

(continued)

Noun (n)	Infinitive/Verb (v) —Past Tense	Adjective (adj)	Adverb (adv)
emphysema; emphysemic		emphysemic; emphysematous	
episode		episodic	episodically
exertion	to exert; exerted	exerted	
exhalation	to exhale; exhaled	exhaled	
exhaustion	to exhaust; exhausted	exhausted; exhausting	
expectorant; expectoration	to expectorate; expectorated		
fever		febrile; fevered; feverish	feverishly
fibrosis		fibrotic	
froth	to froth; frothed	frothy	frothily
influenza		influenzal	
inhalation; inhalant; inhaler	to inhale; inhaled		
persistence	to persist; persisted	persistent	persistently
perspiration	to perspire; perspired	perspiring; perspiratory	
pertussis		pertussal	
pleurisy		pleuritic	
pneumonia		pneumonic	
		pulmonary; pulmonic	
obstruction; obstructor; obstructiveness	to obstruct; obstructed	obstructive; obstructing;	obstructively
shakiness	to shake; shook	shaking; shaky; shaken; shakable	shakily
shallowness		shallow	shallowly
sharpness	to sharpen	sharp; sharpened	sharply
shiver	to shiver; shivered	shivery	
spit	to spit; spit		
tightness	to tighten; tied	tight	
wheezer	to wheeze; wheezed	wheezing; wheezy	wheezingly

Word Forms Exercise

Read the following sentences carefully. Then indicate the word form of the bolded word(s), choosing from v, n, adj, or adv.

1. A **bronchial** infection can be either sudden or **acute,** which means it will last for a short time, or it can be **chronic,** which means it **recurs** often.

   bronchial _____   acute _____   chronic _____   recurs _____

2. Asthma is a respiratory infection that is **triggered** by **allergens** or exercise and results in **labored** breathing, **coughing,** and chest **constriction.**

triggered _____   allergens _____   labored _____   coughing _____   constriction _____

3. Common symptoms experienced by people with **tuberculosis** include, but are not limited to, **tiredness, fever,** night **sweats,** and weight loss.

tuberculosis _____   tiredness_____   fever _____   sweats _____

4. Various **treatments** for people who **suffer** from **emphysema** include antibiotics, **inhalers,** and **bronchodilators.**

treatments _____   suffer _____   emphysema _____   inhalers _____   bronchodilators _____

5. Children with **cystic fibrosis,** a lung disease, are **treated** with **breathing** treatments and **chest** percussions.

cystic fibrosis _____   treated _____   breathing _____   chest _____

6. **Pneumothorax,** or a **collapsed** lung, can be caused by a variety of lung diseases or by injury to the chest as a result of a broken rib, a **stabbing,** or a gunshot **wound.**

pneumothorax _____   collapsed _____   stabbing _____   wound _____

7. Emphysema, which **affects** smokers, is a lung disease that causes the **air sacs** in the lungs to **burst,** making breathing, coughing, and **expelling** mucus **difficult.**

affects _____   air sacs _____   burst _____   expelling _____   difficult _____

8. Asthma can cause the **bronchial tubes** to become narrow, **inflamed, swollen,** and **irritated.**

bronchial tubes _____   inflamed _____   swollen _____   irritated _____

9. **Cigarette,** pipe, and cigar **smoking** can cause **lung cancer.**

cigarette _____   smoking _____   lung cancer _____

10. People with **walking pneumonia** may experience headaches, a dry **cough** without blood or phlegm, a **sore** throat, and **excessive sweating.**

walking pneumonia _____   cough _____   sore _____   excessive _____   sweating _____

11. Children with **croup** will have a loud, **barking cough** and experience **labored** and noisy breathing as a result of swollen **vocal** chords and a swollen **windpipe.**

croup _____   barking cough _____   labored _____   vocal _____   windpipe _____

12. An **asthmatic** will experience **tightness** in the chest and **wheezing,** a sound like a whistle, when **inhaling** and **exhaling.**

asthmatic _____   tightness _____   wheezing _____   inhaling _____   exhaling _____

13. Cystic fibrosis can cause **lung damage, infection,** and **inflammation.**

lung damage _____   infection _____   inflammation _____

14. Bronchitis **affects** the nose, **throat,** and **sinuses.**

affects _____   throat _____   sinuses _____

15. **Expectorate** means to **cough up** or **spit up** phlegm and mucus.

expectorate _____   cough up _____   spit up _____

How did you do? Check your answers against the Answer Key online.

Typical Medical Conditions and Patient Complaints

The sentences below contain vocabulary that describes and explains typical medical conditions, diseases, symptoms, and patient complaints that a pharmacist encounters. Read the sentences carefully.

Then indicate the word form of the bolded word(s), choosing from v, n, adj, or adv. Look up words you do not know in your bilingual or first-language dictionary.

1. An **expectorant** is a **cough medicine** that will help reduce the thick, **sticky** secretions that you may experience when you have the flu or a **cold.**

   expectorant _____   cough medicine _____   sticky _____   cold _____

2. The patient complained he was **fatigued,** had no **appetite,** was having night sweats, had a **low-grade** fever, was coughing **frequently,** and sometimes was spitting up blood.

   fatigued _____   appetite _____   low-grade _____   frequently _____

3. **Chest percussion,** also referred to as chest clapping, is a way to help empty the lungs of unwanted **secretions** that accumulate in the lungs and is often used with patients who **suffer** from cystic fibrosis.

   chest percussion _____   secretions _____   suffer _____

4. People with **pleurisy,** which is an inflammation of the membrane that surrounds the lungs, will experience a **sharp** pain in the chest when they **cough,** inhale, **exhale,** and **sneeze.**

   pleurisy _____   sharp _____   cough _____   exhale _____   sneeze _____

5. If you are suffering from chronic bronchitis, your doctor may **prescribe** a **bronchodilator,** which is a medicine that is **breathed** through the mouth to open up the **air passages,** or the **bronchial tubes,** of the lungs.

   prescribe _____   bronchodilator _____   breathed _____   air passages _____   bronchial tubes _____

6. In addition to **allergens** such as dander, pollen, and mold spores, **triggers** of asthma include respiratory infections and **exercise.**

   allergens _____   triggers _____   exercise _____

7. Children with cystic fibrosis may develop bronchitis, a collapsed lung, and pneumonia as a result of the **thick** and **sticky** mucus that **clogs** the respiratory system and **allows** bacteria to grow within it.

   thick _____   sticky _____   clogs _____   allows _____

8. Symptoms of a pulmonary embolism include chest pain, **sudden shortness of breath,** blood-streaked sputum, excessive **perspiration,** and, in **severe** cases, loss of **consciousness.**

   sudden _____   shortness of breath _____   perspiration _____   severe _____   consciousness _____

9. Early signs of COPD include a **persistent** cough, **respiratory** infections, and shortness of breath with **exertion.**

   persistent _____   respiratory _____   exertion _____

10. Treatment for people who suffer from emphysema includes **smoking cessation,** drug **therapies,** and **supplemental** oxygen designed for home use.

    smoking cessation _____   therapies _____   supplemental _____

11. A child with **whooping cough,** which is a contagious respiratory infection also known as **pertussis,** may initially exhibit symptoms such a **runny nose, sneezing,** and a **mild** cold.

    whooping cough _____   pertussis _____   runny nose _____   sneezing _____   mild _____

12. Croup is a respiratory infection that affects the vocal chords of children and infants and causes a loud, **barking,** hoarse, coughing **sound** and is treated by breathing **moist air** or by **medication** to open the airways.

    barking _____   sound _____   moist _____   air _____   medication _____

13. Some people with **pneumonia** will experience a **sharp** pain when they take deep **breaths.**

    pneumonia _____   sharp _____   breaths _____

14. Emphysema and **chronic bronchitis** are two examples of **COPD**, or chronic **obstructive pulmonary** disease.

    chronic _____   bronchitis _____   COPD _____   obstructive _____   pulmonary _____

15. Tuberculosis is **highly contagious,** affects the lungs, and is **transmitted** to others through sneezing and **mucus.**

    highly _____   contagious _____   transmitted _____   mucus _____

16. Cystic fibrosis is a **hereditary** disease that affects the pancreas and the respiratory system, causing thick and **sticky mucus,** respiratory infections, and **impaired pancreatic** function.

    hereditary _____   sticky _____   mucus _____   impaired _____   pancreatic _____

17. Chronic bronchitis, which is inflammation and **thickening** of the **airways** inside the lungs, is caused by cigarette **smoke,** allergies, **irritants,** and pollutants.

    thickening _____   airways _____   smoke _____   irritants _____

18. Pneumonia is an infection and inflammation of the lung caused by a **bacterium,** virus, or fungus that **enters** the body through the nose and through **inhalation.**

    bacterium _____   enters _____   inhalation _____

19. **Wheezing** is **experienced** by people who **suffer** from asthma, bronchitis, and emphysema.

    wheezing _____   experienced _____   suffer _____

20. **Nasal flaring refers** to the enlargement of the nostrils during breathing and is a sign of breathing **difficulty** in children who are experiencing croup, asthma, or other airway **obstruction.**

    nasal flaring _____   refers _____   difficulty _____   obstruction _____

How did you do? Check your answers against the Answer Key online.

Medical Vocabulary Comprehension

Now that you have read sentences 1 through 20 describing language regarding the chest, lung, and respiratory system, assess your understanding by doing the exercises below.

Multiple Choice Questions

Choose the answer that correctly completes each sentence below.

1. _____ A **bronchodilator:**
a. treats croup
b. is prescribed for chronic bronchitis
c. supplies supplemental oxygen

2. _____ Patients with **pneumonia** may:
a. feel a sharp pain in the chest when they take deep breaths
b. feel a mild pain when they take shallow breaths
c. have labored breathing

3. _____ Thick, sticky mucous secretions caused by the flu or a cold can be reduced by:
a. wheezing
b. taking an expectorant
c. chest percussions

4. _____ A **collapsed lung** can be caused by:
a. a stabbing and gunshot wounds only
b. lung diseases only
c. lung diseases and physical injury such as a broken rib cage, a stabbing, or a gunshot wound

5. _____ Dyspnea refers to:

a. labored breathing

b. shortness of breath

c. exhalation

6. _____ An early sign of **COPD** includes:

a. emphysema

b. shortness of breath with exertion

c. shortness of breath without exertion

7. _____ A **chronic infection:**

a. is sudden and lasts a short time

b. recurs often

c. is sudden and lasts a long time

8. _____ Pertussis is:

a. an infection of the respiratory system

b. an inflammation of the bronchial tubes

c. another word for wheezing

9. _____ **Bronchial tubes** refer to:

a. nasal passages

b. air passages

c. the windpipe

10. _____ An example of chronic obstructive pulmonary disease is:

a. walking pneumonia

b. asthma

c. emphysema

11. _____ Pertussis is another term for:

a. hacking cough

b. wheezing

c. whooping cough

12. _____ Children with **croup:**

a. are having an asthma attack

b. produce a loud, barking sound

c. have suffered a collapsed lung

13. _____ **Expectorate** means to:

a. swallow

b. take a deep breath

c. spit up

14. _____ Asthma can cause the bronchial tubes to:

a. become clogged

b. get inflamed and irritated

c. collapse

15. _____ A treatment for **emphysema** is:

a. moist air

b. smoking cessation

c. lack of oxygen

True/False Questions

Indicate whether each sentence below is true (T) or false (F).

1. _____ Chest percussion is a treatment for asthma.
2. _____ A person who has tuberculosis will wheeze.
3. _____ Irritants and pollutants can cause chronic bronchitis.
4. _____ Pneumonia is an infection and inflammation of the lung caused by cigarette smoke.
5. _____ If a child is suffering from croup, the vocal chords are affected, and the child's voice will be hoarse and produce a loud, barking sound.
6. _____ Bacteria, viruses, and fungi cause asthma.
7. _____ The word "asthmatic" is both a noun and an adjective.
8. _____ Whooping cough is not a contagious disease.
9. _____ Symptoms of COPD include a persistent cold, nausea, and shallow breathing.
10. _____ The word "exhausted" is both an adjective and a noun.

How did you do? Check your answers against the Answer Key online.

Writing Exercise

An important part of communication is the ability to write about what you read, to write correctly, and to spell correctly. In the exercises below, write your understanding of the meaning of the bolded words.

1. Describe in writing what **asthma, emphysema,** and **chronic bronchitis** are.

_____

_____

_____

_____

2. Describe in writing what **croup** and **whooping cough** are.

_____

_____

_____

_____

3. Describe in writing what **cystic fibrosis, tuberculosis,** and **pneumonia** are.

_____

_____

_____

_____

Check what you have written with acceptable answers that appear in the Answer Key online.

LISTENING AND PRONUNCIATION

The ability to listen and understand what is being said and heard, and the ability to pronounce words clearly, is extremely important. A word misheard and a word mispronounced will lead to poor communication and can seriously put both the pharmacist and patient in danger. Therefore, it is very important that one hear clearly what another person has said, and that one speak clearly with correct pronunciation.

Listen carefully to the pharmacy-related words presented in Chapter 5 on thePoint (thePoint.lww.com/diaz-gilbert), and then pronounce them as accurately as you can. Listen and then repeat. You will listen to each word once and then you will repeat it. You will do this twice for each word. Listening and pronunciation practice will increase your listening and speaking confidence.

Many languages do not produce or emphasize certain sounds produced and emphasized in English, so pay careful attention to the pronunciation of each word.

 Pronunciation Exercise

Listen to the audio files found in Chapter 5 on thePoint (thePoint.lww.com/diaz-gilbert). Listen and repeat the words. Then say the words aloud for additional practice.

1. acute	ə-kyo͞ot′	
2. airway	âr′wā′	
3. asthma	ăz′mə	
4. blood-streaked	blŭd strēkt	
5. blood-tinged	blŭd tĭnjd	
6. bluish color	blo͞o′ĭsh kŭl′ər	
7. bronchitis	brŏn-kī′tĭs	
8. chills	chĭls	
9. chronic obstructive pulmonary disease	krŏn′ĭk əb-strŭkt′ĭf pŭl′mə-nĕr′ē dĭ-zēz′	
10. clammy	klăm′ē	
11. collapsed lung	kə-lăpst lŭng	
12. crackles	krăk′əls	
13. creaking	krēkng	
14. croup	kro͞op	
15. cystic fibrosis	sĭs′tĭk fī-brō′sĭs	
16. diphtheria	dĭpthîr′ē-ə	
17. dyspnea	dĭsp-nē′ə	
18. edema	ĭ-dē′mə	
19. episodic	ĕp′ĭ-sŏd′ĭk	
20. exertion	ĭg-zûr′shən	
21. exhale	ēks-hāl′	
22. expectorate	ĭk-spĕk′tə-rāt′	
23. febrile	fē′brəl	
24. frothy	frô′thē	
25. hacking cough	hăkng kôf	
26. influenza	ĭn′flo͞o-ĕn′zə	
27. inhale	ĭn-hāl′	
28. knife-like pain	nīf-līk pān	
29. labored breathing	lā′bərd brē′thĭng	
30. nasal flaring	nā′zəl flârng	
31. persistent cough	pər-sĭs′tənt kôf	
32. perspiration	pûr′spə-rā′shən	
33. pertussis	pər-tŭs′ĭs	
34. pleurisy	plo͞or′ĭ-sē	
35. puffs	pŭfs	
36. pulmonary embolism	pŭl′mə-nĕr′ē ĕm′bə-lĭz′əm	
37. rapid breathing	răp′ĭd brē′thĭng	
38. shaking chills	shākng chĭls	
39. shallow breathing	shăl′ō brē′thĭng	
40. sharp pain	shärp pān	
41. shivering	shĭv′ərng	
42. shortness of breath	shôrt nĕs ŏv brēth	
43. spit	spĭt	
44. tightness	tītĕns	

45. walking pneumonia   wôkng n$\widetilde{oo}$-m$\breve{o}$n′y$\ni$
46. wheezing   w$\bar{e}$z ng,
47. whooping cough   w$\overline{oo}$′p$\breve{i}$ng kôf

Which words are easy to pronounce? Which are difficult to pronounce? Use the space below to write in the words that you find difficult to pronounce. These are words you should practice saying often.

_____

_____

_____

_____

_____

_____

_____

Listen to the audio files found in Chapter 5 on thePoint (thePoint.lww.com/diaz-gilbert) as many times as you need to increase your pronunciation ability of the difficult words. Pronounce these words with a friend or a colleague who speaks English.

English Sounds That Are Difficult for Speakers of Other Languages to Pronounce

Spanish

In Spanish, there is no English "v" sound, but the "v" consonant in Spanish is pronounced like the English "b." The vowel "i" is pronounced like a long "e." Pay careful attention to the "v" sound in English when pronouncing words that begin with "v." Also pay careful attention to English words that begin with "s;" do not use the Spanish "es" sound when pronouncing English words that begin with "s."

For example, in English,

bronchitis is not pronounced bronkeetees
shivering is not pronounced esheebereeng

Vietnamese

In Vietnamese, the "t" consonant is pronounced "s," but in English the "t" is pronounced "t" and "s" is pronounced "s." Be careful with English words that begin with "t". In Vietnamese, the "b" consonant is pronounced "p," but in English "p" is pronounced "p" and "b" is pronounced " b."

In Vietnamese, words do not end in "b," "ch," "f," "d," "j," "l," "p," "r," "s," "sh," "v," and "z." In English, words end in these letters. Pay special attention to pronouncing these English sounds. In Vietnamese, there is no "dzh" or "zh" sound, so English words like "judge" (dzh) and rupture (zh) will be hard for Vietnamese speakers to pronounce.

For example, in English,

bronchitis is not pronounced pronchiti
asthma is not pronounced atma
pertussis is not pronounced pertussih

Gujarati

In Gujarati, "v" is pronounced "w," "f" is pronounced "p," "p" is pronounced "f," and "z" is pronounced "j." Short "i" is pronounced long "e," "x" is pronounced "ch," and "th" is pronounced "s." In English, "v" is pronounced "v," "f" is pronounced "f," "z" is pronounced "z" or

(continued)

"s," "j" is pronounced "j," and "x" is pronounced "x." Pay careful attention when pronouncing these sounds.

For example, in English,

febrile is not pronounced pebrile
croup is not pronounced crouf
spit is not pronounced speet

Korean

In Korean, the "v" consonant is pronounced "b" and the "f" consonant is pronounced "p." In English, the "v" is pronounced "v," the "f" is pronounced "f," and the "p" is pronounced "p." Pay special attention when pronouncing these sounds.

For example, in English,

febrile is not pronounced peprile
wheezing is not pronounced veezing

Chinese

In Chinese, the "r" consonant is pronounced "l" or "w," and "b," "d," "g," and "ng" are not pronounced at all. Pay careful attention to English words that begin with "r" because the "r" is not pronounced "l" or "w," and "b," "d," "g," and "ng" are pronounced in English.

For example, in English,

breathing is not pronounced bleatin

Russian

The "w" consonant is pronounced like a "v" and the "v" sounds like a "w." Pay careful attention to the English "th." It is not pronounced "s."

For example, in English,

wheezing is not pronounced veezing

DICTATION

 ### Listening/Spelling Exercise: Word and Word Pairs

Listen to the words or word pairs on the audio files found in Chapter 5 on thePoint (thePoint.lww.com/diaz-gilbert) and then write them down on the lines below.

1. _____
2. _____
3. _____
4. _____
5. _____
6. _____
7. _____
8. _____

9. _____

10. _____

11. _____

12. _____

13. _____

14. _____

15. _____

Listening/Spelling Exercise: Sentences

Listen to the sentences on the audio files found in Chapter 5 on thePoint (thePoint.lww.com.gilbert-diaz) and then write them down on the lines below.

1. _____
_____

2. _____
_____

3. _____
_____

4. _____
_____

5. _____
_____

6. _____
_____

7. _____
_____

8. _____
_____

9. _____
_____

10. _____
_____

Now, check your sentences against the correct answers in the Answer Key online. If there are any new words that you do not know or that you spelled incorrectly, make a list of those words and study them for meaning and spelling.

PHARMACIST/PATIENT DIALOGUES

The ability to orally communicate effectively with your professors, colleagues, and especially with patients is very important. As a pharmacist, you will be counseling patients; patients will come to you for advice. They will have questions about a condition and symptoms they may experience and will ask you to help treat the condition. Therefore, it is extremely important that you understand what they are saying and that you respond to them and their questions appropriately. Your patients will speak differently. For example, some may speak very quickly, others too low, and yet others may speak angrily. To help you improve your listening skills, listen to the following dialogues, or short conversations, between a pharmacist and a patient and between a pharmacy technician and a patient.

Listening and Comprehension Exercises

Dialogue #1

Listen to Dialogue #1, stop, listen again and take notes. Listen to the dialogue as many times as you need or until you feel you have written sufficient notes and feel confident. You can use your notes to answer the multiple choice questions at the end of the dialogue.

Notes _____

_____

_____

_____

_____

Answer the questions below by selecting the answer that correctly completes each sentence.

1. _____ The prescription the mother brings to the pharmacy is for:
a. herself
b. her 16-year-old daughter
c. her 6-year-old daughter

2. _____ The mother tells the pharmacist the prescription is for:
a. Endep
b. Entex
c. Endex

3. _____ The mother tells the pharmacist her daughter has:
a. broncholilitis
b. bronchitis
c. a lung infection

4. _____ The patient's name is:
a. Aurea Cueva
b. Area Cuevas
c. Aurea Cuevas

5. _____ The patient's date of birth is:
a. August 19, 1990
b. August 9, 1999
c. August 19, 1999

6. _____ When the patient was younger, she was treated for:
a. a ruptured eardrum
b. ear infections
c. eye infections

7. _____ The patient is allergic to:
a. bacitracin
b. Bactrim
c. Benadryl

8. _____ The patient's address is:
a. 111 Morningside Drive
b. 11 Morningside Terrace
c. 11 Morningside Road

6. _____ The adjective form of **bronchitis** is:

a. bronchial and bronchitic

b. bronchial, bronchitic, and bronchiolar

c. bronchial only

7. _____ An expectorant is:

a. mucus

b. sputum

c. cough medicine

8. _____ If a person is a **breath of fresh air,** he or she:

a. is breathing better

b. needs fresh air to breathe

c. has new ideas and ways of doing things

9. _____ Acute bronchitis:

a. lasts for a short time

b. recurs

c. does not affect the nose, throat, and sinuses

10. _____ In the sentence, "Asthma results in labored breathing," the word **labored** is:

a. an adjective

b. a verb

c. a noun

11. _____ The word **persistent** is:

a. an adjective

b. a verb

c. a noun

12. _____ Another word for **shortness of breath** is:

a. diphtheria

b. dyspnea

c. delirium

13. _____ Chest percussion treatment is used with patients who suffer from:

a. asthma

b. a collapsed lung

c. cystic fibrosis

14. _____ The word **tightness** is:

a. a noun, a verb, and an adjective

b. a noun

c. an adjective

15. _____ In the sentence, "The patient complained he was fatigued," **fatigued** is:

a. an adjective

b. a past tense verb

c. a noun

Listening and Comprehension Exercises

Dialogue #1

Listen to Dialogue #1, stop, listen again and take notes. Listen to the dialogue as many times as you need or until you feel you have written sufficient notes and feel confident. You can use your notes to answer the multiple choice questions at the end of the dialogue.

Notes _____

_____

_____

_____

_____

Answer the questions below by selecting the answer that correctly completes each sentence.

1. _____ The patient is picking up a prescription to treat her

a. chronic bronchitis

b. emphysema

c. acute bronchitis

2. _____ The spelling of the patient's first name is

a. Felicity

b. Felicidad

c. Felicita

3. _____ The spelling of the patient's last name is

a. Casstro

b. Castro

c. Kastro

4. _____ The patient lives at

a. 23 Pin Road

b. 23 Penn Road

c. 23 Pen Road

5. _____ The patient stated she has

a. no insurance

b. the same insurance

c. new insurance

6. _____ The patient's birth date is

a. 1/2/49

b. 1/2/09

c. 12/5/09

7. _____ The patient's doctor ordered

a. albuterol

b. Atrovent

c. atropine

8. _____ The doctor prescribed

a. 2 puffs 2 times a day

b. 4 puff 2 times a day

c. 2 puffs 4 times a day

9. _____ The patient told the pharmacist that

a. Atrovent gives her dry mouth

b. albuterol gives her dry mouth

c. both give her dry mouth

10. _____ The pharmacist instructs the patient

a. to rinse her mouth with water to prevent dry mouth

b. not to rinse her mouth

c. to rinse her inhaler

Dialogue #2

Listen to Dialogue #2, stop, listen again and take notes. Listen to the dialogue as many times as you need or until you feel you have written sufficient notes and feel confident. You can use your notes to answer the multiple choice questions at the end of the dialogue.

Notes _____

_____

_____

_____

_____

Answer the questions below by selecting the answer that correctly completes each sentence.

1. _____ The customer is picking up a prescription for

a. her daughter

b. her son

c. herself

2. _____ The patient's name is

a. Jeremy Menbeck

b. Jeremy Manback

c. Jeremy Manbeck

3. _____ The patient has

a. never been to the pharmacy

b. been to the pharmacy once

c. been to the pharmacy many times

4. _____ The prescription is for

a. Pulmicort

b. promethazine

c. Pulmozyme

5. _____ The patient is

a. 8 years old

b. 8 months old

c. 7 years old

6. _____ The patient's birth date is

a. March 3, 1999

b. March 30, 1999

c. March 3, 1990

7. _____ Pulmozyme is a colorless solution used with

a. an inhaler

b. a vaporizer

c. a nebulizer

8. _____ Pulmozyme will

a. produce thick, sticky mucus in the lungs

b. clog the lungs with mucus

c. help to break up thick, sticky mucus that clogs the lungs

9. _____ A side effect of Pulmozyme is

a. shortness of breath

b. hoarseness and laryngitis

c. a scratchy throat

10. _____ The co-pay amount is

a. $20.00

b. $25.00

c. $5.00

Dialogue #3

Listen to Dialogue #3, stop, listen again and take notes. Listen to the dialogue as many times as you need or until you feel you have written sufficient notes and feel confident. You can use your notes to answer the multiple choice questions at the end of the dialogue.

Notes _____

_____

_____

_____

_____

Answer the questions below by selecting the answer that correctly completes each sentence.

1. _____ The customer is getting

a. two asthma medications for his daughter

b. one asthma medication for his son

c. two asthma medications for his son

2. _____ The patient's first name, middle initial, and last name are

a. Jamie B. Griffin

b. Jaime B. Griffith

c. Jaime B. Griffin

3. _____ The patient

a. has no allergies

b. likes peanut butter

c. is allergic to peanut butter

4. _____ The patient's birth date is

a. November 19, 1998

b. November 9, 1999

c. November 19, 1999

5. _____ The patient's address is

a. 1124 Moonriver Street

b. 11 Moonriver Court

c. 1124 Moonriver Court

6. _____ The doctor has ordered
a. Advair only
b. albuterol and Advair
c. albuterol only

7. _____ The patient is covered by
a. Northeastern Medical
b. Northeast Medical
c. Northern Health Plan

8. _____ The pharmacist explains to the patient's parent that
a. Advair and albuterol are bronchodilators
b. Advair is a powder inhaler and albuterol is a bronchodilator
c. albuterol is a an aerosol spray and Advair is a bronchodilator

9. _____ The pharmacist tells the patient's parent that
a. albuterol may cause nausea, headaches, and dizziness
b. Advair might cause hoarseness, throat irritation, and dry mouth
c. both a and b

10. _____ The cost for both prescriptions is
a. $50.00
b. $25.00
c. $100.00

How did you do on the Post-Assessment in Chapter 5? Check your answers in the Answer Key online.

Heart and Cardiovascular System | 6

True/False Questions

Indicate whether each sentence below is true (T) or false (F).

1. _____ Myocardial infarction is another term for **stroke.**
2. _____ Daily activities such as shopping, climbing stairs, and walking are difficult for people with **heart failure.**
3. _____ A warning sign of a **heart attack** is a squeezing sensation and uncomfortable pressure and pain in the center of the chest.
4. _____ Some people with **angina** complain that they have indigestion, heartburn, cramping, and shortness of breath.
5. _____ The adjective forms of **congestion** is congestive and congested.
6. _____ A person who is obese is at risk for peripheral artery disease.
7. _____ Another word for irregular heartbeat is **angina.**
8. _____ Causes of a **stroke** include clogging of the arteries and bleeding within the brain.
9. _____ High cholesterol is not a risk factor for heart disease.
10. _____ The noun form of **obese** is obesity.
11. _____ Cardiovascular accident or **CVA** refers to a stroke.
12. _____ If your **cholesterol** level is 240 or higher, you are not at risk for a heart attack or stroke.
13. _____ Persistent coughing or wheezing, and coughing blood-tinged mucus, can be symptoms of **heart failure.**
14. _____ **TIA** refers to transient ischemic attack.
15. _____ The adjective forms of **failure** are failing and failed.

Multiple Choice Questions

Choose the correct answer from a, b, and c.

1. _____ An **aneurysm:**
a. is a bulge in the eyes
b. is a bulge in a blood vessel
c. occurs in the brain only

2. _____ **Palpitations** are the result of:
a. normal heartbeats
b. abnormal heart rhythms
c. heartburn

3. _____ A **pacemaker** is used to help:

a. heart patients walk at a brisk pace

b. the patient's heart beat in a regular rhythm

c. heart patients pick up the pace

4. _____ **Congestive heart failure** will result in the:

a. heart's failure to be able to properly pump blood

b. heart's failure to be able to beat properly

c. inability to sweat

5. _____ Weakness and **paralysis** on one side of the body or the other, drooling, and speech problems might indicate the person is experiencing:

a. enlargement of the heart

b. high blood pressure

c. a stroke

6. _____ **Angina** is one of the many causes of:

a. chest pain

b. angioplasty

c. stroke

7. _____ A **blood pressure** of 140/90 is considered to be:

a. normal

b. prehypertension

c. hypertension

8. _____ The word **flutter** is:

a. a noun and a verb

b. a verb only

c. a noun only

9. _____ **Congenital heart disease:**

a. Is present at birth

b. occurs later in life

c. is a result of obesity

10. _____ The expression **"my heart goes out to you"** means:

a. I will donate my heart

b. I feel sympathy toward another person

c. I feel no sympathy toward another person

How did you do? Check your answers in the Answer Key online.

MEDICAL VOCABULARY

A good understanding of vocabulary words in pharmacy is very important for communication with professors, fellow students, patients, and coworkers. Knowledge and understanding of vocabulary leads to successful communication and success as a pharmacy student, as a pharmacy technician, and as a practicing pharmacist. You may already know many of the vocabulary words in this chapter, but for words that are unfamiliar, pay careful attention to them and make every effort to know their correct spelling, meaning, and pronunciation. It is a good idea to keep a list of new words and to look up these new words in a bilingual dictionary or dictionary in your first language. A good command of pharmacy-related vocabulary and good pronunciation of vocabulary will help to prevent embarrassing mistakes and increase effective verbal communication skills.

Heart and Circulatory System Vocabulary

adrenaline
aneurysm
angina
angioplasty
anxiety
arrhythmia
artery
atherosclerosis
blood clot
bradycardia
cardiac catheterization
cerebral hemorrhage
cerebrovascular accident
cholesterol
clot
coagulate
congenital
cramping
crushing sensation
diuretics

echocardiogram
edema
electrocardiogram
embolism
epinephrine
exacerbation
faint
flushed
fluttering
gasping
hardening
heartburn
heart failure
high blood pressure
hypertension
intermittent claudication
irregular heartbeat
ischemia
mitral valve prolapse
myocardial infarction

nitroglycerin
palpitations
paralysis
peripheral artery disease
peripheral vascular
  disease
plaque
pump
shining skin
skipping heart beat
spasm
squeezing sensation
stroke
syncope
tachycardia
thickening
throbbing
thrombosis
vein
vomiting

PARTS OF SPEECH

A good understanding of parts of speech, such as verbs, nouns, adjectives, and adverbs, is important for successful communication when speaking or writing. It is equally important to know the various forms of words and to use them appropriately.

Word Forms

The table below lists the main forms of some terms that you will likely encounter in pharmacy practice. Review the table and then do the exercises that follow to assess your understanding.

Noun (n)	Infinitive/Verb (v) —Past Tense	Adjective (adj)	Adverb (adv)
aneurysm		aneurysmal	
angina		anginal; anginose	
anxiety; anxiousness		anxious	anxiously
aorta		aortal; aortic	
artery		arterial	
atherosclerosis		atherosclerotic	atherosclerotically
a beat	to beat; beat	beaten	
bradycardia		bradycardic	
		cerebral	cerebrally
cholesterol		cholesteric	
circulation	to circulate; circulated	circulatory	
a clot	to clot; clotted		

(continued)

Noun (n)	Infinitive/Verb (v) —Past Tense	Adjective (adj)	Adverb (adv)
coagulation; coagulability; coagulator	to coagulate; coagulated	coagulable; coagulative	
		congenital	congenitally
cramps	to cramp; cramped	cramped; cramping	
	to crush; crushed	crushing; crushed	
diuretic		diuretic	diuretically
edema		edematous	
embolism		embolismic	
exacerbation	to exacerbate; exacerbated	exacerbated; exacerbating	
faintness; fainter	to faint; fainted	faint	faintly
flushness; flusher	to flush; flushed	flushed	
flutterer	to flutter; fluttered	fluttering; fluttered	fluttery
hardening	to harden; hardened	hard	
hypertension		hypertensive	
intermittence		intermittent	intermittently
		irregular	irregularly
ischemia		ischemic	
palpitation	to palpitate; palpitated	palpitating	
paralysis; paralytic	to paralyze; paralyzed	paralyzed; paralyzing	
		peripheral	peripherally
pulse; pulsation	to pulsate; pulsated	pulsating	
spasm		spastic; spasmodic	
squeezing; squeezer	to squeeze; squeezed	squeezable	
syncope		syncopal; syncopic	
tachycardia; tachycardic		tachycardic	
thickening	to thicken; thickened	thick; thickened	
a throb	to throb; throbbed	throbbing	throbbingly
vein		venial; veined	
vessel		vascular; vasculitis	vascularly
vomit; vomiter	to vomit; vomited		

Word Forms Exercise

Read the following sentences carefully. Then indicate the word form of the bolded word(s), choosing from v, n, adj, or adv.

1. **Hardening** and **thickening** of the **arteries,** also called **arteriosclerosis,** causes coronary heart disease.

    hardening _____   thickening _____   arteries _____   arteriosclerosis _____

2. **Peripheral** artery disease is also called peripheral **vascular disease.**

   peripheral _____   vascular _____   disease _____

3. The most common cause of a **stroke** is **thrombosis,** which is **blockage** of an artery in the brain by a blood **clot.**

   stroke _____   thrombosis _____   blockage _____   clot _____

4. Warning signs of a heart attack include **uncomfortable pressure** and **squeezing** in the chest and **discomfort** in other areas of the body such as the neck, arms, legs, stomach, and jaw.

   uncomfortable _____   pressure _____   squeezing _____   discomfort _____

5. Patients with type I and type II **diabetes, hypertension,** a family history of **atherosclerotic** disease, and who are **obese** are at risk for peripheral artery disease.

   diabetes _____   hypertension _____   atherosclerotic _____   obese _____

6. A person with heart failure may experience **palpitations** and feel like the heart is **throbbing** and racing, and may experience **swelling** in the feet, legs, and **abdomen.**

   palpitations _____   throbbing _____   swelling _____   abdomen _____

7. **Ischemia** is the term used to describe what happens to the part of the body that is not able to get enough oxygen as a result of a **narrow** or **blocked** artery.

   ischemia _____   narrow _____   blocked _____

8. A **common** symptom of a stroke, which **deprives** the brain of blood and oxygen, is **paralysis** or **weakness** on one side of the body.

   common _____   deprives _____   paralysis _____   weakness _____

9. Feelings of **heaviness, tightening,** and squeezing pressure or aching across the chest and behind the **breastbone** are possible symptoms of **angina,** also called angina pectoris.

   heaviness _____   tightening _____   breastbone _____   angina _____

10. Warning signs of a **stroke,** which is caused by **blockage** of an artery or **rupture** of an artery, include **numbness** on one side of the body, **confusion,** and difficulty talking and walking.

    stroke _____   blockage _____   rupture _____   numbness _____   confusion _____

11. In addition to atherosclerosis, other **causes** of peripheral vascular disease include blood **clots,** diabetes, **inflammation** of the arteries, and **infection.**

    causes _____   clots _____   inflammation _____   infection _____

12. Though not typical and quite rare, it is possible for a patient with peripheral artery disease to develop **gangrene,** ulcers, and open **sores** that will not **heal** as a result of poor **circulation.**

    gangrene _____   sores _____   heal _____   circulation _____

13. Diabetes, smoking, **hypertension,** and high **cholesterol** can cause the arteries to **harden** and **thicken.**

    hypertension _____   cholesterol _____   harden _____   thicken _____

14. Some symptoms of heart failure include **breathlessness** while sleeping or at **rest,** and feeling **tired** and **restless.**

    breathlessness _____   rest _____   tired _____   restless _____

15. Pain from angina can **radiate** to the back, neck, arms, jaw, and teeth, and can give patients **heartburn** and **indigestion.**

    radiate _____   heartburn _____   indigestion _____

How did you do? Check your answers in the Answer Key online.

Typical Medical Conditions and Patient Complaints

The sentences below contain vocabulary that describes and explains typical medical conditions, diseases, symptoms, and patient complaints that a pharmacist encounters. Read the sentences carefully. Then indicate the word form of the bolded word(s), choosing from v, n, adj, or adv. Look up words you do not know in your bilingual or first-language dictionary.

1. Before he was diagnosed with heart failure, the patient had complained that he was very **fatigued** and experiencing **dyspnea** while sleeping and that he needed two pillows to rest his head, and that his feet, ankles, and **abdomen** were **swollen.**

   fatigued _____   dyspnea _____   abdomen _____   swollen _____

2. **Clogging** of the arteries in the brain or the **hardening** of the arteries leading to the brain, or an **embolism** from the heart or an artery to the brain, can **cause** a stroke, which is also referred to as CVA or **cerebrovascular** accident.

   clogging _____   hardening _____   embolism _____   cause _____   cerebrovascular _____

3. Individuals with **advanced** atherosclerosis will **suffer** heart attacks and strokes, have **difficulty** walking, and have leg ulcers and **wounds** that will not **heal.**

   advanced _____   suffer _____   difficulty _____   wounds _____   heal _____

4. The term used to describe **pain** while walking or exercising, or pain that causes a person to **limp,** is **claudication.**

   pain _____   limp _____   claudication _____

5. Tests conducted after the patient complained that she was having pain in her **lower extremities,** especially her feet, during the night when she was lying down and when her legs were **resting indicated** she had peripheral artery disease, also known as PAD.

   lower _____   extremities _____   resting _____   indicated _____

6. **Congestive heart failure,** also know as CHF, can lead to kidney **failure** and pulmonary **edema.**

   congestive heart failure _____   failure _____   edema _____

7. Breaking out in a **sweat, feelings** of nausea, and **feeling lightheaded** are **warning** signs of a heart attack.

   sweat _____   feelings _____   feeling _____   lightheaded _____   warning _____

8. A cerebral **hemorrhage,** which is caused by a **vessel** in the brain that **bursts** and **bleeds,** can **deprive** the brain of oxygen and blood and result in a stroke.

   hemorrhage _____   vessel _____   bursts _____   bleeds _____   deprive _____

9. Another name for a **transient ischemic attack,** or TIA, which is a temporary **loss** of blood to the brain, is **mini-stroke.**

   transient _____   ischemic _____   attack _____   loss _____   mini-stroke _____

10. A person with a total **cholesterol level** of 240 or higher is at increased **risk** of having a heart attack or a stroke.

    cholesterol level _____   risk _____

11. Most people do not know that they are experiencing an **aortic** aneurysm, and their symptoms may include **abdominal,** chest, and back pain and a **pulsating** sensation in the **navel.**

    aortic _____   abdominal _____   pulsating _____   navel _____

12. Atherosclerosis and arteriosclerosis, or hardening of the arteries, are terms that are used **interchangeably** and can **lead** to an aneurysm, TIA, angina, and **circulatory** problems in the arms and legs.

    interchangeably _____   lead _____   circulatory _____

13. A common heart **rhythm** problem is atrial **fibrillation,** which can cause shortness of **breath,** fatigue, **palpitations,** and a stroke.

   rhythm _____   fibrillation _____   breath _____   palpitations _____

14. After complaining of suffering from **fatigue,** feeling **faint,** dizzy, and lightheaded, having swelling in the lower extremities, and experiencing breathlessness while at rest or during physical **exertion,** the patient was **diagnosed** with cardiomyopathy, which is a disease of the heart muscle and affects the heart's ability to **pump** blood.

   fatigue _____   faint _____   exertion _____   diagnosed _____   pump _____

15. Whereas men having a heart attack will experience **shortness** of breath and shoulder pain, and feel a **crushing sensation** in their chest, women might **experience** nausea and jaw and back pain.

   shortness _____   crushing _____   sensation _____   experience _____

16. Patients with **severe** heart failure may need to have an **artificial** heart **device** or require a heart **transplantation.**

   severe _____   artificial _____   device _____   transplantation _____

17. Another name for mitral valve **prolapse,** which is a **disorder** in which the **valve** in the heart does not close **correctly,** is click-murmur syndrome.

   prolapse _____   disorder _____   valve _____   correctly _____

18. A **typical** symptom of pericarditis, which is **swelling** and **irritation** of the membrane that surrounds the heart, is a **sharp, stabbing** pain felt behind the breastbone and in the left shoulder and neck.

   typical _____   swelling _____   irritation _____   sharp _____   stabbing _____

19. A person experiencing heart failure may **exhibit** a **lack** of appetite and feel **full** because the digestive system is receiving **less** blood.

   exhibit _____   lack _____   full _____   less _____

20. Although one cannot control **heredity** as a cause of high cholesterol, **diet, physical** activity, maintaining **appropriate** weight, and treatment can help to **manage** it.

   heredity _____   diet _____   physical _____   appropriate _____   manage _____

How did you do? Check your answers against the Answer Key online.

Medical Vocabulary Comprehension

Now that you have read sentences 1 through 20 describing language regarding the heart and cardiovascular system, assess your understanding by doing the exercises below.

Multiple Choice Questions

Choose the answer that correctly completes each sentence below.

1. _____ **Arteriosclerosis** is also called:

a. thrombosis

b. hypertension

c. hardening and thickening of the arteries

2. _____ A **stroke** can be caused by:

a. palpitations

b. blockage or rupture of an artery

c. blockage or rupture of a vein

3. _____ Pain from **angina** can cause:

a. heartburn

b. heartburn and indigestion

c. fatigue

4. _____ People with **type I and type II diabetes** are at risk for developing:

a. peripheral artery disease

b. dyspnea

c. congestive heart failure

5. _____ Another word for **mini-stroke** is:

a. blockage

b. click-murmur syndrome

c. transient ischemic attack

6. _____ A person experiencing **heart failure** may have loss of appetite because:

a. he or she is fatigued

b. less blood is going into the digestive system

c. more blood is going into the digestive system

7. _____ **Pericarditis** can cause:

a. click-murmur syndrome

b. mitral valve prolapse

c. a sharp, stabbing pain behind the breastbone

8. _____ If a man is experiencing a squeezing sensation and pressure in his chest, and discomfort in his neck, arms, leg, stomach, and jaw, he is most likely having:

a. a stroke

b. an aneurysm

c. a heart attack

9. _____ **Ischemia** occurs when the body:

a. has high cholesterol

b. cannot receive enough oxygen because of a narrow or blocked artery

c. starts to palpitate

10. _____ Causes of **peripheral vascular disease** include:

a. atherosclerosis

b. blood clots, diabetes, inflammation of the arteries, and infection

c. blockage and rupture of an artery

11. _____ **Atrial fibrillation** is a:

a. heart failure problem

b. heart rhythm problem

c. swelling of the membrane that surrounds the heart

12. _____ A person with severe **heart failure** may need:

a. to lose weight and exercise more

b. to lower his or her cholesterol

c. an artificial heart device or a heart transplantation

13. _____ Fatigue, dizziness, lightheadedness, swelling of the lower extremities, and breathlessness are symptoms of:

a. cardiomyopathy

b. mini-stroke

c. angina

14. _____ Patients with **peripheral artery disease** can:

a. develop open sores that won't heal, and gangrene

b. have TIA

c. have pulmonary edema

15. _____ Feeling breathless while sleeping or at rest is a symptom of:

a. heart failure

b. hypertension

c. angina

True/False Questions

Indicate whether each sentence below is true (T) or false (F).

1. _____ Hardening of the arteries can lead to circulatory problems in the arms and legs.

2. _____ A person diagnosed with atrial fibrillation may experience shortness of breath, palpitations, fatigue, and a stroke.

3. _____ Women who are having a heart attack are more likely than men to experience a crushing sensation in their chest and shortness of breath.

4. _____ Possible symptoms of angina include feelings of heaviness, tightening, and squeezing pressure on the chest and behind the breastbone.

5. _____ Diabetes, high cholesterol, smoking, and hypertension do not cause arteriosclerosis.

6. _____ The word "paralyzed" is both an adjective and a verb.

7. _____ An embolism from the heart or artery to the brain can cause cardiomyopathy.

8. _____ The words "breathlessness" and "breathe" are nouns.

9. _____ As a cause of high cholesterol, heredity can be controlled, but diet and exercise cannot be controlled.

10. _____ Hardening of the arteries causes coronary heart disease.

How did you do? Check your answers against the Answer Key online.

Writing Exercise

An important part of communication is the ability to write about what you read, to write correctly, and to spell correctly. In the exercises below, write your understanding of the meaning of the bolded words.

1. Describe in writing what **peripheral artery disease** is.

_____

_____

_____

_____

2. Describe in writing what a **stroke** is.

_____

_____

_____

_____

3. Describe in writing what **heart attack, heart failure,** and **angina** are.

_____

_____

_____

_____

4. Describe in writing what **cardiomyopathy** and **atrial fibrillation** are.

_____

_____

_____

Check what you have written with acceptable answers that appear in the Answer Key online.

LISTENING AND PRONUNCIATION

The ability to listen and understand what is being said and heard, and the ability to pronounce words clearly, is extremely important. A word misheard and a word mispronounced will lead to poor communication and can seriously put both the pharmacist and patient in danger. Therefore, it is very important that one hear clearly what another person has said, and that one speak clearly with correct pronunciation.

Listen carefully to the pharmacy-related words presented in the audio files found in Chapter 6 on thePoint (thePoint.lww.com/diaz-gilbert), and then pronounce them as accurately as you can. Listen and then repeat. You will listen to each word once and then you will repeat it. You will do this twice for each word. Listening and pronunciation practice will increase your listening and speaking confidence. Many languages do not produce or emphasize certain sounds produced and emphasized in English, so pay careful attention to the pronunciation of each word.

Pronunciation Exercise

Listen to the audio files found in Chapter 6 on thePoint (thePoint.lww.com-diaz-gilbert). Listen and repeat the words. Then say the words aloud for additional practice.

1. adrenaline ə-drĕn′ə-lĭin
2. aneurism ăn′yə-rĭz′əm
3. angina ăn-jī′nə
4. angioplasty ăn′jē-ə-plăs′tē
5. anxiety ăng-zī′ĭ-tē
6. aorta ā-ôr′tə
7. arrhythmia ə-rĭth′mē-ə
8. artery är′tə-rē
9. atherosclerosis ăth′ə-rō-sklə-rō′sĭs
10. atrial fibrillation ā′trē-əl fĭb′rə-lā′shən
11. blood clot blŭd klŏt
12. bradycardia brăd′ĭ-kär′dē-ə
13. cardiac catheterization kär′dē-ăk′ kath′ĕ-ter-ī-zā′shŭn
14. cerebral hemorrhage sĕr′ə-brəl, sə-rē′- hĕm′ə r-ĭj
15. cerebrovascular accident ser′ĕ-brō-vas′kŭ-lăr ăk′sĭ-dənt
16. cholesterol kə-lĕs′tə-rôl
17. circulatory sûr′kyə-lə-tôr′ē
18. coagulate kō-ăg′yə-lāt′

19. congenital	kən-jĕn′ĭ-tl
20. cramping	krămpng
21. crushing sensation	krŭshng sĕn-sā′shən
22. diuretic	dī′ə-rĕt′ĭk
23. echocardiogram	ĕk′ō-kär′dē-ə-grăm′
24. edema	ĭ-dē′mə
25. electrocardiogram	ĭ-lĕk′trō-kär′dē-ə-grăm′
26. embolism	ĕm′bə-lĭz′əm
27. epinephrine	ĕp′ə-nĕf′rĭn
28. exacerbation	eg-zas-er-bā′shūn
29. faint	fānt
30. flush	flŭsh
31. fluttering	flŭt′ərng
32. gasping	gāspng
33. hardening	här′dn-ĭng
34. heart failure	härt fāl′yər
35. heartburn	härt′bûrn′
36. high blood pressure	hī blŭd prĕsh′r
37. hypertension	hī′pər-tĕn′shən
38. intermittent claudication	ĭn′tər-mĭt′nt klô′dĭ-kā′shən
39. irregular heartbeat	ĭ-rĕg′yə-lər härt-bēt
40. ischemia	ĭ-skē′mē-ə
41. mitral valve prolapse	mī′trəl vălv prō-lăps′
42. myocardial infarction	mī-ō-kar′dē-əl ĭn-färk′shən
43. nitroglycerin	nī′trō-glĭs′ər-ĭn
44. palpitation	păl′pĭ-tā′shən
45. paralysis	pə-răl′ĭ-sĭs
46. peripheral artery disease	pə-rĭf′ər-əl är′tə-rē dĭ-zēz′
47. peripheral vascular disease	pə-rĭf′ər-əl văs′kyə-lər dĭ-zēz′
48. plaque	plăk
49. pulse	pŭls
50. pump	pŭmp
51. shining skin	shī′nng skĭn
52. skipping heart beat	skĭpng härt bēt
53. spasm	spăz′əm
54. squeezing sensation	skwēzng sĕn-sā′shən
55. stroke	strōk
56. syncope	sĭn′kə-pē
57. tachycardia	tăk′ĭ-kär′dē-ə
58. thickening	thĭk′ə-nĭng
59. throbbing	thrŏbng
60. thrombosis	thrŏm-bō′sĭs
61. vein	vān
62. vomiting	vŏm′ĭtng

Which words are easy to pronounce? Which are difficult to pronounce? Use the space below to write in the words that you find difficult to pronounce. These are words you should practice saying often.

_____

_____

_____

_____

_____

_____

_____

_____

Listen to the audio files found in Chapter 6 on thePoint (thePoint.lww.com/diaz-gilbert) as many times as you need to increase your pronunciation ability of the difficult words. Pronounce these words with a friend or a colleague who speaks English.

English Sounds That Are Difficult for Speakers of Other Languages to Pronounce

Spanish

In Spanish, there is no English "v" sound, but the "v" consonant in Spanish is pronounced like the English "b." The vowel "i" is pronounced like a long "e." Pay careful attention to the "v" sound in English when pronouncing words that begin with "v." Also pay careful attention to English words that begin with "s;" do not use the Spanish "es" sound when pronouncing English words that begin with "s."

For example, in English,

skipping is not pronounced eskeepeeng
vein is not pronounced bein

Vietnamese

In Vietnamese, the "t" consonant is pronounced "s," but in English the "t" is pronounced "t" and "s" is pronounced "s." Be careful with English words that begin with "t." In Vietnamese, the "b" consonant is pronounced "p," but in English "p" is pronounced "p" and "b" is pronounced "b."

In Vietnamese, words do not end in "b," "ch," "f," "d," "j," "l," "p," "r," "s," "sh," "v," and "z." In English, words end in these letters. Pay special attention to pronouncing these English sounds. In Vietnamese, there is no "dzh" or "zh" sound, so English words like "judge" (dzh) and "rupture" (zh) will be hard for Vietnamese speakers to pronounce.

For example, in English,

faint is not pronounced fain
intermittent is not pronounced intehmihin
paralysis is not pronounced pahrahlih

Gujarati

In Gujarati, "v" is pronounced "w," "f" is pronounced "p," "p" is pronounced "f," and "z" is pronounced "j." Short "i" is pronounced long "e," "x" is pronounced "ch," and "th" is pronounced "s." In English, "v" is pronounced "v," "f" is pronounced "f," "z" is pronounced "z" or "s," "j" is pronounced "j," and "x" is pronounced "x." Pay careful attention when pronouncing these sounds.

For example, in English,

pulse is not pronounced fulse
faint is not pronounced paint

(continued)

Korean

In Korean, the "v" consonant is pronounced "b" and the "f" consonant is pronounced "p." In English, the "v" is pronounced "v," the "f" is pronounced "f," and the "p" is pronounced "p." Pay special attention when pronouncing these sounds.

For example, in English,

faint is not pronounced paint

Chinese

In Chinese, the "r" consonant is pronounced "l" or "w," and "b," "d," "g," and "ng" are not pronounced at all. Pay careful attention to English words that begin with "r" because the "r" is not pronounced "l" or "w," and "b," "d," "g," and "ng" are pronounced in English.

For example, in English,

rash is not pronounced lash
stroke is not pronounced stloke

Russian

The "w" consonant is pronounced like a "v" and the "v" sounds like a "w." Pay careful attention to the English "th." It is not pronounced "s."

For example, in English,

thick is not pronounced sick

DICTATION

 ### Listening/Spelling Exercise: Word and Word Pairs

Listen to the words or word pairs on the audio files found in Chapter 6 on thePoint (thePoint.lww.com/diaz-gilbert) and then write them down on the lines below.

1. _____
2. _____
3. _____
4. _____
5. _____
6. _____
7. _____
8. _____
9. _____
10. _____
11. _____
12. _____
13. _____
14. _____
15. _____

Listening/Spelling Exercise: Sentences

Listen to the sentences on the audio files found in Chapter 6 on thePoint (thePoint.lww.com/diaz-gilbert) and then write them down on the lines below.

1. _____
   _____
2. _____
   _____
3. _____
   _____
4. _____
   _____
5. _____
   _____
6. _____
   _____
7. _____
   _____
8. _____
   _____
9. _____
   _____
10. _____
    _____

Now, check your sentences against the correct answers in the Answer Key online. If there are any new words that you do not know or that you spelled incorrectly, make a list of those words and study them for meaning and spelling.

PHARMACIST/PATIENT DIALOGUES

The ability to orally communicate effectively with your professors, colleagues, and especially with patients is very important. As a pharmacist, you will be counseling patients; patients will come to you for advice. They will have questions about a condition and symptoms they may experience and will ask you to help treat the condition. Therefore, it is extremely important that you understand what they are saying and that you respond to them and their questions appropriately. Your patients will speak differently. For example, some may speak very quickly, others too low, and yet others may speak angrily. To help you improve your listening skills, listen to the following dialogues, or short conversations, between a pharmacist and a patient and between a pharmacy technician and a patient.

Listening and Comprehension Exercises

Dialogue #1

Listen to Dialogue #1, stop, listen again and take notes. Listen to the dialogue as many times as you need or until you feel you have written sufficient notes and feel confident. You can use your notes to answer the multiple choice questions at the end of the dialogue.

Notes _____

_____

_____

Answer the questions below by selecting the answer that correctly completes each sentence.

1. _____ The patient is in the pharmacy to:
a. pick up a prescription for Lipitor
b. get a prescription refill for captopril
c. buy over-the-counter multivitamins

2. _____ She has been prescribed this medication because she recently had:
a. an asthma attack
b. a heart transplant
c. a heart attack

3. _____ The patient's name is:
a. Margaret Peters
b. Margaret Peterson
c. Margaret Peter

4. _____ The pharmacist's name is:
a. Sam Morgan
b. Samantha Morgan
c. Morgan Sam

5. _____ The patient tells the pharmacist she stopped taking:
a. vitamins only
b. Lipitor
c. captopril

6. _____ The patient is also taking:
a. prescription vitamins
b. over-the-counter multivitamins with iron and minerals
c. over-the-counter vitamins with calcium

7. _____ The patient tells the pharmacist she stopped taking Lipitor after her heart attack because:
a. it didn't prevent her heart attack
b. her cholesterol level did not improve
c. medicine can be expensive, even with insurance

8. _____ The patient tells the pharmacist that:
a. captopril made her very dizzy and lightheaded
b. captopril still makes her dizzy and lightheaded
c. captopril made her feel dizzy and lightheaded when she first took it

9. _____ The pharmacist asks the patient if she has:
a. had a change in urine and a fast heartbeat
b. been dizzy
c. been feeling tired

10. _____ The patient tells the pharmacist she wants a refill for captopril because:
a. it's not expensive
b. it's making her feel better and she wants to continue to feel better
c. her doctor told her to get a refill

11. _____ The pharmacist refills the prescription for captopril and reminds the patient:

a. to take the one pill three times a day on a full stomach

b. to take two pills two times a day 1 hour before eating

c. to take one pill three times a day 1 hour before eating

12. _____ The patient must also avoid:

a. potassium supplements and salt substitutes

b. potassium supplements only

c. salt substitutes only

Check your answers in the Answer Key online. How did you do? Are there new words you do not know? Take the time now to look them up in your bilingual or first-language dictionary.

Dialogue #2

Listen to Dialogue #2, stop, listen again and take notes. Listen to the dialogue as many times as you need or until you feel you have written sufficient notes and feel confident. You can use your notes to answer the multiple choice questions at the end of the dialogue.

Notes _____

_____

_____

_____

_____

Answer the questions below by selecting the answer that correctly completes each sentence.

1. _____ The patient's name is:

a. Mr. Jack

b. Mr. Jackson

c. Mr. Janson

2. _____ The pharmacist's name is:

a. Linda Riley

b. Linda Wiley

c. Lynne Riley

3. _____ The patient has been diagnosed with:

a. congestion

b. congestive heart failure

c. edema

4. _____ The patient is taking:

a. one medication

b. two medications

c. three medications

5. _____ The patient's medications include:

a. valsartan

b. valsartan, Lotemax, and Lasix

c. Lotemax

6. _____ The patient is taking valsartan:

a. for his heart, Lotemax for his edema, and Lasix for his eye

b. for his edema, Lasix for his heart, and Lotemax for his edema

c. for his heart, Lasix for his edema, an Lotemax for his eye

7. _____ The patient had a cataract removed from his:

a. right eye

b. left eye

c. both eyes

8. _____ After the pharmacist asked the patient if he is having any problems with his medications, the patient said:

a. sometimes he feels dizzy when he gets up after sitting

b. sometimes he feels dizzy when he sits down

c. sometimes he feels dizzy when he gets up from sitting, and he goes to the bathroom a lot

9. _____ The pharmacist tells the patient that a common side effect of valsartan:

a. is dizziness, and a common side effect Lasix is urinating more frequently

b. and Lasix is dizziness, and a common side effect of Lasix is urinating more frequently

c. is frequent urination and dizziness during the night

10. _____ The patient tells the pharmacist he tries:

a. not to take the Lasix pills at night

b. to take the Lasix pills before 4 o'clock in the afternoon

c. to take the Lasix pills after 6 o'clock at night

11. _____ The pharmacist asks the patient if he exercises, and the patient replies that:

a. he tries to go for walks in the evenings and on weekends if the weather is nice

b. he goes for walks on weekends only

c. he can't go for walks because he has a patch on his eye

Check your answers in the Answer Key online. How did you do? Are there new words you do not know? Take the time now to look them up in your bilingual or first-language dictionary.

Dialogue #3

Listen to Dialogue #3, stop, listen again and take notes. Listen to the dialogue as many times as you need or until you feel you have written sufficient notes and feel confident. You can use your notes to answer the multiple choice questions at the end of the dialogue.

Notes _____

_____

_____

_____

_____

Answer the questions below by selecting the answer that correctly completes each sentence.

1. _____ The pharmacist is speaking to the patient in:

a. a pharmacy

b. the hospital

c. the patient's home

2. _____ The pharmacist's name is:

a. Larry Brand

b. Eva Gonzalez

c. Eva Branch

3. _____ The patient's name is:

a. Eva Gonzalez

b. Eva Branch

c. Eve Gonzalez

4. _____ The patient is:

a. 50 years old

b. 51 years old

c. 15 years old

5. _____ The patient is in the hospital because:

a. she is diabetic

b. she is visiting a family member

c. she had a stroke

6. _____ The patient's doctor has prescribed:

a. Aggrenox

b. NovoLog

c. Aggrastat

7. _____ Aggrenox will:

a. treat the patient's diabetes

b. help to prevent blood clots in the brain and decrease the risk of another stroke

c. cause another stroke

8. _____ Aggrenox is a:

a. tablet that contains aspirin

b. capsule that contains dipyridamole

c. capsule that contains aspirin and dipyridamole

9. _____ Aggrenox can only:

a. be chewed

b. be swallowed whole

c. be crushed first and then swallowed

10. _____ The pharmacy instructs the patient to drink:

a. 1–8 ounces of water with the capsule

b. 8 ounces of water with the capsule

c. 8 ounces of water after lying down for 30 minutes

11. _____ Common side effects of Aggrenox include:

a. difficulty breathing

b. nausea, dizziness, heartburn, diarrhea, and sleepiness

c. nausea and vomiting

12. _____ The pharmacist tells the patient:

a. she can take ibuprofen while she's taking Aggrenox

b. she can take naproxen while she's taking Aggrenox

c. she should not take ibuprofen and naproxen while she's taking Aggrenox

Check your answers in the Answer Key online. How did you do? Are there new words you do not know? Take the time now to look them up in your bilingual or first-language dictionary.

IDIOMATIC EXPRESSIONS

Idioms and idiomatic expressions are made up of a group of words that have a different meaning from the original meaning of each individual word. Native speakers of the English language use such expressions comfortably and naturally. However, individuals who are new speakers of English or who have studied English for many years may still not be able to use idioms and idiomatic expressions as comfortably or naturally as native speakers. As pharmacy students, pharmacy technicians, and practicing pharmacists, you will hear many different idiomatic expressions. Some of you will understand and know how to use these expressions correctly. At times, however, you may not understand what your professors, colleagues, and patients are saying. This of course can lead to miscommunication, embarrassment, and possibly dangerous mistakes.

To help you improve your knowledge of idioms and idiomatic expressions, carefully read the following idiomatic expressions that contain the body word heart.

 ## Idiomatic Expressions using "Heart"

1. *from the bottom of one's heart* means you say or do something with sincerity and great feeling.

    For example: The patient thanked the pharmacist *from the bottom of her heart* for saving her life after the pharmacist noticed that the doctor had ordered a medication that could have potentially killed her if the medication had interacted with medication she was taking for hypertension.

2. *heart-to-heart* means to speak seriously and freely about a private matter.

    For example: After receiving several complaints from patients about the pharmacy technician's poor customer service skills, the pharmacy manager had a *heart-to-heart* talk with him.

3. *to have a heart* means to be nice and not be so strict.

    For example: *Have a heart!* I've been working 5 straight hours without a break.

4. *to have a heart of gold* means to be kind, generous, and forgiving.

    For example: Patients were saddened to learn that their favorite pharmacist, Sam, who has *a heart of gold,* had been transferred to another pharmacy.

5. *not have the heart to do something* means not be able to say or do something that will hurt another person.

    For example: I *don't have the heart* to tell her that she did not get the promotion.

6. *heart skips a beat* means a person is very afraid, excited, or surprised.

    For example: Her *heart skipped a beat* when she opened the letter from the pharmacy school announcing that she had been accepted.

7. *to have a heart of stone* means to be mean, cruel, and unsympathetic.

    For example: Many students felt the professor had *a heart of stone* and made all his exams especially difficult.

8. *to have one's heart in the right place* means the person is kind, well-meaning, or sympathetic even though they don't appear to be.

    For example: Even though her boss was not happy with her because she was late, his *heart was in the right place* when he advised her that it's unprofessional to be late for work.

9. *to have a heavy heart* means to be very sad.

    For example: The pharmacy staff worked with *a heavy heart* the day they learned that one of their long-time patients died after her long illness.

10. **to wear one's heart on one's sleeve** means to show one's true feelings openly.

> For example: While some patients are very private and don't discuss many personal matters with their doctors and pharmacists, others will **wear their heart on their sleeve.**

11. **one's heart sank** means to suddenly lose hope and become sad.

> For example: The patient's **heart sank** when the doctor told her that her cancer had returned.

12. **to sing/dance one's heart out** means to sing and dance with a lot of energy.

> For example: The students **danced their hearts** out at their graduation party.

Mini Dialogues Listening Exercise

How much did you understand? Listen to the following mini dialogues on the audio files found in Chapter 6 on thePoint (thePoint.lww.com/diaz-gilbert), read the questions below, and then choose the correct answer.

 ### Mini Dialogue #1

1. _____ To have **a heart-to-heart** talk means:

a. to talk about a heart transplantation

b. to express one's love to another person

c. to speak about a serious matter in private

 ### Mini Dialogue #2

2. _____ To have **a heart of stone** means:

a. to have a heavy heart

b. to feel cold

c. to be mean and unsympathetic

 ### Mini Dialogue #3

3. _____ **My heart sank** means:

a. the person is drowning

b. to lose hope and become very sad

c. the heart stopped beating

 ### Mini Dialogue #4

4. _____ **Wear my heart on my sleeve** means:

a. to wipe my tears on my sleeve

b. to show my true feelings privately

c. to show my true feelings openly

 ### Mini Dialogue #5

5. _____ **Heart's in the right place** means:

a. relationships with other people are important

b. to be well-meaning

c. to be generous and forgiving

 ### Mini Dialogue #6

6. _____ To have **a heart of gold** means:

a. to wear a gold heart

b. to be kind and generous

c. to be excited and surprised

How did you do? Check your answers against the Answer Key online.

POST-ASSESSMENT

True/False Questions

Indicate whether each sentence below is true (T) or false (F).

1. _____ The idiom **to have a heavy heart** means to be kind and sympathetic.

2. _____ The noun form of **hard** is hardening.

3. _____ Another word for hypertension is arteriosclerosis.

4. _____ Paralytic and paralysis are both nouns.

5. _____ If a person's **heart is made of stone,** the person is scared and frightened.

6. _____ Another word for transient ischemic attack or TIA is mini-stroke.

7. _____ Paralysis or weakness in one side of the body is caused by peripheral artery disease.

8. _____ The adjective form of **ischemia** is ischemic.

9. _____ Diabetes, smoking, hypertension, and high cholesterol will not cause the arteries to harden.

10. _____ Congestive heart failure occurs when the heart pumps too much blood throughout the body.

11. _____ If a person has a **heart of gold,** he or she is very wealthy and has lots of money.

12. _____ If a patient complains that he gets cramping in his legs or arms while exercising or walking, he may have peripheral artery disease.

13. _____ Warning signs of a stroke include sudden numbness on one side of the body and the inability to speak.

14. _____ Angina is caused by a bulge in the blood vessels to the brain.

15. _____ If a person's **heart skips a beat** after being surprised or excited, it means he or she has arrhythmia.

Multiple Choice Questions

Choose the correct answer from a, b, and c.

1. _____ The adjective form of **anxiety** is:

a. anxious

b. anxiousness

c. anxiously

2. _____ A person with congestive heart failure may:

a. feel fatigued and cold

b. feel fatigued and have edema of the legs or ankles

c. experience loss of coordination

3. _____ If a person has **a heart of stone,** he or she is:

a. friendly

b. worried and anxious

c. mean and unsympathetic

4. _____ A person with angina will experience:

a. claudication

b. a squeezing sensation in the chest

c. a severe headache

5. _____ In the sentence: "Some symptoms of heart failure include breathlessness while sleeping or at rest, and feeling tired and restless," **rest** is:

a. a verb and a noun

b. an adjective

c. a noun

6. _____ The adjective form of **to crush** is:

a. crushing and crushed

b. crush

c. crushed

7. _____ Aggrenox is used to:

a. decrease strokes

b. help improve paralysis

c. help improve speaking

8. _____ The idiomatic expression that means "to be sad" is:

a. to wear your heart on your sleeve

b. to have a heavy heart

c. to dance your heart out

9. _____ Valsartan is used to treat:

a. patients with congestive heart failure

b. patients with cataracts

c. patients with edema

10. _____ In the sentence, "Paralysis or weakness in one side of the body is caused by peripheral artery disease," the word **paralysis** is:

a. an adjective

b. a verb

c. a noun

11. _____ The words pulse and pulsation are:

a. both a verb and noun

b. an adjective

c. a noun

12. _____ A person with cardiac arrest may experience:

a. chest discomfort, shortness of breath, and cold sweats

b. no warning signs, but will experience sudden loss of consciousness and abnormal breathing

c. a squeezing sensation in the chest

13. _____ Captopril is used to treat:

a. diabetic patients

b. heart attack patients

c. stroke patients

14. _____ The word **exacerbated** is:

a. both a verb and an adjective

b. a past tense verb only

c. an adjective only

15. _____ In the sentence, "Warning signs of a heart attack include uncomfortable pressure and squeezing in the chest, and discomfort in other areas of the body such as the neck, arms, legs, stomach, and jaw," **squeezing** is:

a. an adjective

b. a past tense verb

c. a noun

Listening and Comprehension Exercises

Dialogue #1

Listen to Dialogue #1, stop, listen again and take notes. Listen to the dialogue as many times as you need or until you feel you have written sufficient notes and feel confident. You can use your notes to answer the multiple choice questions at the end of the dialogue.

Notes _____

_____

_____

_____

_____

Answer the questions below by selecting the answer that correctly completes each sentence.

1. _____ The pharmacist's name is:

a. Frederica Cullens

b. Frederica Collins

c. Frederica Collings

2. _____ The patient's name is:

a. Art Jennings

b. Arthur Jennings

c. Arthur Jenkins

3. _____ When the pharmacist asks the patient how he's feeling, the patient states that:

a. it's hard for him to walk and that his back hurts

b. it's hard for him to walk and that his legs hurt

c. he's feeling much better and that his legs do not hurt when he walks

4. _____ The patient tells the pharmacist that his doctor told him:

a. he has bad arteries, which are hard

b. he has good arteries, which are hard

c. he will always have difficulty walking because he has bad arteries

5. _____ The pharmacist tells the patient that he has:

a. peripheral artery disease

b. edema in his legs

c. plaque in his arteries due to cholesterol

6. _____ The pharmacist explains to the patient that:

a. he is having difficulty walking and moving because he is obese

b. he is having difficulty walking and moving because the fatty material in his arteries is blocking the blood from flowing

c. he is having difficulty walking because his feet are numb

7. _____ The patient tells the pharmacist that:

a. his legs feel tight, his calf muscles are tired, and the pain is constant

b. his butt hurts and that his legs feel numb, but that his feet don't ache

c. the pain in his tight legs and tired muscles comes and goes, and sometimes his butt hurts, his legs have a numb and tingling feeling, and his feet ache

8. _____ The patient has been prescribed:

a. Petal

b. Pletal

c. Pedal

9. _____ The pharmacist explains to the patient that the medication will help:

a. him walk faster without pain

b. to reduce his symptoms only

c. to reduce his symptoms, help him walk farther distances with less pain, and improve oxygen and blood flow to his legs

10. _____ The patient needs to take:

a. 1 tablet 30 minutes after breakfast or dinner

b. 1 tablet twice a day 30 minutes before breakfast and dinner or 2 hours after breakfast and dinner

c. 1 tablet daily either 30 minutes before breakfast and dinner or 2 hours after breakfast and dinner

11. _____ The patient should start to feel the benefits of the medication:

a. after 2 weeks

b. after 4 weeks

c. as early as 2 to 4 weeks or as late as 12 weeks

12. _____ The pharmacist tells the patient not to eat:

a. grapes and not to take ibuprofen and naproxen

b. grapefruit and not to take ibuprofen, naproxen, and aspirin

c. grapes and fruit and not to take ibuprofen, naproxen, and aspirin

Dialogue #2

Listen to Dialogue #2, stop, listen again and take notes. Listen to the dialogue as many times as you need or until you feel you have written sufficient notes and feel confident. You can use your notes to answer the multiple choice questions at the end of the dialogue.

Notes _____

_____

_____

_____

_____

Answer the questions below by selecting the answer that correctly completes each sentence.

1. _____ The patient's name is:

a. Brett Long, and the pharmacist's name is Helen Davis

b. Brett Davis, and the pharmacist's name is Helen Long

c. Helen Davis, and the pharmacist's name is Brett Long

2. _____ The patient was hospitalized after suffering:

a. heart attack

b. angina

c. a stroke

3. _____ The patient is:

a. a 49-year-old smoker with high cholesterol and high blood pressure

b. a 49-year-old nonsmoker with high cholesterol

c. a 40-year-old smoker with high blood pressure

4. _____ The patient's angina is being treated with:

a. nitroglycerin tablets

b. a nitroglycerin patch called Nitro-Dur

c. a nitroglycerin patch called Nitrodisc

5. _____ The patient has been:

a. using the nitroglycerin patch as prescribed

b. removing the patch when she should

c. removing the patch when she shouldn't

6. _____ The patient told the pharmacist she:

a. removes the patch because it irritates her skin and she removes the patch in the shower

b. removes the patch in the shower

c. removes the patch because it irritates her skin

7. _____ The pharmacist instructs the patient to:

a. keep the patch on for 12 to 14 hours, and then wait about 10 to 12 hours before she can put a new patch on

b. to keep the patch on for 10 to 12 hours, and then wait about 12 to 14 hours before she can put a new patch on

c. keep the patch on for 12 to 14 hours, and then wait about 10 to 12 hours before she can put on the same patch

8. _____ The patient is allergic to:

a. sulfa

b. ampicillin

c. penicillin

9. _____ The patient is taking:

a. Zocor once a night every night as prescribed to treat her cholesterol even if she's not at home

b. Diovan for her cholesterol but sometimes forgets to take it, especially when she's not at home

c. Zocor for her cholesterol but forgets to take it every night, especially when she's not at home

10. _____ The patient does not take:

a. Diovan, her blood pressure medication, on a daily basis as she should, even though her doctor adjusted the medication, because it made her itchy and irritated

b. Diovan, her blood pressure medication, on a daily basis as she should, even though her doctor adjusted the medication, because it made her lightheaded and dizzy

c. Diovan, her blood pressure medication, on a daily basis because she forgets

11. _____ According to the patient's chart, her doctor has also recommended:

a. physical activity, weight loss, and smoking cessation

b. weight loss, but no physical activity

c. weight loss and smoking fewer cigarettes

12. _____ The pharmacist explains to the patient that she has:

a. COPD

b. angina, caused by coronary heart disease

c. coronary heart disease as a result of not taking her medications as prescribed

13. _____ The pharmacist explains to the patient that:

a. it's difficult for blood and oxygen to get to her heart

b. as a result of coronary heart disease, it's difficult for the blood and oxygen to get to her heart and that cholesterol has hardened her arteries

c. as a result of not taking her medications, blood and oxygen cannot get to her heart

14. _____ The patient was not aware that:

a. high blood pressure is the number one killer in women

b. cancer is the number one killer in women

c. heart disease is the number one killer in women

15. _____ The pharmacist informs the patient that the hospital offers:

a. smoking cessation classes not covered by insurance

b. exercise and smoking cessation classes that some insurance companies cover and that are reasonably priced

c. exercise, weight loss, and smoking cessation classes that are reasonably priced and covered by most insurance companies

How did you do on the Post-Assessment in Chapter 6? Check your answers in the Answer Key online.

The Abdomen and Gastrointestinal System

7

True/False Questions

Indicate whether each sentence below is true (T) or false (F).

1. _____ **Gastroesophageal reflux disease (GERD)** is a chronic stomach condition.
2. _____ **Heartburn** is a burning pain usually felt in the middle of the chest.
3. _____ **Regurgitant** and **regurgitative** are adjective forms.
4. _____ Some individuals with **diverticular disease** may experience bloating, diarrhea, constipation, and cramping.
5. _____ The adjective form of rectum is **rectal.**
6. _____ **Fecal impaction** occurs when the stool in the rectum is soft and causes diarrhea.
7. _____ One cause of **abdominal pain** is inflammation.
8. _____ People with **irritable bowel syndrome (IBS)** do not experience **bloating, constipation, flatulence,** abdominal pain, cramping, and diarrhea.
9. _____ Some people suffering from constipation experience **straining** and will not have difficulty passing **stool.**
10. _____ The adjective form of **esophagus** is esophageal.
11. _____ A person with **diverticulitis,** which occurs when the diverticula in the colon ruptures, experience a fever, **tenderness,** and abdominal pain.
12. _____ A **hiatal hernia** is a protrusion at the opening of the diaphragm where the food pipe meets the stomach that will not allow food to back up into the esophagus.
13. _____ Symptoms of **appendicitis** include abdominal pain, nausea, vomiting, and loss of appetite.
14. _____ Long-term GERD can lead to **Barrett's esophagus,** which in turn can lead to esophageal cancer.
15. _____ The word **urgency** is an adjective and the word **urgent** is a noun.

Multiple Choice Questions

Choose the correct answer from a, b, and c.

1. _____ "It was difficult for the students **to stomach** the poor results on their exams" means:
   a. it was easy for the students to reject the results
   b. it was easy for the students to accept the results
   c. it was difficult for the students to accept the results

2. _____ If a dissection of a fetal pig in your biology class **turns your stomach,** you will:

a. experience sharp pains in your stomach

b. feel sick and upset

c. become hungry

3. _____ Ulcerative colitis and Crohn's disease are examples of:

a. inflammatory bowel disease (IBD)

b. gastroesophageal reflux disease (GERD)

c. diverticular disease

4. _____ Abdominal pain can be caused by:

a. cramping

b. loss of blood supply to an organ, distension of an organ, or inflammation

c. a diet poor in fiber

5. _____ If a patient complains of a burning sensation in the chest, a sour taste in the mouth, and chest pain when lying down, especially at night, he or she is probably suffering from:

a. angina

b. GERD

c. diverticulitis

6. _____ Another word that means difficulty swallowing is:

a. dyspnea

b. dysphagia

c. reflux

7. _____ Constipation is a digestive condition in which a person will:

a. experience severe abdominal pains

b. experience inflammation and loss of blood to an organ

c. pass hard stool, strain during a bowel movement, or have infrequent bowel movements

8. _____ The word impaction is:

a. a noun

b. a verb

c. an adjective

9. _____ Diarrhea is characterized as:

a. hard stool

b. tarry stool

c. loose stool

10. _____ The patient complained that she was experiencing abdominal cramps, diarrhea, blood in her stool, loss of appetite, and weight loss. This could indicate she has:

a. gallstones

b. appendicitis

c. Crohn's disease

How did you do? Check your answers in the Answer Key online.

MEDICAL VOCABULARY

A good understanding of vocabulary words in pharmacy is very important for communication with professors, fellow students, patients, and coworkers. Knowledge and understanding of vocabulary leads to successful communication and success as a pharmacy student, as a pharmacy technician, and as a practicing pharmacist. You may already know many of the vocabulary words in this chapter, but for words that are unfamiliar, pay careful attention to them and make every effort to know their correct spelling, meaning, and pronunciation. It is a good idea to keep a list of new words and to look up these new words in a bilingual dictionary or dictionary in your first language. A good command of pharmacy-related vocabulary and good pronunciation of vocabulary will help to prevent embarrassing mistakes and increase effective verbal communication skills.

Abdomen and Gastrointestinal System Vocabulary

abdomen	digestion	indigestion
absorb	diverticula	intestinal tract
anus	diverticulitis	lower esophageal sphincter
appendix	diverticulosis	moderate
backwash	dysphagia	navel
belch	epigastric	obstruction
belly button	erode	occult blood
bile	esophageal	pancreas
bloating	esophagus	peptic ulcer
bout	expel	pouches
bowel	feces	rectum
bowel movement	flare	reflux
burp	flatulence	regurgitation
colon	gallbladder	Schatzki's ring
colostomy	gas	stomach acid
constipation	gastritis	stool
contractions	gastroenteritis	strain
cramping	heartburn	swallow
diaphragm	hemorrhoid	tenderness
diarrhea	hiatal hernia	

PARTS OF SPEECH

A good understanding of parts of speech, such as verbs, nouns, adjectives, and adverbs, is important for successful communication when speaking or writing. It is equally important to know the various forms of words and to use them appropriately.

Word Forms

The table below lists the main forms of some terms that you will likely encounter in pharmacy practice. Review the table and then do the exercises that follow to assess your understanding.

Noun (n)	Infinitive/Verb (v) —Past Tense	Adjective (adj)	Adverb (adv)
abdomen		abdominal	abdominally
absorption; absorptivity	to absorb; absorbed	absorptive	
anus		anal	anally
appendix; appendectomy; appendicitis			

(continued)

Noun (n)	Infinitive/Verb (v) —Past Tense	Adjective (adj)	Adverb (adv)
belch; belching	to belch; belched		
bellyache; bellyacher	to bellyache; bellyached		
bloating	to bloat; bloated	bloating; bloated	
colon		colonic	
constipation		constipated	
contraction; contract	to contract; contracted		contractually
cramp; cramping	to cramp; cramped		
diaphragm		diaphragmatic	diaphragmatically
diarrhea		diarrheal; diarrheic; diarrhetic	
digestion	to digest; digested	digestive; digestible	
dysphagia		dysphagic	
epigastrium		epigastric	
erodibility	to erode; eroded	erodible	
esophagus		esophageal	
expeller	to expel; expelled	expellable	
feces		fecal	
gas		gaseous	
hemorrhoid		hemorrhoidal	
incontinence		incontinent	
indigestion		indigestible	
intestine		intestinal	intestinally
moderation; moderateness	to moderate; moderated	moderate	moderately
obstruction; obstructor; obstructiveness	to obstruct; obstructed	obstructive; obstructing;	obstructively
pancreas		pancreatic	
rectum		rectal	rectally
regurgitation	to regurgitate; regurgitated	regurgitant; regurgitative	
swallow; swallower	to swallow; swallowed		
tenderness		tender	tenderly

Word Forms Exercise

Read the following sentences carefully. Then indicate the word form of the bolded word(s), choosing from v, n, adj, or adv.

1. **Heartburn** can be characterized as a **burning** pain in the middle of the chest.

   heartburn _____   burning _____

2. A patient with **diverticulosis** has **bulging pouches,** known as **diverticula,** in the **digestive** tract including the stomach, esophagus, and the large and small intestine.

   diverticulosis _____   bulging _____   pouches _____   diverticula _____   digestive _____

3. Heartburn and chest pain can be caused by a large **hiatal hernia,** which **allows** food and **acid** to **back up** into the esophagus.

   hiatal hernia _____   allows _____   acid _____   back up _____

4. People who are **constipated** will either **strain** during a **bowel movement,** pass hard **stool,** or have **infrequent** bowel movements.

   constipated _____   strain _____   bowel movement _____   stool _____   infrequent _____

5. A **clogged** and **obstructed** appendix can **burst** if it becomes **inflamed** and filled with **pus.**

   clogged _____   obstructed _____   burst _____   inflamed _____   pus _____

6. Patients with **GERD** experience **constant backwash** of food and **bile** into their esophagus and this can lead to **irritation** and inflammation of the esophagus.

   GERD _____   constant _____   backwash _____   bile _____   irritation _____

7. Symptoms of **irritable** bowel syndrome (IBS) include abdominal **cramps, bloating, constipation,** diarrhea, and **gas.**

   irritable _____   cramps _____   bloating _____   constipation _____   gas _____

8. **Peptic ulcers** are **open sores** in the **lining** of the stomach or the esophagus and can be caused by **bacterial** infection or certain medications.

   peptic ulcers _____   open _____   sores _____   lining _____   bacterial _____

9. Long-term GERD can lead to **Barrett's esophagus,** a **condition** that can lead to **esophageal** cancer.

   Barrett's esophagus _____   condition _____   esophageal _____

10. The **inability** to control one's bowel movement, thus causing **feces** to suddenly **leak** from the **rectum,** is referred to as fecal or bowel **incontinence.**

    inability _____   feces _____   leak _____   rectum _____   incontinence _____

11. One way to **expel excessive gas** from the stomach, which can be caused by **carbonated** drinks, eating too fast, or talking while eating, is to **belch.**

    expel _____   excessive _____   gas _____   carbonated _____   belch _____

12. **Bloating,** which is the **buildup** of gas in the stomach or intestines, causes the **abdomen** to **swell** and **increase** in size.

    bloating _____   buildup _____   abdomen _____   swell _____   increase _____

13. Patients with Crohn's disease and **ulcerative** colitis, both of which are **inflammatory** bowel diseases, can suffer **severe** abdominal pain and **bouts** of **watery** or bloody stool.

    ulcerative _____   inflammatory _____   severe _____   bouts _____   watery _____

14. Patient's with celiac disease are not able to **tolerate gluten,** which is found in foods such as pizza, breads, cookies, and much more and that can **damage** the small **intestine.**

    tolerate _____   gluten _____   damage _____   intestine _____

15. **Fecal impaction,** which is the result of **chronic** constipation, results in fecal matter being **manually** removed.

    fecal _____   impaction _____   chronic _____   manually _____

How did you do? Check your answers against the Answer Key online.

Typical Medical Conditions and Patient Complaints

The sentences below contain vocabulary that describes and explains typical medical conditions, diseases, symptoms, and patient complaints that a pharmacist encounters. Read the sentences carefully. Then indicate the word form of the bolded word(s), choosing from v, n, adj, or adv. Look up words you do not know in your bilingual or first-language dictionary.

1. In addition to **heartburn,** people with GERD can also experience chest pain, especially at night and when they lie down, and experience **dysphagia** and **regurgitation** of food and **liquids.**

   heartburn _____   dysphagia _____   regurgitation _____   liquids _____

2. Pain in the **epigastric area,** or the upper middle part of the abdomen, may **indicate** a problem with the stomach, the gallbladder, the **upper** small intestine, or the pancreas.

   epigastric _____   area _____   indicate _____   upper _____

3. The **burning** pain experienced by patients with peptic **ulcers** is caused when stomach **acid** comes in contact with the **ulcerated** area.

   burning _____   ulcers _____   acid _____   ulcerated _____

4. Eating a high-fiber diet and drinking plenty of **fluids** can help **prevent** diverticulitis **attacks** because the **fiber** and water will help to **soften waste** and prevent constipation.

   fluids _____   prevent ____   attacks ____   fiber ____   soften ____   waste ____

5. Hemorrhoids, which are **inflamed** veins in the rectum and **anus,** can occur as a result of **straining** during a bowel movement and can **bleed** and cause **itchiness** and irritation.

   inflamed _____   anus _____   straining _____   bleed _____   itchiness _____

6. Large hiatal hernias can cause **belching,** stomach acid to back up into the esophagus, chest pain, and **difficulty swallowing,** and moreso while **straining,** lying down, or lifting heavy objects.

   belching _____   difficulty _____   swallowing _____   straining _____

7. Patients with ulcerative colitis can experience a **range** of symptoms that include **rectal bleeding,** the inability to move their **bowels** despite the **urge** to do so, abdominal **cramping,** bloody diarrhea, weight loss, and even night sweats.

   range ____   rectal ____   bleeding ____   bowels ____   urge ____   cramping ____

8. In some patients, **gastroesophageal** reflux disease can cause **esophagitis,** which is **inflammation** of the **esophagus;** whereas in other patients, GERD may affect the throat and larynx and cause **hoarseness,** coughing, and a sore throat.

   gastroesophageal ___   esophagitis ___   inflammation ___   esophagus __   hoarseness __

9. Irritable bowel syndrome is a **chronic** condition whose symptoms vary from person to person but can be **disabling,** including **bouts** of both diarrhea and constipation, a feeling of being **bloated,** abdominal cramping, **flatulence,** and **mucus** in the stool.

   chronic ____   disabling ___   bouts ___   bloated ___   flatulence _____   mucus ___

10. **Indigestion** is a **feeling** of **discomfort** in the upper abdomen characterized by **various** symptoms, including bloating, belching, nausea, and a **burning** sensation.

    indigestion _____   feeling ____   discomfort _____   various _____   burning ___

11. Factors such as age, a diet **low** in fiber, **living** a **sedentary** life, **inadequate** fluid **intake,** and pregnancy can **contribute** to constipation.

    low ____   living ___   sedentary ___   inadequate _____   intake _____   contribute ___

12. A person with **gastroenteritis,** also called stomach **flu** because it is caused by a **viral** infection in the **lining** of the stomach, may experience **vomiting,** nausea, diarrhea, and indigestion.

    gastroenteritis _____   flu _____   viral _____   lining _____   vomiting _____

13. **Gastritis** is inflammation of the stomach caused by **bacterium** and can cause nausea, **bloating,** belching, and a burning **sensation** in the upper abdomen.

    gastritis _____   bacterium _____   bloating _____   sensation _____

14. People who have a **Schatzki's ring,** also known as a lower **esophageal** ring because **abnormal** tissue forms where the lower esophagus meets the stomach, will experience difficulty **swallowing** and pain under the **sternum,** also known as the breastbone.

    Schatzki's ring _____   esophageal _____   abnormal _____   swallowing _____   sternum _____

15. Constipation, diarrhea, **rectal** bleeding, **blood** in the stool, abdominal **pain** during a bowel movement, and **weight loss** are some symptoms associated with **colon** cancer.

    rectal _____   blood _____   pain _____   weight loss _____   colon _____

16. **Fecal** incontinence can affect **diabetics,** women after giving **birth,** patient's with Alzheimer's disease, and some patients who have become **physically disabled.**

    fecal _____   diabetics _____   birth _____   physically _____   disabled _____

17. **Eating** too much **fatty** or **spicy** food can lead to **indigestion.**

    eating _____   fatty _____   spicy _____   indigestion _____

18. A **gastric** ulcer, which is a peptic ulcer that can be found in the lining of the stomach, and a **duodenal** ulcer, also a peptic ulcer found in the **first** part of the small intestine, can be caused by pain **relievers,** the *Helicobacter pylori* bacteria, nicotine, **excessive** alcohol **consumption,** and stress.

    gastric _____   duodenal _____   first _____   relievers _____   excessive _____   consumption _____

19. Because people with celiac disease are not able to **absorb** certain **nutrients** from the foods they eat, they may have **fatty, oily** stool that is **grayish** in color, and they may experience weight loss.

    absorb _____   nutrients _____   fatty _____   oily _____   grayish _____

20. Crohn's disease, which begins with small **sores** on the **surface** of the intestine, and that can become large ulcers, can also affect a person's **appetite** and the ability to **digest** and **absorb** food.

    sores _____   surface _____   appetite _____   digest _____   absorb _____

How did you do? Check your answers against the Answer Key online.

Medical Vocabulary Comprehension

Now that you have read sentences 1 through 20 describing language regarding the abdomen and gastrointestinal system, assess your understanding by doing the exercises below.

Multiple Choice Questions

Choose the answer that correctly completes each sentence below.

1. _____ **Diverticula** are:
   a. bulging pouches in the digestive tract
   b. peptic ulcer sores
   c. bulging pouches that cause bloating

2. _____ **Dysphagia** means:
   a. regurgitation
   b. difficulty swallowing
   c. backwash

3. _____ **Fecal impaction** is the result of:

a. diarrhea

b. loose stool

c. chronic constipation

4. _____ **GERD** can cause:

a. heartburn only

b. dysphagia, regurgitation, and heartburn

c. inflammation of the small intestine

5. _____ **Hemorrhoids** can be caused by:

a. belching

b. straining during a bowel movement

c. bloody stool

6. _____ A person with a **Schatzki's ring** may experience:

a. pain behind the breastbone and dysphagia

b. weight loss

c. belching and bloating

7. _____ People with **celiac disease:**

a. can tolerate gluten

b. are able to eat food such as pizza and bread

c. cannot tolerate gluten

8. _____ Symptoms found in **ulcerative colitis** include:

a. rectal bleeding, hemorrhoids, and weight gain

b. rectal bleeding, abdominal cramping, weight loss, and the inability to have a bowel movement

c. belching, weight loss, and indigestion

9. _____ Factors such as a sedentary lifestyle and a low-fiber diet can contribute to:

a. hemorrhoids

b. constipation

c. GERD

10. _____ Another term for **gastroenteritis** is:

a. stomach flu

b. abdominal cramps

c. indigestion

11. _____ An example of a **peptic ulcer** includes:

a. a gastric ulcer only

b. a duodenal ulcer only

c. a gastric ulcer and a duodenal ulcer

12. _____ Crohn's disease can affect a person's:

a. indigestion

b. hiatal hernia

c. appetite and ability to digest and absorb food

13. _____ Fatty and spicy foods can lead to:

a. indigestion

b. gastric ulcers

c. bouts of constipation and diarrhea

14. _____ **Irritable bowel syndrome** symptoms include:

a. bouts of diarrhea and constipation only

b. feeling bloated, abdominal cramping, and bouts of diarrhea and constipation

c. belching, nausea, and a burning sensation

15. _____ Symptoms associated with **colon cancer** include:

a. rectal bleeding and hemorrhoids

b. rectal bleeding, blood in the stool, and abdominal pain during a bowel movement

c. constipation and diarrhea only

True/False Questions

Indicate whether each sentence below is true (T) or false (F).

1. _____ Heartburn can be characterized as a burning sensation behind the sternum.

2. _____ Peptic ulcers are open sores in the lining of the stomach or esophagus.

3. _____ Barrett's esophagus is a condition that can lead to colon cancer.

4. _____ Pain in the epigastric area may indicate a problem with the stomach, gallbladder, the upper intestines, or the pancreas.

5. _____ Esophagitis is inflammation of the esophagus.

6. _____ Gastritis is caused by a viral infection in the lining of the stomach.

7. _____ The word "indigestible" is a noun.

8. _____ Crohn's disease and ulcerative colitis are inflammatory bowel diseases.

9. _____ One way to expel excessive gas from the stomach is to belch.

10. _____ Bloating, which is the reduction of gas in the stomach or intestines, causes the abdomen to decrease in size.

How did you do? Check your answers against the Answer Key online.

Writing Exercise

An important part of communication is the ability to write about what you read, to write correctly, and to spell correctly. In the exercises below, write your understanding of the meaning of the bolded words.

1. Describe in writing what **gastroesophageal reflux disease** is.

_____

_____

_____

_____

2. Describe in writing what **constipation** and **fecal impaction** are.

_____

_____

_____

_____

3. Describe in writing what **bloating** and **belching** are.

_____

_____

_____

_____

4. Describe in writing what **celiac disease, ulcerative colitis,** and **irritable bowel syndrome** are.

_____

_____

_____

_____

5. Describe in writing what **gastritis, gastroenteritis,** and **indigestion** are.

_____

_____

_____

_____

Check what you have written with acceptable answers that appear in the Answer Key online.

LISTENING AND PRONUNCIATION

The ability to listen and understand what is being said and heard, and the ability to pronounce words clearly, is extremely important. A word misheard and a word mispronounced will lead to poor communication and can seriously put both the pharmacist and patient in danger. Therefore, it is very important that one hear clearly what another person has said, and that one speak clearly with correct pronunciation.

Listen carefully to the pharmacy-related words presented in the audio files found in Chapter 7 on thePoint (thePoint.lww.com/diaz-gilbert), and then pronounce them as accurately as you can. Listen and then repeat. You will listen to each word once and then you will repeat it. You will do this twice for each word. Listening and pronunciation practice will increase your listening and speaking confidence. Many languages do not produce or emphasize certain sounds produced and emphasized in English, so pay careful attention to the pronunciation of each word.

 Pronunciation Exercise

Listen to the audio files found in Chapter 7 on thePoint (thePoint.lww.com/diaz-gilbert). Listen and repeat the words. Then say the words aloud for additional practice.

1.	abdominal	ăb-dŏm′ə-nəl
2.	absorption	əb-sôrp′shən
3.	anus	ā′nəs
4.	appendix	ə-pĕn′dĭks
5.	backwash	băk′wŏsh′
6.	belch	bĕlch
7.	bellyache	bĕl′ē-āk′
8.	belly button	bĕl′ē bŭt′n
9.	bile	bīl
10.	bloating	blō′tng
11.	bout	bout
12.	bowel	bou′əl
13.	bowel movement	bou′əl mōōv′mənt
14.	burp	bûrp
15.	colon	kō′lən
16.	colostomy	kə-lŏs′tə-mē
17.	constipation	kŏn′stə-pā′shən
18.	contractions	kən-trăk′shəns

19. cramping — krămp ng
20. diaphragm — dī'ə-frăm'
21. diarrhea — dī'ə-rē'ə
22. digestion — dī-jĕs'chən
23. diverticula — dī'vûr-tĭk'yə-lə
24. diverticulitis — dī'vûr-tĭk'yə-lī'tĭs
25. diverticulosis — dī'vûr-tĭk'yə-lō'sĭs
26. dysphagia — dĭs-fā'jē-ə
27. epigastric — ĕp'ĭ-găs trĭk
28. erode — ĭ-rōd'
29. esophageal — ĭ-sŏf'ə jē'əl
30. esophagus — ĭ-sŏf'ə-gəs
31. expel — ĭk-spĕl'
32. feces — fē'sēz
33. flare — flâr
34. flatulence — flăch'ə-ləns
35. gallbladder — gôl blăd'ər
36. gas — găs
37. gastric ulcer — gă-strī'tĭs ŭl'sər
38. gastritis — gă-strī'tĭs
39. gastroenteritis — găs'trō-ĕn'tə-rī'tĭs
40. heartburn — härt'bûrn'
41. hemorrhoid — hĕm'ə-roid'
42. hiatal hernia — hī-ā'tāl hûr'nē-ə
43. incontinence — ĭn-kŏn'tə-nəns
44. indigestion — ĭn'dĭ-jĕs'chən
45. intestinal tract — ĭn-tĕs'tə-nəl trăkt
46. lower esophageal sphincter — lō'ər ĭ-sŏf'ə jē'əl sfĭngk'tər
47. moderate — mŏd'ə-rāt
48. navel — nā'vəl
49. obstruction — əb-strŭk'shən
50. occult blood — ə-kŭlt blŭd
51. pancreas — păng'krē-əs
52. peptic ulcer — pĕp't ĭk ŭl'sər
53. pouch — pouch
54. rectum — rĕk'təm
55. reflux — rē'flŭks
56. regurgitation — rē-ger'ji-tā'-shŭn
57. Schatzki's ring — shaht'skez rĭng
58. stomach acid — stŭm'ək ăs'ĭd
59. stool — sto͞ol
60. strain — strān
61. swallow — swŏl'ō
62. tender — tĕn'dər

Which words are easy to pronounce? Which are difficult to pronounce? Use the space below to write in the words that you find difficult to pronounce. These are words you should practice saying often.

_____

_____

_____

_____

_____

_____

_____

_____

_____

_____

Listen to the audio files found in Chapter 7 on thePoint (thePoint.com/diaz-gilbert) as many times as you need to increase your pronunciation ability of the difficult words. Pronounce these words with a friend or a colleague who speaks English.

English Sounds That Are Difficult for Speakers of Other Languages to Pronounce

Spanish

In Spanish, there is no English "v" sound, but the "v" consonant in Spanish is pronounced like the English "b." The vowel "i" is pronounced like a long "e." Pay careful attention to the "v" sound in English when pronouncing words that begin with "v." Also pay careful attention to English words that begin with "s;" do not use the Spanish "es" sound when pronouncing English words that begin with "s."

For example, in English,

swallow is not pronounced eswallow

Vietnamese

In Vietnamese, the "t" consonant is pronounced "s," but in English the "t" is pronounced "t" and "s" is pronounced "s." Be careful with English words that begin with "t." In Vietnamese, the "b" consonant is pronounced "p," but in English "p" is pronounced "p" and "b" is pronounced "b."

In Vietnamese, words do not end in "b," "ch," "f," "d," "j," "l," "p," "r," "s," "sh," "v," and "z." In English, words end in these letters. Pay special attention to pronouncing these English sounds. In Vietnamese, there is no "dzh" or "zh" sound, so English words like "judge" (dzh) and "rupture" (zh) will be hard for Vietnamese speakers to pronounce.

For example, in English,

bowel movement is not pronounced pow momen
esophagus is not pronounced ehfaguh
tenderness is not pronounced tenerneh

Gujarati

In Gujarati, "v" is pronounced "w," "f" is pronounced "p," "p" is pronounced "f," and "z" is pronounced "j." Short "i" is pronounced long "e," "x" is pronounced "ch," and "th" is pronounced "s." In English, "v" is pronounced "v," "f" is pronounced "f," "z" is pronounced "z" or "s," "j" is pronounced "j," and "x" is pronounced "x." Pay careful attention when pronouncing these sounds.

For example, in English,

feces is not pronounced peces
peptic is not pronounced fepteek

(continued)

Korean

In Korean, the "v" consonant is pronounced "b" and the "f" consonant is pronounced "p." In English, the "v" is pronounced "v," the "f" is pronounced "f," and the "p" is pronounced "p." Pay special attention when pronouncing these sounds.

For example, in English,

febrile is not pronounced peprile
wheezing is not pronounced veezing

Chinese

In Chinese, the "r" consonant is pronounced "l" or "w," and "b," "d," "g," and "ng" are not pronounced at all. Pay careful attention to English words that begin with "r" because the "r" is not pronounced "l" or "w," and "b," "d," "g," and "ng" are pronounced in English.

For example, in English,

diarrhea is not pronounced dialeeah
cramp is not pronounced clamp

Russian

The "w" consonant is pronounced like a "v" and the "v" sound like a "w." Pay careful attention to the English "th." It is not pronounced "s."

For example, in English,

swallow is not pronounced svallow

DICTATION

Listening/Spelling Exercise: Word and Word Pairs

Listen to the words or word pairs on the audio files found in Chapter 7 on thePoint (thePoint.lww.com/diaz-gilbert), and then write them down on the lines below.

1. _____
2. _____
3. _____
4. _____
5. _____
6. _____
7. _____
8. _____
9. _____
10. _____
11. _____
12. _____
13. _____
14. _____
15. _____

Listening/Spelling Exercise: Sentences

Listen to the sentences on the audio files found in Chapter 7 on thePoint (thePoint.lww.com/diaz-gilbert), and then write them down on the lines below.

1. _____
   _____

2. _____
   _____

3. _____
   _____

4. _____
   _____

5. _____
   _____

6. _____
   _____

7. _____
   _____

8. _____
   _____

9. _____
   _____

10. _____
    _____

Now, check your sentences against the correct answers in the Answer Key online. If there are any new words that you do not know or that you spelled incorrectly, make a list of those words and study them for meaning and spelling.

PHARMACIST/PATIENT DIALOGUES

The ability to orally communicate effectively with your professors, colleagues, and especially with patients is very important. As a pharmacist, you will be counseling patients; patients will come to you for advice. They will have questions about a condition and symptoms they may experience and will ask you to help treat the condition. Therefore, it is extremely important that you understand what they are saying and that you respond to them and their questions appropriately. Your patients will speak differently. For example, some may speak very quickly, others too low, and yet others may speak angrily. To help you improve your listening skills, listen to the following dialogues, or short conversations, between a pharmacist and a patient and between a pharmacy technician and a patient.

Listening and Comprehension Exercises
 Dialogue #1

Listen to Dialogue #1, stop, listen again and take notes. Listen to the dialogue as many times as you need or until you feel you have written sufficient notes and feel confident. You can use your notes to answer the multiple choice questions at the end of the dialogue.

Notes _____
_____
_____
_____
_____

Answer the questions below by selecting the answer that correctly completes each sentence.

1. _____ The patient's doctor is:
a. Chris Meloni, and the patient's pharmacist is Gary Lubin
b. Gary Lubin, and the patient's pharmacist is Chris Meloni
c. Chris Lubin, and the patients' pharmacist is Gary Meloni

2. _____ The patient's name is:
a. Amanda Adam
b. Adam Amanda
c. Amanda Adams

3. _____ The patient's medical condition is:
a. conjunctivitis
b. dysphagia
c. GERD

4. _____ The patient noticed she was:
a. having heartburn about 3 months ago
b. choking on her food about 3 months ago
c. having heartburn about 2 weeks ago

5. _____ The patient stated she:
a. eats spicy food
b. does not eat spicy food
c. eats spicy foods sometimes

6. _____ The patient took:
a. Mylanta, Maalox, and Tums for her GERD
b. Mylanta, Maalox, and Tums for heartburn
c. Mylanta, Maalox, and Tums to prevent choking

7. _____ The patient's husband took her to the:
a. emergency room about 2 weeks ago because she was choking and gagging on her food
b. emergency room about 3 months ago because she was choking and gagging on her food
c. doctor about 2 weeks ago because she was choking and gagging on her food

8. _____ The hospital referred the patient to:
a. a gastroenterologist
b. an endocrinologist
c. a gastrologist

9. _____ The doctor performed:
a. a colonoscopy 3 days ago and found an inflamed esophagus
b. an endoscopy 3 weeks ago and found a hiatal hernia
c. an endoscopy 3 days ago and found a hiatal hernia and an inflamed esophagus

10. _____ At the patient's request, the doctor prescribed:
a. Zantac because it's a generic drug and the patient refuses to buy brand-name drugs
b. ranitidine because it's a brand-name drug and the patient refuses to buy generic drugs
c. ranitidine because it's a generic drug and the patient refuses to buy a brand-name drug

11. _____ Since the endoscopy, the patient has been:
a. eating Jell-O and soup, has had a sore throat, and is starting to feel better
b. eating Jell-O, has had a sore throat, and is feeling worse
c. choking on food and has been having difficulty swallowing

12. _____ The pharmacist tells the patient that the medication:

a. reduces the amount of stomach acid and the inflammation in the esophagus

b. will decrease the size of her hiatal hernia

c. will stop her from choking and gagging

13. _____ The pharmacist tells the patient to take:

a. a capsule in the morning and a capsule in the evening with food

b. a teaspoon in the morning with food and a teaspoon in the evening without food

c. a teaspoon in the morning and a teaspoon in the evening with or without food

14. _____ The patient tells the pharmacist that about:

a. 2 weeks ago she was taking Tobramycin for her pink eye and that it hasn't cleared up

b. 1 week ago she was taking Tobramycin for her pink eye and that it has cleared up

c. 2 weeks ago she was taking Tobramycin for her pink eye and that it has cleared up

15. _____ The pharmacist told the patient that:

a. although unlikely, ranitidine may cause dizziness, constipation, and headaches

b. although unlikely, ranitidine may cause swelling, difficulty breathing, and a rash

c. ranitidine may cause swelling, dizziness, and headaches

16. _____ The patient tells the pharmacist that when she was a:

a. college student she almost died during a CAT scan because she's allergic to Benadryl

b. high school student she almost died during a CAT scan because she was allergic to iodine

c. college student she almost died during a CAT scan because she was allergic to iodine

Check your answers in the Answer Key online. How did you do? Are there new words you do not know? Take the time now to look them up in your bilingual or first-language dictionary.

Dialogue #2

Listen to Dialogue #2, stop, listen again and take notes. Listen to the dialogue as many times as you need or until you feel you have written sufficient notes and feel confident. You can use your notes to answer the multiple choice questions at the end of the dialogue.

Notes _____

_____

_____

_____

_____

Answer the questions below by selecting the answer that correctly completes each sentence.

1. _____ The patient's name is:

a. Gerry Wade, and the pharmacist's name is Alex Hardy

b. Gary Hardy, and the pharmacist's name is Alex Wade

c. Alex Hardy, and the pharmacist's name is Gerry Wade

2. _____ The patient's doctor's name is:

a. Dr. Fink, and he prescribed Asacol

b. Dr. Finko, and he prescribed albuterol

c. Dr. Finkel, and he prescribed Asacol

3. _____ The patient's medical condition is:

a. gastric ulcer

b. peptic ulcer

c. ulcerative colitis

4. _____ The patient tells the pharmacist he has:

a. abdominal swelling and diarrhea

b. diarrhea and rectal bleeding and is always going to the bathroom

c. diarrhea and rectal bleeding and sometimes can't go to the bathroom even though he feels he has to

5. _____ The pharmacist explains to the patient that he has:

a. ulcerative colitis, which causes inflammation of the rectum and difficulty moving his bowels

b. ulcerative colitis, which causes inflammation of the colon and difficulty moving his bowels

c. ulcerative colitis, which causes inflammation of the intestine and diarrhea

6. _____ The patient:

a. has a history of ulcerative colitis

b. is experiencing ulcerative colitis for the first time

c. has had bouts of ulcerative colitis

7. _____ The patient's birth date is:

a. December 12, 1961

b. December 2, 1961

c. December 1, 1961

8. _____ The patient is allergic to:

a. ampicillin

b. penicillin

c. Nizoral

9. _____ According to the patient's chart, the patient has had a problem with:

a. fungal infection of the toe that has not cleared up

b. jock itch, a fungal infection, in his groin area, arms, and legs, which has cleared up

c. jock itch, a fungal infection, which did not clear up

10. _____ For his fungal infection, the patient:

a. took Nizoral, which cleared it up about 3 weeks after he started taking it, and he is no longer taking it

b. took Nizatine, which cleared it up about 2 weeks after he started taking it, and he is still taking it

c. is still taking Nix because the fungal infection has not cleared up

11. _____ The doctor has prescribed the patient to take:

a. three Asacol tablets twice a day with food

b. two Asacol tablets three times a day, unchewed and uncrushed, with or without food

c. one crushed Asacol tablet a day with food

12. _____ The pharmacist explains to the patient that the possible side effects of Asacol include:

a. flu-like symptoms, abdominal and back pain, and gas, but that if he experiences very bad stomach and abdominal pain, worsening bloody diarrhea or constipation, or a fever he should call the doctor

b. very bad stomach and abdominal pain, worsening bloody diarrhea or constipation, or a fever, but that if he experiences flu-like symptoms and abdominal and back pain, he should call the doctor

c. worsening diarrhea or constipation, but that if he experiences flu-like symptoms and gas, he should call the doctor

13. _____ The pharmacist tells the patient that:
  a. it's possible to see part of or the whole tablet in his stool
  b. Asacol will cure his ulcerative colitis
  c. it's okay to have a beer once in a while

14. _____ If the patient misses a dose, the patient should:
  a. double up the next time he is scheduled to take his medicine
  b. skip the dose
  c. try to take it as soon as he remembers, but if he remembers right as he's coming to his next dose, he should skip the dose he forgot

Check your answers in the Answer Key online. How did you do? Are there new words you do not know? Take the time now to look them up in your bilingual or first-language dictionary.

Dialogue #3

Listen to Dialogue #3, stop, listen again and take notes. Listen to the dialogue as many times as you need or until you feel you have written sufficient notes and feel confident. You can use your notes to answer the multiple choice questions at the end of the dialogue.

Notes _____

_____

_____

_____

_____

Answer the questions below by selecting the answer that correctly completes each sentence.

1. _____ The patient's name is:
  a. Lily Oliver, and the pharmacist's name is Chaz Soto
  b. Lily Soto, and the pharmacist's name is Chaz Oliver
  c. Chaz Oliver, and the pharmacist's name is Lily Soto

2. _____ The pharmacist is reviewing the patient's:
  a. chart
  b. chart and reviewing her new prescription
  c. complaints

3. _____ The patient's states the new prescription is for her:
  a. high blood pressure
  b. pregnancy
  c. constipation

4. _____ The patient tells the pharmacist:
  a. she feels bloated, her pants don't fit, and she's pregnant
  b. she feels bloated, her pants don't fit, and she feels like she's pregnant
  c. she's tearing her hair out because she's pregnant

5. _____ According to the chart, the patient was in the clinic:
  a. 4 weeks ago for her blood pressure medicine refill
  b. 4 weeks ago for a prescription for constipation
  c. 4 weeks ago because she was bloated

6. _____ The patient states she can't take it any more because:

a. she has diarrhea

b. she tore out her hair

c. she has not had a bowel movement

7. _____ The patient is taking:

a. Dulcolax for her high blood pressure

b. Telmisartan for her high blood pressure

c. Temazepam for anxiety

8. _____ The patient tells the pharmacist that:

a. high blood pressure runs in her family

b. high blood pressure does not run in her family, but that constipation does

c. high blood pressure and constipation run in her family

9. _____ The patient's doctor:

a. has prescribed Dulcolax pills for her constipation

b. has prescribed Dulcolax capsules for her constipation

c. has prescribed Dulcolax suppositories for her constipation

10. _____ The patient has:

a. never used suppositories

b. used suppositories in the past to treat constipation

c. used suppositories in the past to treat hemorrhoids

11. _____ The pharmacist instructs the patient:

a. not to have a bowel movement 10 to 15 minutes before she inserts the suppository

b. to have a bowel movement 10 to 15 minutes after she inserts the suppository

c. not to have a bowel movement 5 to 10 minutes before she inserts the suppository

12. _____ The pharmacist tells the patient to:

a. insert one suppository in the morning before breakfast or bedtime

b. insert one suppository in the morning before breakfast and one before bedtime

c. insert one suppository at bedtime only

13. _____ The patient needs to call the doctor:

a. if she is no longer experiencing constipation

b. if she has a bowel movement immediately

c. immediately if she does not have a bowel movement after taking the suppositories

14. _____ The pharmacist explains to the patient that:

a. she cannot continue taking her blood pressure medication

b. that she can continue taking her blood pressure medication after she is no longer constipated

c. she can continue taking her blood pressure medication

15. _____ The pharmacist tells the patient she may experience:

a. irritation in her rectal area and watery diarrhea

b. irritation in her rectal area and bloody diarrhea

c. irritation in her rectal area, cramping, and diarrhea

Check your answers in the Answer Key online. How did you do? Are there new words you do not know? Take the time now to look them up in your bilingual or first-language dictionary.

IDIOMATIC EXPRESSIONS

Idioms and idiomatic expressions are made up of a group of words that have a different meaning from the original meaning of each individual word. Native speakers of the English language use such expressions comfortably and naturally. However, individuals who are new speakers of English or who have studied English for many years may still not be able to use idioms and idiomatic expressions as comfortably or naturally as native speakers. As pharmacy students, pharmacy technicians, and practicing pharmacists, you will hear many different idiomatic expressions. Some of you will understand and know how to use these expressions correctly. At times, however, you may not understand what your professors, colleagues, and patients are saying. This of course can lead to miscommunication, embarrassment, and possibly dangerous mistakes.

To help you improve your knowledge of idioms and idiomatic expressions, carefully read the following idiomatic expressions that contain the word stomach.

Idiomatic expressions using "stomach"

1. **hard to stomach** means that the person dislikes something or someone else very much.

   For example: I really **can't stomach** my new boss.

2. **to have butterflies in one's stomach** means to have anxiety and feelings of fear.

   For example: The patient **had butterflies in her stomach** as she waited for the doctor to give her the results of her endoscopy.

3. **to be difficult to stomach** means to be unable to accept someone or endure something that is unpleasant or wrong.

   For example: Sometimes it's **difficult to stomach** patients who demand that their prescription be filled immediately and who think they are the only patients waiting for their prescriptions.

4. **turn one's stomach** means to disgust someone or to make one feel sick.

   For example: The film of the war on the TV nightly news really **turns my stomach.**

5. **eyes are bigger than one's stomach** means to eat more food than one can eat.

   For example: My **eyes were bigger than my stomach** when I put so much food on my plate.

6. **not have the stomach for** means the person has no desire for something he or she feels is wrong or unpleasant.

   For example: She **doesn't have the stomach** to listen to her roommate talk about her boyfriend problems.

7. **can't stomach** means to dislike someone or something very much.

   For example: Most patients **can't stomach** the increasing cost of prescription medicines.

Mini Dialogues Listening Exercise

How much did you understand? Listen to the following mini dialogues on the audio files found in Chapter 7 on thePoint (thePoint.lww.com/diaz-gilbert), read the questions below, and then choose the correct answer.

 Mini Dialogue #1

1. _____ **Butterflies in my stomach** means:

a. to be happy

b. to be anxious

c. to be disgusted

Mini Dialogue #2

2. _____ ***Can't stomach them*** means:

a. can't digest them

b. can't accept them

c. to like them very much

Mini Dialogue #3

3. _____ ***Don't have the stomach*** for means:

a. to feel nauseous

b. to have no desire

c. to have an upset stomach

Mini Dialogue #4

4. _____ ***Turned my stomach*** means:

a. to turn the intestines

b. to disgust

c. to make someone scream

Mini Dialogue #5

5. _____ ***Difficult to stomach*** means:

a. unable to accept

b. unable to eat

c. unable to digest

Mini Dialogue #6

6. _____ ***Hard to stomach*** means:

a. to accept behavior that is wrong

b. difficult to digest

c. unable to accept

How did you do? Check your answers against the Answer Key online.

POST-ASSESSMENT

True/False Questions

Indicate whether each sentence below is true (T) or false (F).

1. _____ The idiom **to turn one's stomach** means to have indigestion.

2. _____ Esophageal is an adjective and esophagus is a noun.

3. _____ Another word for difficulty swallowing is regurgitation.

4. _____ Tender is an adjective form of tenderness.

5. _____ If a person's **eyes are bigger than his or her stomach,** the person is still very hungry and needs to eat more.

6. _____ Spicy foods can help treat indigestion.

7. _____ Crohn's disease and ulcerative colitis are both inflammatory bowel diseases.

8. _____ Regurgitant and regurgitative are adjective forms.

9. _____ An appendix clogged with pus will not burst.

10. _____ Peptic ulcers are caused by viral infection.

11. _____ If a person **has butterflies in the stomach,** they are very hungry.

12. _____ Fiber and water can help to soften waste and prevent constipation.

13. _____ People with celiac disease are able to eat gluten.

14. _____ Patients with GERD can experience dysphagia and dyspnea.

15. _____ Hemorrhoids are inflamed veins in the rectum and anus.

Multiple Choice Questions

Choose the correct answer from a, b, and c.

1. _____ The adjective form of **digestion** is:
a. digestible
b. digestive
c. digestible and digestive

2. _____ If a person is constipated, he or she has:
a. watery stool
b. bloody stool
c. difficulty having a bowel movement

3. _____ If a person **can't stomach someone or something,** the person:
a. likes another person or thing
b. dislikes another person or thing
c. has a feeling of anxiety

4. _____ Stress and diet can trigger:
a. irritable bowel syndrome
b. gas
c. belching

5. _____ In this sentence, "Fecal impaction is the result of chronic constipation," the word **fecal** is:
a. an adjective and a noun
b. an adjective
c. a noun

6. _____ Dulcolax is used to treat:
a. constipation
b. blood pressure
c. GERD

7. _____ Bloating is the buildup of:
a. mucus
b. sputum
c. gas

8. _____ If a person is **difficult to stomach,** he or she:
a. has dysphagia
b. is nervous
c. is hard for others to accept

9. _____ Another term for lower esophageal ring is:

a. Schatzki's ring

b. peptic ring

c. diverticula

10. _____ In the sentence, "Rectal bleeding is associated with colon cancer," the word **rectal** is:

a. an adjective

b. a verb

c. a noun

11. _____ The word **gastric** is:

a. an adjective

b. a verb

c. a noun

12. _____ Another word for difficulty swallowing is:

a. dysphagia

b. dyspnea

c. delirium

13. _____ A diet low in fiber and with inadequate fluid intake can lead to:

a. belching

b. GERD

c. constipation

14. _____ Ranitidine is used to treat:

a. GERD

b. ulcerative colitis

c. constipation

15. _____ In the sentence, "The patient complained he was bloated," the word **bloated** is:

a. an adjective

b. a past tense verb

c. a noun

Listening and Comprehension Exercises

Dialogue #1

Listen to Dialogue #1, stop, listen again and take notes. Listen to the dialogue as many times as you need or until you feel you have written sufficient notes and feel confident. You can use your notes to answer the multiple choice questions at the end of the dialogue.

Notes _____

_____

_____

_____

_____

Answer the questions below by selecting the answer that correctly completes each sentence.

1. _____ The patient is embarrassed because she:

a. forgot her prescription

b. is constipated

c. has hemorrhoids

2. _____ The pharmacist tells the patient:

a. she needs a prescription

b. she can get over-the-counter treatment

c. she needs to see her doctor

3. _____ The patient is allergic to:

a. birth control pills

b. milk

c. milk and onions

4. _____ The patient states she has been constipated for:

a. 3 days

b. about 3 months

c. about 3 weeks

5. _____ The pharmacist recommends:

a. Sani-Supp glycerin suppositories to treat hemorrhoids

b. Sani-Supp glycerin suppositories that should be moistened with lukewarm water before use to treat her constipation

c. Preparation H glycerin suppositories to treat her hemorrhoids

6. _____ The pharmacist also recommends:

a. Metamucil or Citrucel for her constipation

b. Citrucel only for her constipation

c. Preparation H for her constipation

7. _____ Metamucil and Citrucel are:

a. pills that must be chewed

b. fiber laxatives that increase the amount of water in the stool, and harden it

c. fiber laxatives that increase the amount of water in the stool, and soften it

8. _____ The suppositories:

a. can be used until the patient gets relief

b. should not be used for more than a week

c. should not be used for more than a month

9. _____ The patient tells the pharmacist that she:

a. feels bloated

b. feels crampy

c. had abdominal pain

10. _____ The pharmacist also recommends that the patient:

a. drink 4 to 6 glasses of water every day and eat fiber and roughage

b. drink 46 glasses of water daily

c. mix 4 to 6 glasses of water with fiber and drink them daily

11. _____ To treat her constipation and her hemorrhoids, the patient purchases:

a. Citrucel powder, Metamucil tablets, and Preparation H

b. Sani-Supp, Citrucel powder, Metamucil wafers, and Preparation H

c. Sani-Supp, Metamucil tablets, and Preparation H

Dialogue #2

Listen to Dialogue #2, stop, listen again and take notes. Listen to the dialogue as many times as you need or until you feel you have written sufficient notes and feel confident. You can use your notes to answer the multiple choice questions at the end of the dialogue.

Notes _____

_____

_____

_____

_____

_____

Answer the questions below by selecting the answer that correctly completes each sentence.

1. _____ The patient's name is:

a. Samuel Torres, and the pharmacist's name is Erin Farrell

b. Samuel Farrell, and the pharmacist's name is Erin Torres

c. Erin Farrell, and the pharmacist's name is Samuel Torres

2. _____ The patient's prescription will treat:

a. his gastric ulcer

b. his colitis

c. his peptic ulcer

3. _____ The patient tells the pharmacist that he's been having a burning pain:

a. in his chest

b. around his belly button and breastbone

c. in his stomach

4. _____ The burning pain:

a. flares up during the day

b. comes and goes, but flares up during the night and he can't sleep

c. is persistent and flares up at night

5. _____ Before the patient saw:

a. Dr. B. J. Lewis, he was taking Pepto-Bismol, Mylanta, and Maalox

b. Dr. B. J. Lewis, he was taking Metamucil, Mylanta, and Maalox

c. Dr. B. J. Lewis, he was taking Pepto-Bismol, Mylanta, and Metamucil

6. _____ Other medications the patient is taking include:

a. Motrin and vitamins

b. Tylenol and vitamins

c. vitamins only

7. _____ The patient:

a. is allergic to penicillin

b. is allergic to all antibiotics

c. is not allergic to penicillin or any antibiotic

8. _____ The doctor prescribed:

a. Prevacid, which will stop bacteria from growing and reduce stomach acid

b. Prevpac, which contains medicine to help block stomach acid and antibiotics to help stop bacteria from growing

c. Prevpac, which will block stomach acid and stop bleeding in the stomach

9. _____ The pharmacist instructs the patient to:

a. take one tablet in the morning and one tablet in the evening for 14 days

b. take two tablets in the morning for 14 days

c. take a total of 14 tablets during 14 days

10. _____ The patient must take the tablets:

 a. with food

 b. before a meal

 c. with water only

11. _____ Side effects of the medication include:

 a. a headache and an abnormal taste in the mouth

 b. dizziness and a tingling sensation in the tongue

 c. bleeding in the stomach

12. _____ The pharmacist advises the patient:

 a. who does not smoke, not to smoke, not to drink excessively, and to avoid Motrin and Aleve

 b. who is trying to quit smoking and drinks beer once in while, not to smoke because smoking can increase stomach acid, and not to drink excessively because alcohol can cause the stomach to bleed

 c. that he should avoid Tylenol, and take Motrin or Aleve when he needs to

How did you do on the Post-Assessment in Chapter 7? Check your answers in the Answer Key online.

The Musculoskeletal System 8

PRE-ASSESSMENT

True/False Questions

Indicate whether each sentence below is true (T) or false (F).

1. _____ **Rheumatoid arthritis** results from wear and tear on the joints.
2. _____ An accumulation of urate crystals causes **gout,** or inflammation of a joint, usually in the big toe.
3. _____ Another word for degenerative joint disease is **osteoporosis.**
4. _____ **Sjögren's syndrome** is a disorder of the immune system that affects the tendons.
5. _____ The adjective form of arthritis is **arthritic.**
6. _____ A risk factor for developing **lupus,** a chronic inflammatory disease, is pregnancy.
7. _____ **Osteoporosis,** which means porous bones, causes bones to be strong and brittle.
8. _____ **Tendonitis,** which is inflammation of the tendon, affects only the wrist and elbow.
9. _____ **Bursitis,** which is inflammation of the fluid that lubricates joints and muscle tendons, can be caused by overuse, infection, arthritis, and gout.
10. _____ The noun form of **stiff** is stiffness and stiff.
11. _____ Osteomyelitis refers to infection of the bone.
12. _____ Symptoms of **Paget's disease,** which is a disease of the bone, includes bowlegs and an enlarged head size.
13. _____ People with **Marfan syndrome** have scoliosis, very loose and flexible joints, and a breast-bone that protrudes outward or is concave.
14. _____ **Scleroderma** is an arthritic condition and a connective tissue disease.
15. _____ The adjective forms of **deteriorate** are deteriorated and deteriorating.

Multiple Choice Questions

Choose the correct answer from a, b, and c.

1. _____ Over time, **arthritis** can lead to:
a. deformity of the joints
b. weak and brittle bones
c. bone infection

2. _____ A risk factor for developing **gout** is:
a. malnutrition
b. excessive urination
c. excess consumption of alcohol

3. _____ The disorder of the immune system that includes symptoms of dry eyes and dry mouth is:

a. scleroderma

b. Sjögren's syndrome

c. Marfan syndrome

4. _____ **Lupus** is a chronic autoimmune inflammatory disease that can affect the:

a. lungs, heart, skin, joints, kidneys, and blood cells

b. skin and joints only

c. skin only

5. _____ Digestive problems can occur in patients with:

a. localized scleroderma

b. systemic scleroderma

c. osteoarthritis

6. _____ **Fibromyalgia** is a chronic condition that affects the:

a. bone marrow

b. muscles

c. tendons

7. _____ A chronic form of inflammation of the spine is:

a. amyloidosis

b. ankylosing spondylitis

c. osteoarthritis

8. _____ The word **mobility** is:

a. a noun and a verb

b. a verb only

c. a noun only

9. _____ People with **osteoporosis** will experience:

a. sensitivity to sun

b. a rash on their face

c. fractures

10. _____ The expression **"I can feel it in my bones"** means:

a. you are having bone pain

b. you feel something will happen, even though you are not sure it will

c. you are very cold

How did you do? Check your answers in the Answer Key online.

MEDICAL VOCABULARY

A good understanding of vocabulary words in pharmacy is very important for communication with professors, fellow students, patients, and coworkers. Knowledge and understanding of vocabulary leads to successful communication and success as a pharmacy student, as a pharmacy technician, and as a practicing pharmacist. You may already know many of the vocabulary words in this chapter, but for words that are unfamiliar, pay careful attention to them and make every effort to know their correct spelling, meaning, and pronunciation. It is a good idea to keep a list of new words and to look up these new words in a bilingual dictionary or dictionary in your first language. A good command of pharmacy-related vocabulary and good pronunciation of vocabulary will help to prevent embarrassing mistakes and increase effective verbal communication skills.

Musculoskeletal System Vocabulary

aching
ankylosing spondylitis
arthritis
autoimmune
bony lumps
brittle
bursitis
carpal tunnel syndrome
cartilage
collagen
connective tissue
debilitating
deformity
degenerative
erythrocyte
   sedimentation rate
fibromyalgia

flexibility
fracture
fusion
gout
immune
joints
knuckles
ligaments
lupus
mobility
nodes
osteoarthritis
osteoporosis
photosensitivity
range of motion
relapse
remission

rheumatism
scleroderma
Sjögren's syndrome
spine
stiffness
stooped posture
stress
stretch
subside
susceptible
synovitis
temporomandibular
   joint
tendonitis
urate crystals
vertebrae
wear and tear

PARTS OF SPEECH

A good understanding of parts of speech, such as verbs, nouns, adjectives, and adverbs, is important for successful communication when speaking or writing. It is equally important to know the various forms of words and to use them appropriately.

Word Forms

The table below lists the main forms of some terms that you will likely encounter in pharmacy practice. Review the table and then do the exercises that follow to assess your understanding.

Noun (n)	Infinitive/Verb (v) —Past Tense	Adjective (adj)	Adverb (adv)
ache; aching	to ache; ached	aching	achingly
arthritis; arthritic		arthritic	arthritically
brittleness	to brittle; brittled	brittle	brittlely
collagen		collagenous; collagenic	
debilitation	to debilitate; debilitated	debilitating; debilitative	
deformity		deformed	
degeneration	to degenerate; degenerated	degenerative	
flexibility; flexibleness	to flex; flexed	flexible	flexibly
fracture	to fracture; fractured		
fusion	to fuse; fused		
gout; goutiness		gouty	
immunization	to immunize; immunized	immune	

(*continued*)

Noun (n)	Infinitive/Verb (v) —Past Tense	Adjective (adj)	Adverb (adv)
joint	to join; joined	jointed	jointly
knuckle	to knuckle; knuckled		
ligament		ligamental; ligamentary; ligamentous	
mobility; mobilization	to mobilize; mobilized	mobile	
osteoarthritis		osteoarthritic	
osteoporosis		osteoporotic	
photosensitivity		photosensitive	
posture; posturer	to posture; postured	postural	
rheumatism		rheumatoid	rheumatoidally
spine		spinal	
stiffness; a stiff	to stiff; stiffed	stiff; stiffish	stiffly
stress	to stress; stressed	stressful	
stretchability	to stretch; stretched	stretchable	
susceptibleness		susceptible	susceptibly
synovitis; synovium; synovia		synovial	

Word Forms Exercise

Read the following sentences carefully. Then indicate the word form of the bolded word(s), choosing from v, n, adj, or adv.

1. Symptoms of **rheumatoid** arthritis include swelling and **deformity** in the **joints** of the hand and feet, loss of **motion** in the joints, and a loss of **strength** in the muscles attached to the joints.

   rheumatoid _____   deformity _____   joints _____   motion _____   strength _____

2. **Gouty arthritis,** also known as **gout,** is a form of arthritis that causes an **intolerable** hot, **tender,** and **swollen** sensation in the big toe.

   gouty _____   arthritis _____   gout _____   intolerable _____   tender _____   swollen _____

3. **Osteoarthritis,** also known as **degenerative** bone disease, is a **common** form of arthritis that results in the **breakdown** of joint **cartilage.**

   osteoarthritis _____   degenerative _____   common _____   breakdown _____   cartilage _____

4. People with Sjögren's **syndrome,** an **autoimmune disorder,** will **experience** dry eyes and dry mouth.

   syndrome _____   autoimmune _____   disorder _____   experience _____

5. People with **osteoporosis,** which causes bones to become **brittle** and weak, are likely to have bone loss, **fractures,** and a **stooped posture.**

   osteoporosis _____   brittle _____   fractures _____   stooped _____   posture _____

6. **Sensitivity** to sunlight is a **typical** symptom of **lupus,** a chronic inflammatory disease that develops when an individual's **immune** system **attacks** its organs and tissues.

   sensitivity _____   typical _____   lupus _____   immune _____   attacks _____

7. Ankylosing spondylitis is a form of **inflammatory** arthritis that causes **inflammation** of the joints between the **vertebrae** of the **spine** and of the joints between the spine and pelvis.

   inflammatory _____   inflammation _____   vertebrae _____   spine _____

8. **Scleroderma,** which means "**hard** skin," is a **connective** tissue disease that leads to **hardening** of the skin as a result of inflammation and the **overproduction** of **collagen,** and can affect other organs in the body.

   scleroderma _____   hard _____   connective _____   hardening _____   overproduction _____   collagen _____

9. Pain throughout the body, fatigue, **interrupted** sleep, headaches, **facial** pain, irritable bowel syndrome, and sensitivity to **bright** lights, noise, **touch,** and odors are some of the signs and symptoms of **fibromyalgia.**

   interrupted _____   facial _____   bright _____   touch _____   fibromyalgia _____

10. It is typical for **arthritic** patients to experience severe fatigue during a **flare-up** and to have **stiff** and **achy** joints and muscles, especially after **periods** of **rest** and sleep.

    arthritic _____   flare-up _____   stiff _____   achy _____   periods _____   rest _____

11. In addition to experiencing **intense** joint pain and a red, swollen, and **tender** big toe, **sufferers** of gout may experience **similar** pain and **discomfort** in their hands, wrists, feet, and ankles.

    intense _____   tender _____   sufferers _____   similar _____   discomfort _____

12. Fingers affected by osteoarthritis can develop **nodes,** or **bony** knobs, and the **bones** along the spine affected by osteoarthritis can **deteriorate, leading** to neck pain and **stiffness.**

    nodes _____   bony _____   bones _____   deteriorate _____   lead _____   stiffness _____

13. In addition to dry eyes and dry mouth, symptoms of Sjögren's syndrome include, but are not limited to, a dry **cough** without sputum, **difficulty** chewing and swallowing, fatigue, **dental cavities,** and swollen and **stiff** joints.

    cough _____   difficulty _____   dental _____   cavities _____   stiff _____

14. Inflammation in the joints in an **arthritic** person occurs when red blood cells attack the **synovial** membrane that **lines** the **movable** joints, which becomes **inflamed.**

    arthritic _____   synovial _____   lines _____   movable _____   inflamed _____

15. Medications and **lifestyle** changes such as weight **reduction,** limiting alcohol intake, which can prevent the **excretion** of uric acid, and drinking plenty of water to **dilute** uric acid in the body can help reduce **attacks** of gout.

    lifestyle _____   reduction _____   excretion _____   dilute _____   attacks _____

How did you do? Check your answers against the Answer Key online.

Typical Medical Conditions and Patient Complaints

The sentences below contain vocabulary that describes and explains typical medical conditions, diseases, symptoms, and patient complaints that a pharmacist encounters. Read the sentences carefully. Then indicate the word form of the bolded word(s), choosing from v, n, adj, or adv. Look up words you do not know in your bilingual or first-language dictionary.

1. Before she was **diagnosed** with lupus, the patient had **complained** of a rash that developed across the cheeks and bridge of her nose, of pain and **stiffness** in her wrists, hips, and knees, of **swelling** in her fingers, and that she could not **tolerate** the sun.

   diagnosed _____   complained _____   stiffness _____   swelling _____   tolerate _____

2. **Sufferers** of ankylosing spondylitis, which can affect other parts of the body such as the joints between the ribs and the **spine,** the joints in the feet, knees, shoulders, and hips, and the

tendons and **ligaments,** may also develop **chronic stooping,** a stiff, **inflexible** spine, and bowel inflammation.

sufferers _____ spine _____ ligaments _____ chronic _____ stooping _____ inflexible _____

3. Scleroderma, which is caused when the body **attacks** itself and **produces** too much collagen, is classified into **localized** scleroderma, a disease that **affects** only the skin, and **systemic** scleroderma, which affects the skin, blood vessels, and **major** organs.

attacks _____ produces _____ localized _____ affects _____ systemic _____ major _____

4. People who **suffer** from fibromyalgia need to reduce **stress** and **avoid overexertion,** get enough sleep to help reduce the fatigue **typical** of fibromyalgia, **exercise,** learn relaxation techniques, and eat healthy foods.

suffer _____ stress _____ avoid _____ overexertion _____ typical _____ exercise _____

5. Arthritis, which comes in many **forms,** is a joint **disorder** accompanied by inflammation and ranges from **rheumatoid** arthritis, which is inflammation from an **overactive** immune system, to osteoarthritis, which is the **wear and tear** of cartilage.

forms _____ disorder _____ rheumatoid _____ overactive _____ wear and tear _____

6. **Aging,** heredity, and injury can cause **osteoarthritis,** also known as **degenerative** arthritis, which is the loss and **degeneration** of cartilage **caused** by inflammation.

aging _____ osteoarthritis _____ degenerative _____ degeneration _____ caused _____

7. Patients with Sjögren's syndrome, an **autoimmune** disease that affects the glands that produce **tears** and saliva and causes dry eye and dry mouth, can be treated with **artificial** tears and eye **lubricant** ointments, plenty of fluids, and **humidifying** air.

autoimmune _____ tears _____ artificial _____ lubricant _____ humidifying _____

8. Quitting smoking, **reducing** alcohol **consumption,** exercising, and eating foods with calcium and vitamin D can help treat the **loss** of bone and loss of bone **strength** caused by osteoporosis, which results in bone **fractures.**

reducing _____ consumption _____ loss _____ strength _____ fractures _____

9. Kidney stones and **decreased** kidney **function** can result from gout, a form of arthritis that is caused by very **high** levels of **uric acid** in the blood.

decreased _____ function _____ high _____ uric _____ acid _____

10. Ankylosing spondylitis, which is **chronic** inflammation of the **spine** and the **sacroiliac** joints that causes **stiffness,** pain, and the loss of **mobility** of the spine, can also **affect** other tissue and organs in the body.

chronic _____ spine _____ sacroiliac _____ stiffness _____ mobility _____ affect _____

11. People suffering from fibromyalgia, a chronic condition that is aggravated by weather **change, emotional** stress, and noise, are **sensitive** to various stimuli, feel pain, stiffness, and **tenderness** throughout their body and may experience sleep **disturbances,** anxiety, depression, fatigue, and irritable bowel syndrome.

change _____ emotional _____ sensitive _____ tenderness _____ disturbances _____

12. Some people with rheumatoid arthritis, which is an autoimmune disease that **causes** the joints to **inflame,** will experience **remission** for weeks, months, or years during which symptoms such as joint pain, fatigue, swelling, stiffness, and muscle and joint **aches disappear.**

causes _____ inflame _____ remission _____ aches _____ disappear _____

13. Scleroderma can be classified into **diffused** scleroderma, which causes **thickening** of the skin on the face, **extremities,** and in **major** organs such as the esophagus, lungs, kidneys, bowels, and heart, and **limited** scleroderma, which affects the skin and fingers.

diffused _____ thickening _____ extremities _____ major _____ limited _____

12. debilitation dĭ-bĭl′ĭ-tā′t′
13. deformity dĭ-fôr′mĭ-tē
14. degenerative dĭ-jĕn′ər-ə-tĭv
15. erythrocyte sedimentation rate ĭ-rĭth′rə-sīt′ sĕd′ə-mən-tā′shən rāt
16. fibromyalgia fī′brō-mī-ăl′jē-ə
17. flexibility flĕk′sə-bəl ĭ-tē
18. fracture frăk′chər
19. fuse fyōōz
20. gout gout
21. immune ĭ-myōōn′
22. joint joint
23. knuckles nŭk′əls
24. ligament lĭg′ə-mənt
25. lupus lōō′pəs
26. mobility mō-bĭl′ĭ-tē
27. node nōd
28. osteoarthritis ŏs′tē-ō-är-thrī′tĭs
29. osteoporosis ŏs′tē-ō-pə-rō′sĭs
30. photosensitivity fō′tō-sĕn′sĭ-tĭv′ĭ-tē
31. range of motion rānj ŭv mō′shən
32. relapse rĭ-lăps
33. remission rĭ-mĭsh′ən
34. rheumatism rōō′mə-tĭz′əm
35. scleroderma sklĭr′ə-dûr′mə
36. Sjögren's syndrome shō′grənz sĭn′drōm′
37. spine spīn
38. stiff stĭf
39. stooped posture stōōpt pŏs′chər
40. stress strĕs
41. stretch strĕch
42. subside səb-sīd′
43. susceptible sə-sĕp′tə-bəl
44. synovitis sĭ′nə-vī′tĭs
45. temporomandibular joint tĕm′pə-rō-măn-dĭb′yə-lər joint
46. tendonitis tĕn′də-nī′tĭs
47. urate crystals yōōr′āt′ krĭs′təls
48. vertebrae vûr′tə brā
49. wear and tear wâr ənd târ

Which words are easy to pronounce? Which are difficult to pronounce? Use the space below to write in the words that you find difficult to pronounce. These are words you should practice saying often.

_____
_____
_____
_____
_____
_____
_____
_____

Listen to the audiofiles found in Chapter 8 on thePoint (thePoint.lww.com/diaz-gilbert) as many times as you need to increase your pronunciation ability of the difficult words. Pronounce these words with a friend or a colleague who speaks English.

English Sounds That Are Difficult for Speakers of Other Languages to Pronounce

Spanish

In Spanish, there is no English "v" sound, but the "v" consonant in Spanish is pronounced like the English "b." The vowel "i" is pronounced like a long "e." Pay careful attention to the "v" sound in English when pronouncing words that begin with "v." Also pay careful attention to English words that begin with "s;" do not use the Spanish "es" sound when pronouncing English words that begin with "s."

For example, in English,

arthritis is not pronounced artreetees

Vietnamese

In Vietnamese, the "t" consonant is pronounced "s," but in English the "t" is pronounced "t" and "s" is pronounced "s." Be careful with English words that begin with "t." In Vietnamese, the "b" consonant is pronounced "p," but in English "p" is pronounced "p" and "b" is pronounced "b."

In Vietnamese, words do not end in "b," "ch," "f," "d," "j," "l," "p," "r," "s," "sh," "v," and "z." In English, words end in these letters. Pay special attention to pronouncing these English sounds. In Vietnamese, there is no "dzh" or "zh" sound, so English words like "judge" (dzh) and "rupture" (zh) will be hard for Vietnamese speakers to pronounce.

For example, in English,

joint is not pronounced join

Gujarati

In Gujarati, "v" is pronounced "w," "f" is pronounced "p," "p" is pronounced "f," and "z" is pronounced "j." Short "i" is pronounced long "e," "x" is pronounced "ch," and "th" is pronounced "s." In English, "v" is pronounced "v," "f" is pronounced "f," "z" is pronounced "z" or "s," "j" is pronounced "j," and "x" is pronounced "x." Pay careful attention when pronouncing these sounds.

For example, in English,

flexibility is not pronounced plexeebeeleetee
vertebrae is not pronounced wertebrae

Korean

In Korean, the "v" consonant is pronounced "b" and the "f" consonant is pronounced "p." In English, the "v" is pronounced "v," the "f" is pronounced "f," and the "p" is pronounced "p." Pay special attention when pronouncing these sounds.

For example, in English,

fibromyalgia is not pronounced pibromyalgia

(continued)

Chinese

In Chinese, the "r" consonant is pronounced "l" or "w," and "b," "d," "g," and "ng" are not pronounced at all. Pay careful attention to English words that begin with "r" because the "r" is not pronounced "l" or "w," and "b," "d," "g," and "ng" are pronounced in English.

For example, in English,

relapse is not pronounced relap

Russian

The "w" consonant is pronounced like a "v" and the "v" sounds like a "w." Pay careful attention to the English "th." It is not pronounced "s."

For example, in English,

"wear and tear" is not pronounced "vear and tear"

DICTATION

 ### Listening/Spelling Exercise: Word and Word Pairs

Listen to the words or word pairs on the audio files found in Chapter 8 on thePoint (thePoint.lww.com/diaz-gilbert) and then write them down on the lines below.

1. _____
2. _____
3. _____
4. _____
5. _____
6. _____
7. _____
8. _____
9. _____
10. _____
11. _____
12. _____
13. _____
14. _____
15. _____

 ### Listening/Spelling Exercise: Sentences

Listen to the sentences on the audio files found in Chapter 8 on thePoint (thePoint.lww.com/diaz-gilbert) and then write them down on the lines below.

1. _____
   _____
2. _____
   _____

3. _____
_____

4. _____
_____

5. _____
_____

6. _____
_____

7. _____
_____

8. _____
_____

9. _____
_____

10. _____
_____

Now, check your sentences against the correct answers in the Answer Key online. If there are any new words that you do not know or that you spelled incorrectly, make a list of those words and study them for meaning and spelling.

PHARMACIST/PATIENT DIALOGUES

The ability to orally communicate effectively with your professors, colleagues, and especially with patients is very important. As a pharmacist, you will be counseling patients; patients will come to you for advice. They will have questions about a condition and symptoms they may experience and will ask you to help treat the condition. Therefore, it is extremely important that you understand what they are saying and that you respond to them and their questions appropriately. Your patients will speak differently. For example, some may speak very quickly, others too low, and yet others may speak angrily. To help you improve your listening skills, listen to the following dialogues, or short conversations, between a pharmacist and a patient and between a pharmacy technician and a patient.

Listening and Comprehension Exercises
Dialogue #1

Listen to Dialogue #1, stop, listen again and take notes. Listen to the dialogue as many times as you need or until you feel you have written sufficient notes and feel confident. You can use your notes to answer the multiple choice questions at the end of the dialogue.

Notes _____
_____
_____
_____
_____

Answer the questions below by selecting the answer that correctly completes each sentence.

1. _____ The pharmacist's name is:
   a. Walter Lipton, and the patient's name is Rachel Cronin
   b. Rachel Lipton, and the patient's name is Walter Lipton
   c. Walter Cronin, and the patient's name is Rachel Lipton

2. _____ The patient has been prescribed:

a. sulfasalazine for her body stiffness

b. sulfasalazine for her rheumatoid arthritis

c. sulfasalazine for her deformed joints

3. _____ The patient's doctor's name is:

a. Dr. Sal Mann

b. Dr. Solomon

c. Dr. Sullyman

4. _____ The patient tells the pharmacist that her:

a. rheumatoid arthritis is getting better and that she does not have swelling or pain

b. rheumatoid arthritis pain and swelling is getting worse, that her fingers are curling and becoming deformed, and that only her knees are stiff

c. rheumatoid arthritis pain and swelling is getting worse, that her fingers are curling and becoming deformed, and that her knees, hips, and feet are stiff

5. _____ When the patient tells the pharmacist, "It's so painful, but I try to keep a stiff upper lip," **keep a stiff upper lip** means:

a. the patient's upper lip is also stiff

b. the patient is trying to be strong even though she is suffering with pain

c. because the patient is in pain, the upper lip is stiff

6. _____ Other medications that the patient tells the pharmacist have not worked are:

a. Aleve only

b. Aleve and prednisone

c. Aleve, prednisone, and Vioxx

7. _____ The pharmacist tells the patient that sulfasalazine:

a. will help to reduce the joint pain and swelling and stiffness, and will help to slow down the progression of the disease and prevent further joint damage

b. will help to reduce the joint pain, swelling, and stiffness but will not help to slow down the progression of the disease and will not prevent further joint damage

c. will slow down the progression of the disease and prevent further joint damage, but will not reduce joint pain, swelling, and stiffness

8. _____ The pharmacist tells the patient that the doctor wants her to take:

a. sulfasalazine with prednisone

b. sulfasalazine with prednisone and Aleve

c. sulfasalazine with Aleve

9. _____ The pharmacist explains to the patients that sulfasalazine is a:

a. yellow, delayed-release 5-milligram tablet that should not be chewed, crushed, or broken because doing so can cause an upset stomach

b. gold, delayed-release 50-milligram tablet that can be chewed, crushed, or broken because doing so will not cause an upset stomach

c. gold, delayed-release 500-milligram tablet that should not be chewed, crushed, or broken because doing so can cause an upset stomach

10. _____ Side effects of sulfasalazine include:

a. nausea, headache, vomiting, ringing in the ears, painful urination, and difficulty breathing, and patients should avoid staying in the sun for extended periods and use sunscreen

b. nausea, headache, vomiting, ringing in the ears, painful urination, and difficulty breathing, but it is not necessary for patients to avoid the sun

c. headaches, vomiting, and sensitivity to sun only

11. _____ When the patient tells the pharmacist, "Sometimes I just want to yell at the top of my lungs, it hurts so bad," **yell at the top of my lungs** means:

a. the patient's lungs are in a lot of pain

b. the patient wants to express how painful she's feeling by yelling

c. the patient is able to yell loudly because she has good lungs

12. _____ The pharmacist tells the patient that she should be feeling better:

a. 1 to 3 weeks after taking the medication

b. 1 to 3 days after taking the medication

c. 1 to 3 months after taking the medication

13. _____ When the patient tells the pharmacist, "That long? I'll be tearing my hair out," **tearing my hair out** means:

a. the patient will lose her hair

b. the patient will become anxious and worried

c. the patient will remain calm

14. _____ The pharmacist tells that patient that along with taking the medications, she should:

a. exercise

b. exercise, have physical therapy, and watch her weight

c. live a sedentary lifestyle

15._____ The patient tells the pharmacist that:

a. sometimes she wraps hot pads around her fingers, puts hot pads on her stiff knees, feet, and muscles, and that Mr. Lipton massages her, and the pharmacist recommends that she also use cold packs

b. sometimes she puts ice packs on her fingers and stiff knees, feet, and muscles and the pharmacist also recommends that she try hot pads

c. she gets relieve only when Mr. Lipton massages her

Check your answers in the Answer Key online. How did you do? Are there new words you do not know? Take the time now to look them up in your bilingual or first-language dictionary.

Dialogue #2

Listen to Dialogue #2, stop, listen again and take notes. Listen to the dialogue as many times as you need or until you feel you have written sufficient notes and feel confident. You can use your notes to answer the multiple choice questions at the end of the dialogue.

Notes _____

_____

_____

_____

_____

Answer the questions below by selecting the answer that correctly completes each sentence.

1. _____ The patient's name is:

a. Steven Washington

b. Steven Brady

c. Brady Washington

2. _____ The patient first saw the pharmacist when he was diagnosed with:

a. COPD

b. ankylosing spondylitis

c. rheumatoid arthritis

3. _____ The patient has a prescription for:

a. Atrovent

b. Rheumatrex

c. Azulfidine

4. _____ The patient's has been recently diagnosed with:

a. chronic bronchitis

b. COPD and ankylosing spondylitis

c. ankylosing spondylitis

5. _____ Dr. Anderson prescribed:

a. Rheumatrex only

b. Rheumatrex, but methotrexate can also be used

c. Methotrexate only

6. _____ The patient told the pharmacist he was having:

a. soreness in his lower back, and pain and tenderness in his spine, rib cage, and shoulders

b. tenderness in his spine and rib cage

c. soreness in his rib cage and shoulders

7. _____ The patient told the pharmacist, "He gave me some blood tests and an MRI and then he told me I had AS. I really got "hit between the eyes." **Hit between the eyes** means the patient:

a. got punched between the eyes

b. was not surprised he was diagnosed with ankylosing spondylitis

c. received some surprising and shocking news

8. _____ The pharmacist tells the patient that ankylosing spondylitis can cause:

a. the rib cage to stiffen and expand lung capacity and function

b. the rib cage to stiffen and restrict lung capacity and function

c. the rib cage to break and collapse the lungs

9. _____ The patient told the pharmacist that:

a. Dr. Anderson also told him he will have difficulty walking and standing and be hunched and stooped over when the joints begin to fuse

b. Dr. Anderson also told him he will have difficulty walking and standing, but will not be hunched and stooped over

c. Dr. Posner also told him he will have difficulty walking and standing, and be hunched and stooped over when the joints begin to fuse

10. _____ The patient is:

a. experiencing breathing difficulty

b. is not really experiencing breathing difficulty

c. experiencing severe breathing difficulty

11. _____ The pharmacist recommends:

a. physical therapy because it will help relieve pain and give the patient physical strength and flexibility

b. that the patient go for walks on weekends only

c. that the patient avoid walking and exercising as the disease progresses and the patient develops a stooped posture

12. _____ The pharmacist tells the patient that:
   a. Rheumatrex is not a strong medication that needs to be taken once a week so it doesn't need to be taken with food or water
   b. Rheumatrex is a potent medication that should only be taken once a month
   c. Rheumatrex is a potent medication that is taken once a week and should be taken with plenty of fluids

13. _____ The pharmacist tells the patient to "keep an eye out" for possible side effects. **Keep an eye out** means:
   a. to look for, watch for, or notice side effects
   b. to make sure the medication has no effect on the eyes
   c. the eyes will definitely be affected by the medication

14. _____ The pharmacist tells the patient that some of the side effects of Rheumatrex include:
   a. sensitivity to sun only
   b. mouth sores and a dry cough
   c. mouth sores, a persistent cough, and black stools

15. _____ The patient:
   a. has a new address, has no new allergies, and will only be taking Rheumatrex
   b. has the same address, has no new allergies, and will not be taking any other medications in addition to Atrovent and Rheumatrex
   c. has a new address, has no allergies, and will not be taking any other medications in addition to Atrovent and Rheumatrex

Check your answers in the Answer Key online. How did you do? Are there new words you do not know? Take the time now to look them up in your bilingual or first-language dictionary.

IDIOMATIC EXPRESSIONS

Idioms and idiomatic expressions are made up of a group of words that have a different meaning from the original meaning of each individual word. Native speakers of the English language use such expressions comfortably and naturally. However, individuals who are new speakers of English or who have studied English for many years may still not be able to use idioms and idiomatic expressions as comfortably or naturally as native speakers. As pharmacy students, pharmacy technicians, and practicing pharmacists, you will hear many different idiomatic expressions. Some of you will understand and know how to use these expressions correctly. At times, however, you may not understand what your professors, colleagues, and patients are saying. This of course can lead to miscommunication, embarrassment, and possibly dangerous mistakes.

To help you improve your knowledge of idioms and idiomatic expressions, carefully read the following idiomatic expressions that contain the body words joint, muscle, spine, stiff, bone and back.

Idiomatic Expressions using "Joint," "Muscle" and "Spine"

1. *to put one's nose out of joint* means to be upset about something.
   For example: Her *nose is out of joint* because we didn't invite her to the party.

2. *muscle one's way in* means to use one's strength to get where you want to go.
   For example: About 10 students tried *to muscle their way in* to the dance club right as the door was closing and not letting in any more customers.

3. *to send chills/shivers up/down one's spine* means to cause someone to feel frightened or excited.
   For example: News that she had received a full scholarship to pharmacy school just *sends shivers up her spine* with excitement.

Idiomatic Expressions using "Stiff"

1. **to be bored stiff** means to be extremely bored.

    For example: The children **became bored stiff** after being home for 3 days because of the snowstorm.

2. **to be scared stiff** means to be extremely scarred.

    For example: When the robber came in to the pharmacy with a gun demanding money, I thought I was going to drop dead from a heart attack. **I was scared stiff.**

3. **a stiff** means a dead body.

    For example: Some professions such as law enforcement and medicine sometimes use the slang term **stiff** to refer to a dead body.

4. **to be stiff-necked** means to be stubborn and to refuse to change or obey.

    For example: **She's so stiff-necked** and refuses to follow the exercises the physical therapist has told her to do.

5. **to be stiffed** means someone is not paid the money they are expected to receive.

    For example: I'll never lend my roommate money again; I loaned her twenty dollars and **she stiffed me.**

Idiomatic Expressions using "Bone"

1. **a bone of contention** refers to something that people disagree about.

    For example: His salary became **a bone of contention** with his boss.

2. **to feel something in one's bones** means to be sure about something even though you have no proof.

    For example: I just know that I'm going pass my licensing exam; I can **feel it in my bones.**

3. **to make no bones about something** means to not feel ashamed or nervous about saying or doing something.

    For example: The patient **made no bones about** how he felt about the pharmacist, who was rude and unpleasant.

4. **work one's fingers to the bone** means to work very hard.

    For example: She really **works her fingers to the bone,** but she is rarely appreciated by her boss.

5. **to have a bone to pick** means to you want to talk to the person who is annoying you.

    For example: **I have a bone to pick** with you! Why did you change my schedule without telling me? I don't want to work this weekend!

Idiomatic Expressions using "Back"

1. **behind one's back** means to say or do something secretly.

    For example: I don't appreciate people who talk about me behind my back.

2. **to get off one's back** means to tell someone to stop criticizing, nagging, or telling them what to do.

    For example: Stop telling me that we're very busy. I'll take care of the patients as soon as I can. Just **get off my back!**

3. **to break one's back** means to work very hard on something.

    For example: **He broke his back** trying to finish his research paper on time.

4. **to give someone a pat on the back** means to congratulate and praise someone.

    For example: You've done nice work this month. Our sales are up. You definitely deserve **a pat on the back.**

5. **to stab someone in the back** means to betray and do something bad to a person who trusts you.

    For example: **She stabbed her roommate in the back** when she cheated with her roommate's boyfriend.

Mini Dialogues Listening Exercise

How much did you understand? Listen to the following mini dialogues on the audio files found in Chapter 8 on thePoint (thePoint.lww.com/diaz-gilbert), read the questions below, and then choose the correct answer.

 ### Mini Dialogue #1

1. _____ Her ***nose is out of joint*** means:

a. she needs nose surgery

b. her nose is tender and sore

c. she is upset

 ### Mini Dialogue #2

2. _____ ***To get off your back*** means:

a. to stop working so hard

b. to stop criticizing

c. to work very hard

 ### Mini Dialogue #3

3. _____ ***Bored stiff*** means:

a. to be extremely bored

b. to become bored because of stiffness in the body

c. to be scared

 ### Mini Dialogue #4

4. _____ ***Muscle their way in*** means:

a. they couldn't get in because their muscles were too big

b. they tried to use their strength to get in

c. they didn't use their strength to get in

 ### Mini Dialogue #5

5. _____ ***Broke my back*** means:

a. writing the research paper caused him to break his back

b. receiving a C+ caused the back to break

c. he worked very hard to write the research paper

 ### Mini Dialogue #6

6. _____ ***Work your fingers to the bone*** means:

a. the person's bones are sore from working too hard

b. the person works very hard

c. the person's fingers and bones are inflamed from working too much

Mini Dialogue #7

7. _____ He **stiffed me** means:

a. he paid back the money he borrowed

b. he will pay back the money he borrowed

c. he did not pay back the money he borrowed

 ### Mini Dialogue #8

8. _____ **Send chills up my spine** means

a. the person is very excited

b. the person's spine is cold

c. the person is feeling very cold

 ### Mini Dialogue #9

9. _____ **Stabbed me in the back** means:

a. I was betrayed

b. I have loyal friends

c. they stabbed me in the back with a knife

 ### Mini Dialogue #10

10. _____ **A stiff-neck** means:

a. the neck is unable to move

b. the person is unable to move

c. the person is stubborn and refuses to change

How did you do? Check your answers against the Answer Key online.

POST-ASSESSMENT

True/False Questions

Indicate whether each sentence below is true (T) or false (F).

1. _____ The idiom **to break one's back** means to talk about someone secretly.

2. _____ The noun and adjective form of the word **synovitis** is synovial.

3. _____ Lupus means "hard skin."

4. _____ Arthritic and arthritis are both nouns.

5. _____ If a person receives a **pat on the back,** he or she receives praise and encouragement.

6. _____ Osteoarthritis caused by aging and repetitive use of the joints over time is called primary osteoarthritis.

7. _____ Discoid lupus affects organs such as the brain, heart, lungs, and heart.

8. _____ The verb form of the word **deterioration** is deteriorate.

9. _____ Losing weight and reducing alcohol consumption will not decrease a gout attack.

10. _____ Scleroderma is caused by an underproduction of collagen.

11. _____ The idiom **to put someone's nose out of joint** means the person is upset about something.

12. _____ If a patient complains that she has dry eyes, dry mouth, fatigue, and swollen and stiff joints, he or she could have ankylosing spondylitis.

13. _____ Rheumatoid arthritis is inflammation caused by wear and tear of cartilage.

14. _____ Kidney stones and decreased kidney function can result from gout.

15. _____ If a person is **stiff necked,** he or she cannot move the neck.

Multiple Choice Questions

Choose the correct answer from a, b, and c.

1. _____ Stooped is:
a. an adjective and verb
b. an adjective only
c. a verb only

2. _____ A person with scleroderma will experience:
a. hardening of the skin
b. inflammation of the spine
c. dry eyes and dry mouth

3. _____ If a person is **scared stiff,** he or she is:
a. afraid to get stiff
b. extremely scared
c. mean and unsympathetic

4. _____ A person with gout will experience:
a. wear and tear on the big toe
b. bony knobs, or nodes, on his or her toes
c. a very hot, tender, and swollen sensation in the big toe

5. _____ In this sentence, "Patients with Sjögren's syndrome can treat their dry eyes with artificial tears and lubricant ointments," the word **lubricant** is:
a. a verb and a noun
b. an adjective
c. a noun

6. _____ The adjective form of **debilitation** is:
a. debilitated, debilitating, debilitative
b. debilitated
c. debilitating

7. _____ Sulfasalazine is used to:
a. reduce collagen production
b. reduce swelling, inflammation, and joint pain
c. increase tear production

8. _____ The idiomatic expression that means to be sure about something even though you have no proof is:
a. a bone of contention
b. to feel something in one's bones
c. to make no bones about something

9. _____ Methotrexate is used to treat:
a. rheumatoid arthritis and ankylosing spondylitis
b. scleroderma
c. fibromyalgia

10. _____ In the sentence, "Sufferers of ankylosing spondylitis can potentially develop chronic stooping and a stiff and inflexible spine," the word **inflexible** is:

a. an adjective

b. a verb

c. a noun

11. _____ The words **mobility** and **mobilization** are:

a. both a verb and noun

b. an adjective

c. a noun

12. _____ A person with fibromyalgia may experience:

a. sensitivity to sun

b. fractures

c. fatigue, emotional stress, and sleep disturbances

13. _____ A person who works very hard:

a. works his fingers to the bone

b. breaks his back

c. both a and b

14. _____ The word **posture** is:

a. a verb

b. a noun

c. an adjective only

15. _____ In the sentence, "Osteoarthritis is also known as degenerative bone disease," the word **degenerative** is:

a. an adjective

b. a past tense verb

c. a noun

Listening and Comprehension Exercises

Dialogue #1

Listen to Dialogue #1, stop, listen again and take notes. Listen to the dialogue as many times as you need or until you feel you have written sufficient notes and feel confident. You can use your notes to answer the multiple choice questions at the end of the dialogue.

Notes _____

_____

_____

_____

_____

Answer the questions below by selecting the answer that correctly completes each sentence.

1. _____ The pharmacist's name is:

a. Elizabeth New, and the patient's name is Eric Gallagher

b. Eric Gallagher, and the patient's name is Elizabeth New

c. Elizabeth Gallagher, and the patient's name is Eric New

2. _____ The patient complaints that:

a. his left toe is inflamed

b. his right toe is inflamed and burning

c. both toes are inflamed and swollen

3. _____ The patient tells the pharmacist that he has:

a. gout, and that he's had it for about 5 years

b. gout, and that this is his first real big flare-up

c. gout, and that he's had it about 10 years

4. _____ The patient tells the pharmacist that he:

a. went to the emergency room 3 hours ago and received a cortisone shot

b. went to the emergency room 3 days ago and the doctor gave him a prescription for probenecid

c. went to the emergency room 3 weeks ago and did not receive a cortisone shot

5. _____ The patient tells the pharmacist that he had:

a. a gout attack about 1 year ago and his doctor prescribed Aleve

b. a gout attack about 1 month ago and his doctor prescribed Probenecid

c. a gout attack about 1 year ago and his doctor gave him a cortisone shot and Probenecid

6. _____ The ER doctor gave the patient:

a. a cortisone shot and a prescription for Aleve

b. a cortisone shot and a prescription for probenecid

c. a prescription for probenecid and over-the-counter Aleve

7. _____ The patient:

a. is visiting the clinic for the first time

b. is a returning clinic patient

c. has visited the clinic twice in the past

8. _____ The patient:

a. is 55 years old, and has a history of swimmer's ear that was treated with Cortisporin

b. is 53 years old, and has a history of a ruptured eardrum that was treated with Neosporin

c. is 53 years old, and has a history of swimmer's ear that was treated with Cortisporin

9. _____ The patient currently takes:

a. multivitamins and Citrucel for diarrhea

b. multivitamins and Metamucil for constipation

c. multivitamins and Cortisporin

10. _____ The patient's medical history:

a. includes an appendectomy 1 year ago and right knee surgery 2 years ago, and a family history of gout

b. includes an appendectomy about 10 years ago and left knee surgery about 15 years ago, and a family history of gout

c. includes an appendectomy 15 years ago and knee surgery on both needs about 10 years ago, and no family history of gout

11. _____ The patient:

a. smokes two packs of cigarettes a day and is allergic to iodine

b. used to smoke two packs of cigarettes a day and has no allergies

c. quit smoking two packs of cigarettes a day about 3 years ago after his friend died from lung cancer, and is allergic to iodine

12. _____ The pharmacist tells the patient that Probenecid:

a. will help to reduce the uric acid in his body and that it is not a pain reliever

b. will relieve the swelling in his right toe

c. is a pain reliever that will help to reduce uric acid in his body

13. _____ The pharmacist warns the patient that:

a. it's possible that he may experience more gout attacks in next month while the Probenecid helps the body remove the extra uric acid in his body, and that he should not stop taking Probenecid if he has another gout attack

b. it's possible that he may experience more gout attacks in the next month while the Probenecid helps the body remove the extra uric acid in his body, and that he should stop taking Probenecid if he has another gout attack

c. that he will definitely experience another gout attack while on Probenecid and that he should discontinue using it immediately

14. _____ The pharmacist tells the patient he needs to take Probenecid:

a. twice a day without food or water

b. twice a day with food and water, and that he should drink eight 8-ounce glasses of fluids during the day

c. once a day with one 8-ounce glass of water

15. _____ When the patient tells the doctor, "This gout is really difficult to stomach," he means:

a. he doesn't know how much longer he can take the medication

b. that the gout causes an upset stomach

c. that it's difficult to endure gout attacks

16. _____ The pharmacist recommends that the patient:

a. avoid or limit alcohol, maintain a good weight, and drink plenty of fluids

b. avoid or limit alcohol to only two drinks per day

c. maintain a good weight and drink plenty of fluids

Dialogue #2

Listen to Dialogue #2, stop, listen again and take notes. Listen to the dialogue as many times as you need or until you feel you have written sufficient notes and feel confident. You can use your notes to answer the multiple choice questions at the end of the dialogue.

Notes _____

_____

_____

_____

_____

Answer the questions below by selecting the answer that correctly completes each sentence.

1. _____ The patient's name is:

a. Anthony Vo, and the pharmacist's name is Vicky Gonzalez

b. Anthony Gonzalez, and the pharmacist's name is Vicky Vo

c. Vicky Vo, and the pharmacist's name is Anthony Gonzalez

2. _____ The patient is visiting the clinic:

a. after being diagnosed with osteoarthritis

b. after being diagnosed with osteoporosis

c. after being diagnosed with osteomalacia

3. _____ The patient had:

a. a cataract removed on October 6, 2005

b. a cataract removed in each eye on October 5, 2006

c. a cataract removed in each eye on October 6, 2005

4. _____ The patient's eye doctor is:

a. Dr. Wu

b. Dr. Woo

c. Dr. Jones

5. _____ The patient was prescribed:

a. Lotemax to treat inflammation after cataract surgery

b. Lotemax to treat her osteoarthritis

c. Fosamax to treat inflammation after cataract surgery

6. _____ The pharmacist tells the patient to:

a. take two Fosamax tablets with her first meal of the day

b. take one Fosamax tablet a day after she gets up in the morning and after she has her first meal of the day and before she has her first drink

c. take one Fosamax tablet a day after she gets up in the morning and before she eats her first meal of the day, has her first drink—for example, tea—and before she takes any other medications she may be on

7. _____ The pharmacist instructs the patient:

a. to chew the tablet and drink water

b. not to chew or suck the tablet and to drink a full glass of water

c. to suck the tablet and then drink a full glass of water

8. _____ The pharmacist instructs the patient:

a. not to lie down after taking Fosamax. Her body must be upright so she should sit on a chair, stand, or walk for 30 minutes. After 30 minutes, she can eat her meal and drink her tea, coffee, or juice; she cannot drink water

b. not to lie down after taking Fosamax. Her body must be upright so she should sit on a chair, or walk for 20 minutes. After 20 minutes she can eat her meal and drink her tea, coffee, juice, or water

c. not to lie down after taking Fosamax. Her body must be upright so she should sit on a chair, stand, or walk for 30 minutes. After 30 minutes, she can eat her meal and drink her tea, coffee, juice, or water

9. _____ The pharmacist tells the patient that:

a. a side effect of Fosamax is stomach pain

b. a side effect of Fosamax is stomach pain, and that he will give her a patient information leaflet to read carefully

c. all the side effects are listed in the patient information leaflet

10. _____ The patient is allergic to:

a. citrus fruit and tomatoes

b. citrus fruit and bees

c. bees

11. _____ The pharmacist tells the patient to avoid eating or drinking:

a. tea, coffee, tomatoes, and citrus fruit

b. coffee, chocolate, soda, peppermint, pepper, citrus fruit, tomatoes, and tomato sauce

c. honey and citrus fruit

12. _____ The patient speaks Vietnamese:

a. but has no one to help her read the patient information leaflet

b. and will use her Vietnamese dictionary and her son to help her read the patient information leaflet carefully

c. and does not need a dictionary to help her understand the patient information leaflet

How did you do on the Post-Assessment in Chapter 8? Check you answers in the Answer Key online.

3. **Trembling, difficulty** walking, and muscle **rigidity** are typical symptoms **found** in Parkinson's disease.

   trembling _____   difficulty _____   rigidity _____   found _____

4. **Slurring** of **speech,** arm or leg weakness, and muscle **twitching** are symptoms of amyotrophic lateral sclerosis, also known as **ALS.**

   slurring _____   speech _____   twitching _____   ALS _____

5. A person suffering from **generalized anxiety** disorder, also known as GAD, often feels **anxious** and very **worried** without a **reason.**

   generalized _____   anxiety _____   anxious _____   worried _____   reason _____

6. Crying **spells,** sadness, **hopelessness,** and losing **interest** in **normal** activities are usually signs of **depression.**

   spells _____   hopelessness _____   interest _____   normal _____   depression _____

7. Seasonal **affective** disorder, also known as SAD, is a type of **depressive** disorder believed to be **caused** by **decreased** daylight in the winter months, and can cause **depression,** lethargy, and fatigue.

   affective _____   depressive _____   caused _____   decreased _____   depression _____

8. **Epileptic** seizures that are the result of **abnormal** activity in one part of the brain are called **partial** or focal seizures, and epileptic seizures that **affect** the **whole** brain are called **generalized** seizures.

   epileptic _____   abnormal _____   partial _____   affect _____   whole _____
   generalized _____

9. Alzheimer's disease is a **progressive,** degenerative disease that **leads** to **irreversible mental impairment.**

   progressive _____   leads _____   irreversible _____   mental _____   impairment _____

10. People with multiple sclerosis, also known as **MS,** a **chronic** and potentially **debilitating** disease that affects the central nervous system, will experience **numbness** and **weakness** in their body.

    MS _____   chronic _____   debilitating _____   numbness _____   weakness _____

11. A **stooped** posture, a slow, **shuffling walk,** and an **unsteady gait** are characteristic of patients with Parkinson's disease.

    stooped _____   shuffling _____   walk _____   unsteady _____   gait _____

12. Symptoms of ALS, a **neurologic** disease that **attacks** the nerve cells that **control** voluntary muscles, include hand weakness, **clumsiness,** and **slurred** speech.

    neurologic _____   attacks _____   control _____   clumsiness _____   slurred _____

13. Patients with generalized **anxiety** disorder will experience a **variety** of symptoms such as **irritability,** restlessness, muscle **tension,** and difficulty concentrating.

    anxiety _____   variety _____   irritability _____   tension _____

14. People who have bipolar disorder, also known as **manic-depressive** disorder, have recurrent **episodes** of **depression** and **elation.**

    manic _____   depressive _____   episodes _____   depression _____   elation _____

15. Because some patients with multiple sclerosis will experience **extreme** muscle weakness resulting from exposure to extreme **heat** such as a sauna, a **hot** bath, or shower, it's recommended that they take **tepid showers** or baths.

    extreme _____   heat _____   hot _____   tepid _____   showers _____

How did you do? Check your answers against the Answer Key online.

Typical Medical Conditions and Patient Complaints

The sentences below contain vocabulary that describes and explains typical medical conditions, diseases, symptoms, and patient complaints that a pharmacist encounters. Read the sentences carefully. Then indicate the word form of the bolded word(s), choosing from v, n, adj, or adv. Look up words you do not know in your bilingual or first-language dictionary.

1. **Epileptics** who experience simple **partial** seizures will not lose consciousness, but those who experience **complex** partial seizures will lose consciousness for a short **period** of time and experience lip **smacking**, hand rubbing, and swallowing.

   epileptics _____　　partial _____　　complex _____　　period _____　　smacking _____

2. Difficulty **recognizing** numbers, finding the right words to **express** thoughts, following conversations, feeling **disoriented,** and becoming **lost** in **familiar** places are symptoms experienced by Alzheimer's patients.

   recognizing _____　　express _____　　disoriented _____　　lost _____　　familiar _____

3. It is important for patients with Parkinson's disease to **improve** their **balance, range** of motion, and **mobility** with **regular** exercise.

   improve _____　　balance _____　　range _____　　mobility _____　　regular _____

4. In patients with ALS, the motor neurons in the brain and spine no longer **control voluntary** muscles that would **normally** move the arms, legs, neck, face, and torso or the muscles to talk, chew, and swallow, and as a result the muscles become **weak** and **atrophy.**

   control _____　　voluntary _____　　normally _____　　weak _____　　atrophy _____

5. Multiple sclerosis, which is an **autoimmune** disease, **results** in slowing or blocking nerve **signals** that **control** strength, sensation, muscle **coordination,** and vision.

   autoimmune _____　　results _____　　signals _____　　control _____　　coordination _____

6. **Certain** medical conditions, coping with and worrying about the medical condition, a **stressful** life, heredity, and an individual's personality **type** can **cause** generalized anxiety disorder.

   certain _____　　coping _____　　stressful _____　　type _____　　cause _____

7. Patients with depression may not only have **negative** thoughts, **behaviors,** and moods but also develop **irregular** eating **habits,** have difficulty sleeping, and experience **crying spells** and a decreased libido.

   negative _____　　behaviors _____　　irregular _____　　habits _____　　crying spells _____

8. The symptoms of people affected by seasonal **affective** disorder in the fall and winter include **trouble** concentrating, **overeating,** fatigue, depression, and crying spells, and the symptoms of people affected by seasonal affective disorder in the spring and summer include poor **appetite,** weight loss, **insomnia,** and crying spells.

   affective _____　　trouble _____　　overeating _____　　appetite _____　　insomnia _____

9. A person with epilepsy who experiences a petit mal **seizure,** also known as an absence seizure, will **stare,** experience **subtle** body movements, and **brief lapses** of **awareness.**

   seizure _____　　stare _____　　subtle _____　　brief _____　　lapses _____　　awareness _____

10. **Feeling** tired, feeling **shaky,** having difficulty getting up after sitting, **speaking** softly, being unable to **speak** words, and feeling **depressed** for no reason are early symptoms of Parkinson's disease, a disorder that affects nerve cells in the part of the brain that control muscle movement.

    feeling _____　　shaky _____　　speaking _____　　speak _____　　depressed _____

11. ALS, also known as Lou Gehrig's disease after the New York Yankee baseball player who died from the motor **neuron** disease, **causes progressive** muscle **wasting** or atrophy, and is a **fatal** disease.

    neuron _____　　causes _____　　progressive _____　　wasting _____　　fatal _____

12. Multiple sclerosis is characterized by seven different patterns of which the most common pattern is relapsing-remitting (RR) MS, in which patients experience a series of attacks followed by **periods** of **remission** when the symptoms **disappear,** until a **relapse** occurs, when the symptoms **reappear.**

    periods _____   remission _____   disappear _____   relapse _____   reappear _____

13. Seasonal affective disorder, which is also referred to as the **winter blues** and winter depression, **causes** some people to **crave sweets** and **starches.**

    winter blues _____   causes _____   crave _____   sweets _____   starches _____

14. **Factors** such as stress, illness, **postpartum** depression, **certain** medications, hormones, and alcohol and drug **abuse** can **contribute** to depression.

    factors _____   postpartum _____   certain _____   abuse _____   contribute _____

15. Patients suffering from ALS, an **irreversible** disease, will require physical therapy to help them with muscle **strength,** speech therapy to help them communicate more **clearly** as the speech muscles begin to **deteriorate,** and breathing assistance as the muscles needed to breathe become **weakened.**

    irreversible _____   strength _____   clearly _____   deteriorate _____   weakened _____

16. **Dementia** and the **inability** to concentrate, remember, think, and **reason** can also **occur** in Parkinson's patients as the disease **progresses.**

    dementia _____   inability _____   reason _____   occur _____   progresses _____

17. **Strengthening exercises** and learning how to use **devices** such as a walking cane, a **motorized** scooter, or a wheelchair can help MS patients maintain their **independence.**

    strengthening _____   exercises _____   devices _____   motorized _____
    independence _____

18. Patients with **advanced** Alzheimer's disease can develop pneumonia as a result of inhaling food and drink into the lungs, **urinary incontinence** and urinary tract infections, and increase their **risk** of falling and **fractures.**

    advanced _____   urinary _____   incontinence _____   risk _____   fractures _____

19. **Complications** and **dangers** from epilepsy include receiving a head **injury** and drowning as a result of a seizure and **losing** control and **awareness** while driving.

    complications _____   dangers _____   injury _____   losing _____   awareness _____

20. Depression is a **serious** illness that can **disable** some people and cause **others** to become **suicidal.**

    serious _____   disable _____   others _____   suicidal _____

How did you do? Check your answers against the Answer Key online.

Medical Vocabulary Comprehension

Now that you have read sentences 1 through 20 describing language regarding the neurologic system, assess your understanding by doing the exercises below.

Multiple Choice Questions

Choose the answer that correctly completes each sentence below.

1. _____ **ALS** is:
   a. a fatal neurologic disease
   b. an autoimmune disease
   c. a depressive disorder

2. _____ **Dementia** develops as the result of:

a. slurred speech

b. manic-depression

c. degeneration of healthy brain tissue

3. _____ **Seasonal affective disorder** is caused by:

a. sensitivity to sun

b. decreased sunlight

c. crying spells

4. _____ **MS:**

a. affects the central nervous system

b. leads to irreversible mental impairment

c. causes petit mal seizures

5. _____ A person with **generalized anxiety disorder:**

a. will slur his or her speech

b. will experience muscle weakness from exposure to extreme heat

c. feels worried and anxious

6. _____ A person suffering from **Parkinson's disease** may experience:

a. trembling and muscle rigidity

b. numbness in the body

c. loss of consciousness

7. _____ Some people with **depression:**

a. have crying spells

b. are always elated

c. have uncontrollable muscle twitching

8. _____ Symptoms of **ALS** include:

a. a stooped posture and trembling

b. muscle twitching and slurring of speech

c. dementia

9. _____ **Epileptic seizures** that affect the whole body are called:

a. focal seizures

b. unsteady seizures

c. generalized seizures

10. _____ Another term for **muscle wasting** is:

a. atrophy

b. voluntary muscle

c. muscle twitching

11. _____ **MS** blocks nerve signals that:

a. improve balance

b. control strength, sensation, and muscle coordination

c. control voluntary muscles

12. _____ A shuffling walk and unsteady gait are characteristics of:

a. Parkinson's disease

b. ALS

c. epilepsy

13. _____ Symptoms of **SAD** in the spring and summer include:

a. poor appetite and insomnia

b. feeling shaky and speaking softly

c. overeating

14. _____ **GAD** can be caused by:

a. a stressful life, worrying about a medical condition, or heredity

b. lethargy and fatigue

c. suicidal thoughts

15. _____ Patients who tend to stare during an attack of their disease are:

a. epilepsy patients

b. ALS patients

c. MS patients

True/False Questions

Indicate whether each sentence below is true (T) or false (F).

1. _____ Early symptoms of Parkinson's disease include feeling tired and shaky and having difficulty getting up after sitting.

2. _____ Multiple sclerosis is a progressive and fatal neurologic disease.

3. _____ Feeling disoriented and becoming lost in familiar places are symptoms of GAD.

4. _____ ALS is also known as Lou Gehrig's disease.

5. _____ Factors such as stress, postpartum depression, and alcohol and drug abuse do not contribute to depression.

6. _____ The word "irreversible" is a noun.

7. _____ A person who experiences a petit mal seizure will stare and will experience subtle body movements and brief lapses of awareness.

8. _____ People with bipolar disorder will experience recurrent episodes of depression and elation.

9. _____ Patients with GAD will not experience irritability, restlessness, or difficulty concentrating.

10. _____ Regular exercise can help patients with Parkinson's disease to improve their balance, range of motion, and mobility.

How did you do? Check your answers against the Answer Key online.

Writing Exercise

An important part of communication is the ability to write about what you read, to write correctly, and to spell correctly. In the exercises below, write your understanding of the meaning of the bolded words.

1. Describe in writing what **epilepsy** is.

_____

_____

_____

_____

2. Describe in writing what **multiple sclerosis** is.

_____

_____

_____

_____

3. Describe in writing what **Parkinson's disease** is.

_____

_____

_____

_____

4. Describe what **amyotrophic lateral sclerosis** and **Alzheimer's disease** are.

_____

_____

_____

_____

5. Describe what **GAD** and **SAD** are.

_____

_____

_____

_____

Check what you have written with acceptable answers that appear in the Answer Key online.

LISTENING AND PRONUNCIATION

The ability to listen and understand what is being said and heard, and the ability to pronounce words clearly, is extremely important. A word misheard and a word mispronounced will lead to poor communication and can seriously put both the pharmacist and patient in danger. Therefore, it is very important that one hear clearly what another person has said, and that one speak clearly with correct pronunciation.

Listen carefully to the pharmacy-related words presented in the audio files found in Chapter 9 on thePoint (thePoint.lww.com/diaz-gilbert), and then pronounce them as accurately as you can. Listen and then repeat. You will listen to each word once and then you will repeat it. You will do this twice for each word. Listening and pronunciation practice will increase your listening and speaking confidence. Many languages do not produce or emphasize certain sounds produced and emphasized in English, so pay careful attention to the pronunciation of each word.

Pronunciation Exercise

Listen to the audio files found in Chapter 9 on thePoint (thePoint.lww.com/diaz-gilbert). Listen and repeat the words. Then say the words aloud for additional practice.

1. Alzheimer's disease
2. amyotrophic lateral sclerosis
3. aspirate
4. atonic
5. balance
6. bipolar disorder
7. dementia
8. depression
9. dexterity
10. disorientation
11. distracted
12. electric shock

13. epilepsy   ĕp′ə-lĕp′sē
14. exacerbation   eg-zas-er-bā′shŭn
15. forgetfulness   fər-gĕt fŏŏl nĕs
16. gait   gāt
17. irreversible   ĭr′ĭ-vûr′sə-bəl
18. isolation   ī′sə-lā′shən
19. jerking movements   jûrking mŏŏv′mənt s
20. lapse   lăps
21. light therapy   līt thĕr′ə-pē
22. mental impairment   mĕn′tl im-pār′ment
23. multiple sclerosis mŭl′tə-pəl sklə-rō′sĭs
24. mumbling speech   mŭm′blŋ spēch
25. myelin sheath   mī′ə-lĭn shēth
26. myoclonic   mī-ō-klon′ik
27. neurology   nŏŏ-rŏl′ə-jē
28. obsessive-compulsive disorder   ŏb-sĕs′ĭv kəm-pŭl′sĭv dĭs-ôr′dər
29. onset   ŏn′sĕt
30. panic attack   păn′ĭk ə-tăk′
31. phobias   fō′bē-əs
32. pill rolling   pil′rōl′ing
33. progressive   prə-grĕs′ĭv
34. rigid   rĭj′ĭd
35. rouse   rouz
36. seizure   sē′zhər
37. shuffling walk   shŭf′lng wôk
38. slurred speech   slûrd spēch
39. spinal tap   spī′nəl tăp
40. staring spells   stârng spĕls
41. suicide   sŏŏĭ-sīd′
42. tremor   trĕm′ər
43. twitch   twĭch
44. unsteady   ŭn-stĕd′ē
45. voluntary muscles   vŏl′ən-tĕr′ē mŭs′əls
46. wandering   wŏn′dərng

Which words are easy to pronounce? Which are difficult to pronounce? Use the space below to write in the words that you find difficult to pronounce. These are words you should practice saying often.

_____

_____

_____

_____

_____

_____

_____

_____

Listen to the audio files found in Chapter 9 on thePoint (thePoint.lww.com/diaz-gilbert) as many times as you need to increase your pronunciation ability of the difficult words. Pronounce these words with a friend or a colleague who speaks English.

English Sounds That are Difficult for Speakers of Other Languages to Pronounce

Spanish

In Spanish, there is no English "v" sound, but the "v" consonant in Spanish is pronounced like the English "b." The vowel "i" is pronounced like a long "e." Pay careful attention to the "v" sound in English when pronouncing words that begin with "v." Also pay careful attention to English words that begin with "s;" do not use the Spanish "es" sound when pronouncing English words that begin with "s."

For example, in English,

chronic is not pronounced crohneek

Vietnamese

In Vietnamese, the "t" consonant is pronounced "s," but in English the "t" is pronounced "t" and "s" is pronounced "s." Be careful with English words that begin with "t." In Vietnamese, the "b" consonant is pronounced "p," but in English "p" is pronounced "p" and "b" is pronounced "b."

In Vietnamese, words do not end in "b," "ch," "f," "d," "j," "l," "p," "r," "s," "sh," "v," and "z." In English, words end in these letters. Pay special attention to pronouncing these English sounds. In Vietnamese, there is no "dzh" or "zh" sound, so English words like "judge" (dzh) and "rupture" (zh) will be hard for Vietnamese speakers to pronounce.

For example, in English,

numbness is not pronounced numneh

Korean

In Korean, the "v" consonant is pronounced "b" and the "f" consonant is pronounced "p." In English, the "v" is pronounced "v," the "f" is pronounced "f," and the "p" is pronounced "p." Pay special attention when pronouncing these sounds.

For example, in English,

forgetfulness is not pronounced porgetpulnes

Gujarati

In Gujarati, "v" is pronounced "w," "f" is pronounced "p," "p" is pronounced "f," and "z" is pronounced "j." Short "i" is pronounced long "e," "x" is pronounced "ch," and "th" is pronounced "s." In English, "v" is pronounced "v," "f" is pronounced "f," "z" is pronounced "z" or "s," "j" is pronounced "j," and "x" is pronounced "x." Pay careful attention when pronouncing these sounds.

For example, in English,

voluntary is not pronounced woluntary

Chinese

In Chinese, the "r" consonant is pronounced "l" or "w," and "b," "d," "g," and "ng" are not pronounced at all. Pay careful attention to English words that begin with "r" because the "r" is not pronounced "l" or "w," and "b," "d," "g," and "ng" are pronounced in English.

For example, in English,

rigid is not pronounced ligih
disoriented is not pronounced disolienteh

Russian

The "w" consonant is pronounced like a "v" and the "v" sound like a "w." Pay careful attention to the English "th." It is not pronounced "s."

For example, in English,

voluntary is not pronounced woluntary

DICTATION

 ### Listening/Spelling Exercise: Word and Word Pairs

Listen to the words or word pairs on the audio files found in Chapter 9 on thePoint (thePoint.lww.com-/diaz-gilbert) and then write them down on the lines below.

1. _____
2. _____
3. _____
4. _____
5. _____
6. _____
7. _____
8. _____
9. _____
10. _____
11. _____
12. _____
13. _____
14. _____
15. _____

 ### Listening/Spelling Exercise: Sentences

Listen to the sentences on the audio files found in Chapter 9 on thePoint (thePoint.lww.com/diaz-gilbert) and then write them down on the lines below.

1. _____
   _____

2. _____
   _____

3. _____
   _____

4. _____
   _____

5. _____
   _____

6. _____
   _____

7. _____
   _____

8. _____
   _____

9. _____
   _____

10. _____
    _____

Now, check your sentences against the correct answers in the Answer Key online. If there are any new words that you do not know or that you spelled incorrectly, make a list of those words and study them for meaning and spelling.

PHARMACIST/PATIENT DIALOGUES

The ability to orally communicate effectively with your professors, colleagues, and especially with patients is very important. As a pharmacist, you will be counseling patients; patients will come to you for advice. They will have questions about a condition and symptoms they may experience and will ask you to help treat the condition. Therefore, it is extremely important that you understand what they are saying and that you respond to them and their questions appropriately. Your patients will speak differently. For example, some may speak very quickly, others too low, and yet others may speak angrily. To help you improve your listening skills, listen to the following dialogues, or short conversations, between a pharmacist and a patient and between a pharmacy technician and a patient.

Listening and Comprehension Exercises

Dialogue #1

Listen to Dialogue #1, stop, listen again and take notes. Listen to the dialogue as many times as you need or until you feel you have written sufficient notes and feel confident. You can use your notes to answer the multiple choice questions at the end of the dialogue.

Notes_____

_____

_____

_____

_____

Answer the questions below by selecting the answer that correctly completes each sentence.

1. _____ The patient's name is:

a. Ari Snow

b. Ariana Snow

c. Arianne Snow

2. _____ The pharmacist name is:

a. Richard Mendez and the doctor's name is Gabby Lucas

b. Gabby Lucas and the doctor's name is Richard Mendez

c. Richard Lucas and the doctor's name is Gabby Mendez

3. _____ The patient is being discharged from the:

a. emergency room

b. clinic

c. hospital

4. _____ The patient has been diagnosed with:

a. epilepsy

b. unexplained seizures

c. two seizures

5. _____ The patient has been prescribed:

a. tegaserod

b. Tegrin

c. Tegretol

6. _____ The medication will help treat:

a. her petit mal seizures

b. her grand mal seizures

c. both kinds of seizures

7. _____ The form of medication the doctor has prescribed:

a. is a chewable red-speckled pink tablet whose generic name is carbamazepine

b. is a liquid whose generic name is carbamazepine

c. is a chewable pink-speckled red tablet that has no generic

8. _____ The patient has a history of:

a. recurrent ear infections that were treated successfully with Ceclor

b. recurrent eye infections

c. recurrent ear infections when she was young and is allergic to Ceclor

9. _____ Serious side effects of Tegretol include:

a. diarrhea and a rash

b. chest pain, swollen ankles, and problems with speech and coordination

c. vomiting, nausea, and swollen ankles

10. _____ The patient is also allergic to:

a. cats and dogs, and has had stitches as a result of a dog bite and wears contacts

b. cats and latex, and has had stitches on her head and chin, has broken her arm, and wears contacts

c. cats and latex, and has broken both arms and wears contacts

11. _____ The patient:

a. plays softball, and the pharmacist told she can continue to play but that she should talk to her doctor and continue to take her medication

b. plays softball, and the pharmacist told her she should stop playing sports

c. plays softball, and the pharmacist told her she should always wear a helmet when she's pitching

12. _____ The pharmacist tells the patient that:

a. she should wear a medical alert bracelet and that she can swim alone

b. she should wear a medical alert bracelet and that she should never swim again

c. she should wear a helmet when participating in recreational activities with a high risk of head injury and wear a medical alert bracelet, and that she never swim alone

13. _____ The pharmacist tells the patient and her mother that when she has a seizure:

a. she should be rolled over and a pillow placed under her head, that no one should put their fingers in her mouth, and that she should not be shaken or yelled at during a seizure

b. she should be aroused and shaken

c. she should not be rolled over and no one should put their fingers in her mouth

14. _____ The pharmacist tells the patient that:

a. people with epilepsy will have seizures for life

b. more than half of children with seizures eventually become seizure-free and no longer need to take medication

c. the seizures will get progressively worse

15. _____ When the patient's mother says the patient is "tough as nails," she means that:

a. the patient is strong and determined

b. the patient only appears to be strong and determined but is not

c. the patient is strong and determined only when she is having a seizure

Check your answers in the Answer Key online. How did you do? Are there new words you do not know? Take the time now to look them up in your bilingual or first-language dictionary.

Dialogue #2

Listen to Dialogue #2, stop, listen again and take notes. Listen to the dialogue as many times as you need or until you feel you have written sufficient notes and feel confident. You can use your notes to answer the multiple choice questions at the end of the dialogue.

Notes_____

_____

_____

_____

_____

Answer the questions below by selecting the answer that correctly completes each sentence.

1. _____ The patient's name is:
a. Lucas Page, and the pharmacist's name is Susan Wilson
b. Susan Page, and the pharmacist's name is Lucas Wilson
c. Susan Wilson, and the pharmacist's name is Lucas Page

2. _____ The patient's doctor's name is:
a. Lena Kasporova, and she prescribed Betaseron
b. Rina Kasporova, and she prescribed Betadine
c. Lena Casper, and she prescribed Betaseron

3. _____ The patient has been diagnosed with:
a. relapsing-remitting multiple sclerosis
b. relapsing multiple sclerosis
c. progressive relapsing multiple sclerosis

4. _____ The pharmacist explains to the patient that the medication:
a. is interferon and it will cure her MS
b. is interferon and it will help to reduce the number of flare-ups and attacks that make her weak, but it will not cure her MS
c. is interferon and it will not slow down the disease

5. _____ The patient:
a. is 44 years old, was born on May 21, 1964, and is allergic to penicillin and latex
b. is 44 years old, was born on May 20, 1964, and is allergic to cats and penicillin
c. is 44 years old, was born on May 21, 1964, and is allergic to wasps and penicillin

6. _____ The patient:
a. is pregnant and has a current history of migraine headaches
b. is not pregnant and used to be on medication 10 years ago for migraine headaches
c. is not pregnant and has no history of migraine headaches

7. _____ Currently the patient:
a. does not work, but has children
b. works as a freelance writer and has no children
c. works as a freelance writer and has children

11. _____ To treat his Parkinson's, the pharmacist instructs the patient to take:

 a. a 5-mg capsule twice a day; one with breakfast and one with dinner

 b. a 10-mg capsule once a day with breakfast

 c. a 5-mg capsule twice a day; one with breakfast and one with lunch

12. _____ Common side effects of the medication include:

 a. dry mouth, dizziness, nausea, and trouble sleeping

 b. dry mouth only

 c. dizziness and trouble sleeping

13. _____ The pharmacist tells the patient to avoid certain foods such as:

 a. red wine, cheese, salami, liverwurst, pickled herring, and soy sauce because they contain sugar and can cause serious high blood pressure

 b. red wine, cheese, salami, liver, pickled herring, and soy sauce because they contain tyramine, which can cause serious high blood pressure

 c. red wine, cheese, salami, liver, pickled herring, and soy sauce because they do not contain tyramine

14. _____ The pharmacist tells the patient to eat healthy foods such as:

 a. fruits, vegetables, and whole grains because they will help to prevent constipation, which is common in patients whose digestive tract is affected by Parkinson's

 b. fruits, vegetables, and whole grains because they will help to improve his walking

 c. fruits, vegetables, and whole grains because they will help to improve his tremors

15. _____The pharmacist advices the patient:

 a. to stop walking and recommends he visit the American Parkinson's Disease Association website

 b. that Parkinson's is curable and that he should continue to walk

 c. that Parkinson's is not curable, but is treatable, that walking and swimming are good forms of exercise, that he should call his doctor if he notices that is having difficulty speaking, chewing, and swallowing, and that he should visit the American Parkinson's Disease Association website for more information about the disease

Dialogue #2

Listen to Dialogue #2, stop, listen again and take notes. Listen to the dialogue as many times as you need or until you feel you have written sufficient notes and feel confident. You can use your notes to answer the multiple choice questions at the end of the dialogue.

Notes_____

_____

_____

_____

_____

Answer the questions below by selecting the answer that correctly completes each sentence.

1. _____ The patient's name is:

 a. Karen Frank, and the pharmacist's name is Eric Manning

 b. Eric Manning, and the pharmacist's name is Karen Frank

 c. Karen Manning, and the pharmacist's name is Eric Frank

2. _____ The patient's prescription is for:

 a. Zantac to treat her generalized anxiety disorder

 b. Xanax to treat her depression

 c. Xanax to treat her generalized anxiety disorder

3. _____ The patient's birth date is:

a. December 31, 1968 and she is 38

b. December 1, 1968 and she is 38

c. December 30, 1968 and she is 38

4. _____ The patient's address is:

a. 37 Marina Drive and her telephone number is 767-1187

b. 37 Marina Drive and her telephone number is 766-1187

c. 37 Marina Drive and her telephone number is 766-1186

5. _____ The patient's doctor's name is:

a. Brian Duncan

b. Ryan Duncan

c. Brian Dunn

6. _____ The patient has:

a. allergies and is currently taking birth control pills and vitamins

b. no allergies and is currently taking only vitamins

c. no allergies and is currently taking birth control pills and vitamins

7. _____ The patient's medical history and conditions include:

a. appendicitis, nail fungal infection, and acid reflux

b. appendicitis and acid reflux

c. nail fungal infection and acid reflux

8. _____ The pharmacist tells the patient that Xanax will:

a. treat her anxiety and produce a sleepy effect

b. cure her anxiety and produce a calming effect

c. treat her anxiety and produce a calming effect

9. _____ The patient tells the pharmacist that her anxiety has been triggered by:

a. her boss and her work, and that she can't sleep and can't concentrate

b. her boss and her work, and that she can't sleep, can't concentrate, feels restless, gets headaches, and sometimes gets diarrhea

c. her boss and her work, and that she hasn't been able to work

10. _____ The pharmacists advices the patient that Xanax:

a. is an anti-anxiety sedative that is not habit-forming

b. is an anti-anxiety sedative that is habit-forming and produces dependency

c. is not an anti-anxiety sedative

11. _____ Side effects of the medication include:

a. drowsiness, dizziness, slurred speech, clumsiness, and difficulty walking

b. dry mouth and dizziness

c. slurred speech

12. _____ The pharmacist advises the patient that if she doesn't feel better:

a. she should double her dosage

b. she should tell her doctor, and that she take care of herself by walking, eating well, and avoiding alcohol, nicotine, and caffeine

c. she should discontinue taking her medication

How did you do on the Post-Assessment in Chapter 9? Check your answers in the Answer Key online.

The Urinary System | 10

PRE-ASSESSMENT

True/False Questions

Indicate whether each sentence below is true (T) or false (F).

1. _____ The voluntary loss of urine is called **incontinence.**
2. _____ Loss of urine caused by coughing, laughing, sneezing, lifting heavy objects, or exercising is called **stress incontinence.**
3. _____ **Interstitial cystitis** is a painful and chronic bladder syndrome.
4. _____ An **overactive bladder,** which is also known as an irritable bladder, causes the sudden urge to hold in urine.
5. _____ The noun forms of **leak** are leak and leakage.
6. _____ A risk factor for developing **urinary tract infection** (UTI) is a kidney stone.
7. _____ Factors that contribute to an **overactive bladder** include, but are not limited to, UTI, an enlarged prostrate, diabetes, and excessive alcohol and caffeine consumption.
8. _____ Obese people have a much lower risk of experiencing **stress incontinence.**
9. _____ Men who experience the urgent need to urinate, who have difficulty urinating, or who experience pain during urination should be tested for **prostate cancer.**
10. _____ The noun form of **urgent** is urge.
11. _____ **Overactive bladder** that includes urge incontinence is called overactive bladder, wet; and overactive bladder that does not include urge incontinence is referred to as overactive bladder, dry.
12. _____ Symptoms of a **kidney infection,** which is a specific type of UTI, include a burning sensation while urinating, pus or blood in the urine, and frequent urination at night.
13. _____ **Urethritis** and **cystitis** are types of bladder control problems.
14. _____ **Urinary incontinence** is the ability to control the release of urine from the bladder.
15. _____ Another word for urinate is **void.**

Multiple Choice Questions

Choose the correct answer from a, b, and c.

1. _____ An untreated kidney infection can lead to:
a. blood poisoning
b. dehydration
c. excessive urination

2. _____ A risk factor for developing **interstitial cystitis** is:
a. obesity
b. excessive urination
c. sexual intercourse

3. _____ To help decrease the risk of **urinary incontinence,** one should:

a. drink as little water as possible

b. maintain a healthy weight and eat more fiber, which helps to prevent constipation, which can cause incontinence

c. avoid alcohol completely

4. _____ **Nocturnal enuresis** is the medical term for:

a. nighttime bed wetting

b. toilet trained

c. uncontrollable leaking

5. _____ Neurologic disorders such as Parkinson's disease can contribute to:

a. prostate cancer

b. overactive bladder

c. stress incontinence

6. _____ Drinking cranberry juice and water can help to reduce the risk of getting:

a. UTI

b. overactive bladder

c. reflex incontinence

7. _____ **Total incontinence** is used to describe:

a. loss of urine without warning

b. periodic large volumes of urine and uncontrollable leaking or continuous leaking of urine

c. wetting the bed at night

8. _____ The word **burning** is:

a. a noun and an adjective

b. a verb only

c. a noun only

9. _____ Benign prostatic hyperplasia (BPH) refers to:

a. inflammation of the prostate

b. a condition that causes the prostate to enlarge and incontinence

c. a condition that causes the prostate to shrink

10. _____ The expression **"I need to take a piss"** means:

a. I need to urinate

b. I need to go away

c. I cannot control my urine

How did you do? Check your answers in the Answer Key online.

MEDICAL VOCABULARY

A good understanding of vocabulary words in pharmacy is very important for communication with professors, fellow students, patients, and coworkers. Knowledge and understanding of vocabulary leads to successful communication and success as a pharmacy student, as a pharmacy technician, and as a practicing pharmacist. You may already know many of the vocabulary words in this chapter, but for words that are unfamiliar, pay careful attention to them and make every effort to know their correct spelling, meaning, and pronunciation. It is a good idea to keep a list of new words and to look up these new words in a bilingual dictionary or dictionary in your first language. A good command of pharmacy-related vocabulary and good pronunciation of vocabulary will help to prevent embarrassing mistakes and increase effective verbal communication skills.

Urinary System Vocabulary

absorbent pads
bed wetting
bladder
bladder training
catheter
contents
contract
cystitis
double voiding
drain
dribbles
emptying
enlarged prostate
flow

hematuria
impede
incontinence
interstitial cystitis
involuntary
   contraction
Kegel exercises
kidney infection
leakage
nocturia
nocturnal enuresis
overactive bladder
overflow
pelvis

pessary
postvoid residual
   urine
septicemia
toilet
urethra
urethral inserts
urethritis
urinalysis
urinary sphincter
urinary tract infection
urinate
urine output
void

PARTS OF SPEECH

A good understanding of parts of speech, such as verbs, nouns, adjectives, and adverbs, is important for successful communication when speaking or writing. It is equally important to know the various forms of words and to use them appropriately.

Word Forms

The table below lists the main forms of some terms that you will likely encounter in pharmacy practice. Review the table and then do the exercises that follow to assess your understanding.

Noun (n)	Infinitive/Verb (v) —Past Tense	Adjective (adj)	Adverb (adv)
absorbency; absorption	to absorb; absorbed	absorbent	
drainage	to drain; drained	draining	
dribble	to dribble; dribbled	dribbling	
emptiness; emptying	to empty; emptied	empty	
enlargement	to enlarge; enlarged	enlarged	
flow	to flow; flowed	flowing	flowingly
hematuria		hematuric	
impediment	to impede; impeded	impedimental; impedimentary	
incontinence		incontinent	
involuntariness		involuntary	involuntarily
leak; leakage	to leak; leaked	leaking	
overactivity		overactive	
residue		residual	
septicemia		septicemic	
urethra		urethral	
urine; urinalysis; urination; urinator	to urinate; urinated	urinative	

Word Forms Exercise

Read the following sentences carefully. Then indicate the word form of the bolded word(s), choosing from v, n, adj, or adv.

1. **Unintentional urine loss** caused by **physical** activity such as sneezing, coughing, laughing, and lifting heavy objects is called **stress incontinence.**

   unintentional _____ urine _____ loss _____ physical _____ stress incontinence _____

2. Symptoms of **urinary** tract infection, or **UTI**, include the **urge** to **urinate,** a **burning** sensation when **urinating,** and passing small amounts of **urine** frequently.

   urinary _____ UTI _____ urge _____ urinate _____ burning _____
   urinating _____ urine _____

3. Loss of **bladder control,** also known as **urinary incontinence,** causes the inability to control the **release** of urine in the form of minor **leaks** or **dribbles** to **wetting** one's clothes.

   bladder control _____ urinary incontinence _____ release _____ leaks _____
   dribbles _____ wetting _____

4. The type of urinary incontinence that makes a person feel like they need to **empty** their **bladder** but can't and continue to **constantly dribble** urine is called **overflow incontinence.**

   empty _____ bladder _____ constantly _____ dribble _____ overflow
   incontinence _____

5. Prostate cancer symptoms include **urgency** of urination, **dribbling** urine **flow,** pain during **urination,** and a **feeling** that the bladder is not **empty.**

   urgency _____ dribbling _____ flow _____ urination _____ feeling _____ empty _____

6. Waking up during the night to **urinate, urinating** more than eight times during a 24-hour period, and experiencing urge incontinence and losing **urine** are symptoms commonly found in **overactive** bladder, also referred to as **irritable** bladder.

   urinate _____ urinating _____ urine _____ overactive _____ irritable _____

7. Several factors contribute to and **exacerbate** stress **incontinence,** including childbirth, prostate surgery, **urinary** tract infection, smoking, which causes coughing, and **diabetes,** which can **cause excessive** urine production.

   exacerbate _____ incontinence _____ urinary _____ diabetes _____ cause _____ excess _____

8. The type of urinary incontinence that **affects** some children, especially boys, is called **nocturnal enuresis,** and is more **commonly** known as **bed wetting** at night.

   affects _____ nocturnal enuresis _____ commonly _____ bed wetting _____

9. **Interstitial cystitis,** also known as **painful** bladder **syndrome,** is chronic inflammation of the bladder that causes a **persistent urge** to urinate, pain and **pressure** around the bladder, and **pain** during sexual intercourse.

   interstitial cystitis _____ painful _____ syndrome _____ persistent _____
   urge _____ pressure _____ pain _____

10. Symptoms of **cystitis,** which is **inflammation** or infection of the bladder and a type of urinary tract infection, include the urge to **urinate,** a burning sensation, and blood in the **urine;** cystitis can become a **serious** health problem if it **spreads** to the kidneys.

    cystitis _____ inflammation _____ urinate _____ urine _____ serious _____
    spreads _____

11. Many cases of overactive bladder occur because the muscles of the bladder **involuntarily contract** when the bladder is still filling or is only half full to create **contractions** and the urgent **need** to **urinate.**

    involuntarily _____ contract _____ contractions _____ need _____ urinate _____

12. An enlarged **prostate** can compress the **urethra** and **impede** urine flow from the bladder, which can cause **retention** and the **need** for **frequent** urination.

    prostate _____   urethra _____   impede _____   retention _____   need _____   frequent _____

13. Nausea, vomiting, **shaking chills,** high fever, and back pain are symptoms of acute pyelonephritis, a type of urinary tract **infection** that **infects** the kidney as a result of a **spreading** bladder infection.

    shaking _____   chills _____   infection _____   infects _____   spreading _____

14. **Complications** of interstitial cystitis include **interrupted** sleep, **emotional** stress, **interference** with social and work activities, and sexual **intimacy.**

    complications _____   interrupted _____   emotional _____   interference _____   intimacy _____

15. People suffering from urge **incontinence** are **susceptible** to **complications** such as anxiety, depression, and **poor concentration.**

    incontinence _____   susceptible _____   complications _____   poor _____   concentration _____

How did you do? Check your answers against the Answer Key online.

Typical Medical Conditions and Patient Complaints

The sentences below contain vocabulary that describes and explains typical medical conditions, diseases, symptoms, and patient complaints that a pharmacist encounters. Read the sentences carefully. Then indicate the word form of the bolded word(s), choosing from v, n, adj, or adv. Look up words you do not know in your bilingual or first-language dictionary.

1. Before he was diagnosed with an **enlarged prostate,** the patient had **complained** that he was unable to **empty** his bladder but that he had the **urgent need** to urinate often.

   enlarged prostate _____   complained _____   empty _____   urgent _____   need _____

2. Cystitis in women whose **bladder** becomes **infected** as a result of **bacteria** being introduced into the bladder through the **urethra** during sexual intercourse is sometimes called **honeymoon cystitis.**

   bladder _____   infected _____   bacteria _____   urethra _____   honeymoon cystitis _____

3. Avoiding **certain** foods, such as caffeine, chocolate, citrus, tomatoes, alcohol, and foods **high** in vitamin C, which can **irritate** the bladder, can **relieve interstitial cystitis.**

   certain _____   high _____   irritate _____   relieve _____   interstitial cystitis _____

4. People who suffer from overactive bladder can help **alleviate** their symptoms by practicing **interventions** such as reducing fluid **intake,** increasing fiber intake, **training** the bladder to delay **voiding,** and double voiding, which means trying to **urinate** again after urinating.

   alleviate _____   interventions _____   intake _____   training _____   voiding _____   urinate _____

5. Types of devices to help women who suffer from stress incontinence include a **urethral plug,** which is a tampon-like **disposable device** inserted in the urethra to prevent **leakage,** and a bladder neck support device **inserted** into the vagina to lift the bladder.

   urethral _____   plug _____   disposable _____   device _____   leakage _____   inserted _____

6. **Urethritis, inflammation** or infection of the bladder, **causes** a **burning** sensation when urinating, and in some men causes a penile **discharge.**

   urethritis _____   inflammation _____   causes _____   burning _____   discharge _____

7. It is important for women to **urinate** as soon as they feel the **urge** and not keep **urine** in the bladder, to **empty** the bladder right after sexual intercourse, and to **wipe** from the front to the back after a bowel movement to **avoid** bacteria from entering the vagina to help **reduce** urinary tract infection.

   urinate _____   urge _____   urine _____   empty _____   wipe _____   avoid _____
   reduce _____

8. Patients with certain **medical** or physical **impairments** such as arthritis or Alzheimer's disease, which **prevents** them from getting to the bathroom on time to **urinate,** will experience a type of urinary incontinence called **functional incontinence.**

medical _____   impairments _____   prevents _____   urinate _____   functional incontinence _____

9. An **enlarged** prostate can **constrict** the urethra and **block urine flow,** which can result in the **urge** to **release** urine, also known as overflow incontinence.

enlarged _____   constrict _____   block _____   urine flow _____   urge _____   release _____

10. To reduce the **risk** of kidney infection, it is important to drink plenty of water and cranberry juice to help remove bacteria from the body during **urination,** to **urinate** frequently and not hold in **urine,** and to **shower** rather than bathe to prevent **moisture** that can cause infection.

risk _____   urination _____   urinate _____   urine _____   shower _____   moisture _____

11. Two types of bladder infection, or **cystitis,** caused by bacteria are **community-acquired** bladder infection, which is not acquired in hospitals and nursing homes, and **hospital-acquired** bladder infection, which occurs as a result of **urinary** catheters inserted in the urethra to **collect** urine.

cystitis _____   community-acquired _____   hospital-acquired _____   urinary _____   collect _____

12. In women, **urethritis** can be caused by **sexually transmitted diseases** such as herpes simplex and **chlamydia,** and in men urethritis can be caused by gonorrhea and chlamydia.

urethritis _____   sexually _____   transmitted _____   diseases _____   chlamydia _____

13. An enlarged prostate can lead to other **complications** such as interrupted **sleep,** the inability to **empty** the bladder, **recurrent** bladder infections, and potential kidney **damage.**

complications _____   sleep _____   empty _____   recurrent _____   damage _____

14. **Diabetics** and people with an **abnormal** urinary tract, an enlarged prostate, low immune systems, and those who have had a **catheter inserted** in their bladder, may be more **prone** to developing urinary tract infections.

diabetics _____   abnormal _____   catheter _____   inserted _____   prone _____

15. Overactive bladder is caused by a **sudden, involuntary** muscle **contraction** in the wall of the bladder that **leads** to **urination urgency.**

sudden _____   involuntary _____   contraction _____   leads _____   urination _____   urgency _____

16. Causes of urinary **incontinence** include pregnancy, childbirth, menopause, **prostate** surgery, **impaired** thinking such as forgetfulness and **senility,** and **various** diseases and medications.

incontinence _____   prostate _____   impaired _____   senility _____   various _____

17. **Ulceration** and bleeding of the bladder, which can lead to **scarring** and bladder **stiffness,** can be caused by interstitial cystitis, a **chronic inflammatory** disease of the bladder.

ulceration _____   scarring _____   stiffness _____   chronic _____   inflammatory _____

18. Symptoms of kidney infection include **pus** and blood in the **urine;** back, side, and **groin** pain, **frequent** urination, a burning **sensation,** nausea, and a **fever.**

pus _____   urine _____   groin _____   frequent _____   sensation _____   fever _____

19. Left **untreated,** cystitis can cause scarring and **formation** of **stones** as a result of holding in **urine** to avoid **painful urination.**

untreated _____   formation _____   stones _____   urine _____   painful _____   urination _____

20. **Regular** exercise, reducing alcohol and caffeine **consumption,** and a **diet** high in fiber can help **reduce** the **risk** of **overactive** bladder.

regular _____   consumption _____   diet _____   reduce _____   risk _____   overactive _____

How did you do? Check your answers against the Answer Key online.

Medical Vocabulary Comprehension

Now that you have read sentences 1 through 15 describing language regarding the urinary system, assess your understanding by doing the exercises below.

Multiple Choice Questions

Choose the answer that correctly completes each sentence below.

1. _____ Unintentional urine loss caused by sneezing, coughing, or heavy lifting is called:
a. overflow incontinence
b. dribbling
c. stress incontinence

2. _____ A symptom of an **enlarged prostate** is:
a. leakage
b. inability to empty the bladder
c. double voiding

3. _____ Another term for loss of bladder control is:
a. urinary incontinence
b. urgency
c. persistent urge

4. _____ A **catheter** in the bladder can cause:
a. involuntary muscle contraction in the wall of the bladder
b. urinary tract infection
c. chronic inflammation of the bladder

5. _____ Another term for **nocturnal enuresis** is:
a. bed wetting at night
b. urethritis
c. retaining urine

6. _____ A person experiencing pus and blood in the urine should be tested for:
a. kidney infection
b. overflow incontinence
c. bacteria

7. _____ **Community-acquired bladder infection** is a type of:
a. overactive bladder
b. functional incontinence
c. cystitis

8. _____ To reduce the risk of **kidney infection,** it is important to:
a. drink plenty of water and cranberry juice to help remove bacteria during urination
b. double void
c. resist the urge to urinate

9. _____ An **enlarged prostate** can:
a. cause overflow incontinence
b. impede urine flow
c. cause inflammation of the bladder

10. _____ Symptoms of **urinary tract infection** include:

a. the urge to urinate and a burning sensation when urinating

b. loss of bladder control

c. excess urine production

11. _____ Chronic inflammation of the bladder that causes a persistent urge to urinate, pain in the bladder, and pain during sexual intercourse can be caused by:

a. an enlarged prostate

b. interstitial cystitis

c. stress incontinence

12. _____ Pregnancy, childbirth, prostate surgery, and diabetes can exacerbate:

a. enuresis

b. cystitis

c. stress incontinence

13. _____ **Cystitis** can be the cause of:

a. scarring and formation of stones resulting from holding in urine to avoid painful urination

b. scarring and formation of stones due to leakage

c. overactive bladder

14. _____ Patients suffering from **urge incontinence** are susceptible to:

a. anxiety and depression

b. kidney infection

c. chlamydia

15. _____ Another term for **overactive bladder** is:

a. irritable bladder

b. empty bladder

c. full bladder

True/False Questions

Indicate whether each sentence below is true (T) or false (F).

1. _____ The type of urinary incontinence that causes a person to constantly dribble urine is called overflow incontinence.

2. _____ Cystitis will not become a serious health problem if it spreads to the kidneys.

3. _____ People who suffer from overactive bladder can help alleviate their symptoms if they reduce the amount of fluid intake and learn how to train their bladder to delay voiding.

4. _____ Urethritis is inflammation of the kidneys and causes a penile discharge in some men.

5. _____ Another word for cystitis that results from sexual intercourse as a result of bacteria being introduced into the bladder through the urethra is honeymoon cystitis.

6. _____ The words "urination" and "urine" are nouns.

7. _____ A type of urinary incontinence that affects children, especially boys, is functional incontinence.

8. _____ Septicemic is the adjective form of septicemia.

9. _____ Urethritis is inflammation or infection of the bladder and causes a burning sensation when urinating.

10. _____ Exercising regularly and reducing alcohol, caffeine, and fiber intake will help decrease the risk of overactive bladder.

How did you do? Check your answers against the Answer Key online.

Writing Exercise

An important part of communication is the ability to write about what you read, to write correctly, and to spell correctly. In the exercises below, write your understanding of the meaning of the bolded words.

1. Describe in writing what **stress incontinence, urge incontinence, overflow incontinence,** and **functional incontinence** are.

_____

_____

_____

_____

2. Describe in writing what **urinary tract infection** is.

_____

_____

_____

_____

3. Describe in writing what **cystitis** and **interstitial cystitis** are.

_____

_____

_____

_____

4. Describe in writing what **enlarged prostate** and **kidney infection** are.

_____

_____

_____

_____

5. Describe in writing what **overactive bladder** and **nocturnal enuresis** are.

_____

_____

_____

_____

Check what you have written with acceptable answers that appear in the Answer Key online.

LISTENING AND PRONUNCIATION

The ability to listen and understand what is being said and heard, and the ability to pronounce words clearly, is extremely important. A word misheard and a word mispronounced will lead to poor communication and can seriously put both the pharmacist and patient in danger. Therefore, it is very important that one hear clearly what another person has said, and that one speak clearly with correct pronunciation.

Listen carefully to the pharmacy-related words presented in the audio files found in Chapter 10 on thePoint (thePoint.lww.com/diaz-gilbert), and then pronounce them as accurately as you can. Listen and then repeat. You will listen to each word once and then you will repeat it. You will do this twice for each word. Listening and pronunciation practice will increase your listening and speaking confidence. Many languages do not produce or emphasize certain sounds produced and emphasized in English, so pay careful attention to the pronunciation of each word.

Pronunciation Exercise

Listen to the audio files found in Chapter 10 on thePoint (thePoint.lww.com/diaz-gilbert). Listen and repeat the words. Then say the words aloud for additional practice.

1. absorbent pad	əb-sôr′bənt păd
2. bed wetting	bĕd wĕt ng
3. bladder	blăd′ər
4. bladder training	blăd′ər trā′nĭng
5. catheter	kăth′ĭ-tər
6. contents	kŏn′tĕnt′s
7. contract	kŏn′trăkt′
8. cystitis	sĭ-stī′tĭs
9. double voiding	dŭb′əl voidng
10. drain	drān
11. dribbles	drĭb′əls
12. empty	ĕmp′tē
13. enlarged prostate	ĕn-lärj′t prŏs′tāt′
14. flow	flō
15. hematuria	hē′mə-to͞or′ē-ə
16. impede	ĭm-pēd′
17. incontinence	ĭn-kŏn′tə-nəns
18. interstitial cystitis	ĭn′tər-stĭsh′əl sĭ-stī′tĭs
19. involuntary contraction	ĭn-vŏl′ən-tĕr′ē kŏn′trăkt′shən
20. Kegel exercises	kē gəl ĕk′sər-sĭz′ĕs
21. kidney infection	kĭd′nē ĭn-fĕk′shən
22. leakage	lē′kĭj
23. nocturia	nŏk-tûreə
24. nocturnal enuresis	nŏk-tûr′nəl ĕn′yə-rē′sĭs
25. overactive bladder	ō′vər-ăk′tĭv blăd′ər
26. overflow	ō′vər-flō′
27. pelvis	pĕl′vĭs
28. pessary	pĕs′ə-rē
29. postvoid residual urine	pōst void rĭ-zĭj′o͞o-əl yo͝or′ĭn
30. septicemia	sĕp′tĭ-sē′mē-ə
31. toilet	toi′lĭt
32. urethra	yo͞o-rē′thrə
33. urethral insert	yo͞o-rē′thrōl ĭn′sûrt′
34. urethritis	yo͝or′ĭ-thrī′tĭs
35. urinalysis	yo͝or′ə-năl′ĭ-sĭs
36. urinary sphincter	yo͝or′ə-nĕr′ē sfĭngk′tər
37. urinary tract infection	yo͝or′ə-nĕr′ē trăkt ĭn-fĕk′shən
38. urinate	yo͝or′ə-nāt′
39. urine output	yo͝or′ĭn out′po͞ot′
40. void	void

Which words are easy to pronounce? Which are difficult to pronounce? Use the space below to write in the words that you find difficult to pronounce. These are words you should practice saying often.

_____

_____

_____

_____

_____

_____

_____

_____

Listen to the audio files found in Chapter 10 on thePoint (thePoint.lww.com/diaz-gilbert) as many times as you need to increase your pronunciation ability of the difficult words. Pronounce these words with a friend or a colleague who speaks English.

English Sounds That Are Difficult for Speakers of Other Languages to Pronounce

Spanish

In Spanish, there is no English "v" sound, but the "v" consonant in Spanish is pronounced like the English "b." The vowel "i" is pronounced like a long "e." Pay careful attention to the "v" sound in English when pronouncing words that begin with "v." Also pay careful attention to English words that begin with "s;" do not use the Spanish "es" sound when pronouncing English words that begin with "s."

For example, in English,

cystitis is not pronounced seesteetees

Vietnamese

In Vietnamese, the "t" consonant is pronounced "s," but in English the "t" is pronounced "t" and "s" is pronounced "s." Be careful with English words that begin with "t." In Vietnamese, the "b" consonant is pronounced "p," but in English "p" is pronounced "p" and "b" is pronounced "b."

In Vietnamese, words do not end in "b," "ch," "f," "d," "j," "l," "p," "r," "s," "sh," "v," and "z." In English, words end in these letters. Pay special attention to pronouncing these English sounds. In Vietnamese, there is no "dzh" or "zh" sound, so English words like "judge" (dzh) and "rupture" (zh) will be hard for Vietnamese speakers to pronounce.

For example, in English,

contents is not pronounced conteh

Gujarati

In Gujarati, "v" is pronounced "w," "f" is pronounced "p," "p" is pronounced "f," and "z" is pronounced "j." Short "i" is pronounced long "e," "x" is pronounced "ch," and "th" is pronounced "s." In English, "v" is pronounced "v," "f " is pronounced "f," "z" is pronounced "z" or "s," "j" is pronounced "j," and "x" is pronounced "x." Pay careful attention when pronouncing these sounds.

For example, in English,

flow is not pronounced plo

Korean

In Korean, the "v" consonant is pronounced "b" and the "f" consonant is pronounced "p." In English, the "v" is pronounced "v," the "f" is pronounced "f," and the "p" is pronounced "p." Pay special attention when pronouncing these sounds.

For example, in English,

void is not pronounced boid

(continued)

Chinese

In Chinese, the "r" consonant is pronounced "l" or "w," and "b," "d," "g," and "ng" are not pronounced at all. Pay careful attention to English words that begin with "r" because the "r" is not pronounced "l" or "w," and "b," "d," "g," and "ng" are pronounced in English.

For example, in English,

impede is not pronounced impee

Russian

The "w" consonant is pronounced like a "v" and the "v" sound like a "w." Pay careful attention to the English "th." It is not pronounced "s."

For example, in English,

void is not pronounced woid

DICTATION

 ### Listening/Spelling Exercise: Word and Word Pairs

Listen to the words or word pairs on the audio files found in Chapter 10 on thePoint (thePoint.lww.com/diaz-gilbert) and then write them down on the lines below.

1. _____
2. _____
3. _____
4. _____
5. _____
6. _____
7. _____
8. _____
9. _____
10. _____
11. _____
12. _____
13. _____
14. _____
15. _____

 ### Listening/Spelling Exercise: Sentences

Listen to the sentences on the audio files found in Chapter 10 on thePoint (thePoint.lww.com/diaz-gilbert) and then write them down on the lines below.

1. _____
_____
2. _____
_____

3. _____
_____

4. _____
_____

5. _____
_____

6. _____
_____

7. _____
_____

8. _____
_____

9. _____
_____

10. _____
_____

Now, check your sentences against the correct answers in the Answer Key online. If there are any new words that you do not know or that you spelled incorrectly, make a list of those words and study them for meaning and spelling.

PHARMACIST/PATIENT DIALOGUES

The ability to orally communicate effectively with your professors, colleagues, and especially with patients is very important. As a pharmacist, you will be counseling patients; patients will come to you for advice. They will have questions about a condition and symptoms they may experience and will ask you to help treat the condition. Therefore, it is extremely important that you understand what they are saying and that you respond to them and their questions appropriately. Your patients will speak differently. For example, some may speak very quickly, others too low, and yet others may speak angrily. To help you improve your listening skills, listen to the following dialogues, or short conversations, between a pharmacist and a patient and between a pharmacy technician and a patient.

Listening and Comprehension Exercises

Dialogue #1

Listen to Dialogue #1, stop, listen again and take notes. Listen to the dialogue as many times as you need or until you feel you have written sufficient notes and feel confident. You can use your notes to answer the multiple choice questions at the end of the dialogue.

Notes _____
_____
_____
_____
_____

Answer the questions below by selecting the answer that correctly completes each sentence.

1. _____ The patient's name is:
a. Lisa Mattson
b. Leeza Matson
c. Leeza Mattson

2. _____ The patient has been prescribed:

a. bacitracin

b. Bactrim

c. Bethaprim

3. _____ The patient's doctor's name is:

a. Dr. Chen

b. Dr. Chang

c. Dr. Chinn

4. _____ The patient's birth date is:

a. March 1, 1982

b. March 2, 1982

c. March 10, 1982

5. _____ The patient's previous address was:

a. 11 Lancaster Road in Summit, and the current address is 1212 Warwick Avenue in Summit

b. 1212 Warwick Road in Lancaster, and the current address is 11 Summit Avenue in Lancaster

c. 1212 Warwick Avenue in Summit, and the current address is 11 Lancaster Road in Summit

6. _____ The patient's phone number is:

a. 332-9376

b. 332-9763

c. 322-9376

7. _____ The patient is allergic to:

a. birth control pills and nuts, and was taking Tylenol for the pressure in her lower abdomen and the burning sensation

b. nuts, is currently on birth control pills, and was taking Tylenol for the pressure in her lower abdomen and the burning sensation

c. nuts, was taking Tylenol for the pain in her lower abdomen, and is not on birth control pills

8. _____ The patient has been prescribed Bactrim because she has:

a. cystitis, an infection of the kidney

b. interstitial cystitis

c. cystitis, an infection of the bladder

9. _____ The pharmacist tells the patient the medication should give her peace of mind. This means:

a. her mind will be peaceful

b. she will experience a feeling of calm and feel less worried

c. she will be free to speak her mind

10. _____ The patient's doctor wants the patient to take the medication:

a. once a day with food only

b. twice a day: once in the morning and once in the evening with a full glass of water

c. twice a day: once in the morning and once in the evening with milk only

11. _____ The pharmacist tells the patient that if the medication upsets her stomach, she can:

a. stop taking the medication

b. take the medicine with milk only

c. take the medicine with milk or food

11. _____ A heating pad can be used to:

a. alleviate lower abdominal pain caused by a bladder infection

b. shrink an enlarged prostate

c. control leakage

12. _____ A person with an overactive bladder should:

a. only learn how to use absorbent pads to control leakage

b. double void to completely empty the bladder

c. drink a lot of water

13. _____ Interstitial cystitis is a:

a. chronic inflammatory disease of the bladder

b. chronic inflammatory disease of the kidney

c. kind of incontinence

14. _____ The word **dribble** is a:

a. verb

b. noun

c. verb and a noun

15. _____ In the sentence, "Losing urine is a symptom of overactive bladder, also known as irritable bladder," the word **overactive** is:

a. an adjective

b. a past tense verb

c. a noun

Listening and Comprehension Exercises
Dialogue #1

Listen to Dialogue #1, stop, listen again and take notes. Listen to the dialogue as many times as you need or until you feel you have written sufficient notes and feel confident. You can use your notes to answer the multiple choice questions at the end of the dialogue.

Notes _____

_____

_____

_____

_____

Answer the questions below by selecting the answer that correctly completes each sentence.

1. _____ The pharmacist's name is:

a. Joan Brown, and the patient's name is Jude Berger

b. Jude Brown, and the patient's name is Joan Brown

c. Jude Berger, and the patient's name is Joan Brown

2. _____ The patient's medical condition is:

a. urinary tract infection

b. overactive bladder

c. stress incontinence

3. _____ The patient's doctor is:

a. Dr. Berger, and she has prescribed Detrol

b. Dr. Hoffman, and she has prescribed Detrol

c. Dr. Brown, and she has prescribed Detrol

4. _____ The patient tells the pharmacist that:

a. she's having problems losing her urine and that she is using Depends absorbent pads

b. she's having problems losing her urine and that she is too embarrassed to use absorbent pads

c. she's having problems losing her urine and is not using absorbent pads

5. _____ The patient tells the pharmacist that she is taking:

a. Amaryl for her type II diabetes

b. Amaryl for her type I diabetes

c. Amoxil for her ear infection

6. _____ The patient is allergic to:

a. Ceclor only

b. Ceclor and latex

c. latex only

7. _____ The patient is:

a. 48 years old, has one fibroid, and has had one breast biopsy that was benign

b. 48 years old, has two fibroids, and has had one breast biopsy that was malignant

c. 48 years old, has three fibroids, and has had two breast biopsies that were benign

8. _____ The pharmacist tells the patient that Detrol will:

a. stop the infection that is causing her overactive bladder

b. help to relax the muscles in the bladder and help to control urination

c. help to relax the muscles and stop the infection in the bladder

9. _____ The patient needs to take Detrol:

a. twice a day with or without food and see her doctor in 6 weeks

b. once a day with or without food and see her doctor in 6 days

c. twice a day with food and see her doctor in 6 months

10. _____ Side effects of the medication include:

a. vomiting, diarrhea, dry eye, and dry mouth

b. dry eye, dry mouth, dizziness, headaches, constipation, drowsiness, and blurred vision

c. dry eye, dry mouth, and constipation

11. _____ The pharmacist advices the patient:

a. to eat a diet rich in fiber and to ask her doctor for a laxative and stool softener if she gets constipated

b. to drink lots of water only

c. to drink lots of water and to eat a diet rich in fiber

12. _____ The pharmacist tells the patient that the medication:

a. will cause her to sweat

b. will cause decreased sweating

c. will cause her to overheat and sweat

13. _____ The pharmacist advices the patient that she can learn to:

a. increase the number of urges to urinate and decrease the number of leakages

b. decrease the number of urges to urinate and decrease the number of leakages

c. decrease the number of urges to urinate and increase the number of leakages

14. _____ The patient should learn how to:

a. delay urination, how to double void, and how to do Kegel exercises

b. retain urination and how to double void

c. hold urine every 10 minutes and double void

15. _____ The pharmacist tells the patient she can find help:

a. in a book entitled *National Association for Continence*

b. from the organization National Association for Continence on the web

c. at a local support group call National Association for Continence

 ### *Dialogue #2*

Listen to Dialogue #2, stop, listen again and take notes. Listen to the dialogue as many times as you need or until you feel you have written sufficient notes and feel confident. You can use your notes to answer the multiple choice questions at the end of the dialogue.

Notes _____

_____

_____

_____

Answer the questions below by selecting the answer that correctly completes each sentence.

1. _____ The patient's name is:

a. Jacqueline Cho, and the pharmacist's name is Leonard Chase

b. Leonard Cho, and the pharmacist's name is Jacklyn Chase

c. Jacklyn Cho, and the pharmacist's name is Leonard Chase

2. _____ The patient has a prescription for Macrodantin to treat:

a. a kidney infection

b. a urinary tract infection

c. an overactive bladder

3. _____ The patient's date of birth is:

a. February 12, 1989, and she is 18 years old

b. February 18, 1989, and she is 8 years old

c. February 18, 1989, and she is 12 years old

4. _____ The patient's address is:

a. 27 Sunset Terrace in Waterville, and her telephone number is 467-4485

b. 27 Sunset Terrace in Watertown, and her telephone number is 476-4485

c. 27 Sunset Terrace in Watertown, and her telephone number is 467-4485

5. _____ The patient is:

a. not covered by her father's insurance, which is Health Choice Medical and Drug Plan

b. covered by her father's insurance, which is Healthy Choice Medical Plan

c. covered by her father's insurance, which is Health Choice Medical and Drug Plan

6. _____ The patient's doctor is:

a. Dr. Varsha Patel

b. Dr. Leonard Chase

c. Dr. Varsha Chase

7. _____ The patient tells the pharmacist that she is:

a. allergic to antibiotics and tomatoes, is lactose intolerant, and is on birth control pills

b. not allergic to medications but gets hay fever, is lactose intolerant, is allergic to tomatoes, and is on birth control pills

c. allergic to medications, gets hay fever, is lactose intolerant, is allergic to tomatoes, and is on birth control pills

8. _____ The patient tells the pharmacist that she is:

a. drinking cranberry juice to treat her urinary tract infection

b. not taking anything to treat her urinary tract infection

c. drinking a lot of water to treat her urinary tract infection

9. _____ The pharmacist tells the patient the prescribed medication is:

a. an antibiotic that will help to relax the muscles in her bladder

b. a muscle relaxant that will help to get rid of bacteria

c. an antibiotic that will help to stop bacteria from growing in her bladder

10. _____ The pharmacist tells the patient to:

a. take the full prescribed amount unless she starts feeling better

b. discontinue taking the medication as soon as the symptoms clear

c. take the full prescribed amount even if she starts to feel better

11. _____ The doctor has prescribed that the patient take:

a. 4 capsules a day, one every 6 hours

b. 6 capsules a day, one every 4 hours

c. 4 capsules at once

12. _____ The pharmacist tells the patient that a side effect of the medication is:

a. dark yellow or brown urine, which is very serious

b. dark yellow or brown urine, which is quite normal

c. dark yellow or brown urine, and that she needs to stop taking the medication

13. _____ The pharmacist tells the patient that she:

a. can continue to drink cranberry juice but to also drink plenty of water to flush out bacteria

b. should stop drinking cranberry juice but drink plenty of water so she doesn't become dehydrated

c. should just drink plenty of water

14. _____ The pharmacist tells the patient she:

a. can drink moderate amounts of alcohol and caffeine

b. should not drink alcohol and caffeine until the infection clears up

c. should not drink alcohol, caffeine, and citrus juice until the infection clears up

15. _____ To prevent future infections, the pharmacist tells the patient to:

a. avoid sexual intercourse

b. drink plenty of water

c. empty the bladder and not hold in urine, to wipe front to back after urinating, and drink plenty of water to flush out bacteria after sexual intercourse

How did you do on the Post-Assessment in Chapter 10? Check your answers in the Answer Key online.

Hepatic System | 11

PRE-ASSESSMENT

True/False Questions

Indicate whether each sentence below is true (T) or false (F).

1. _____ Reversible scarring of the liver is called **cirrhosis.**
2. _____ One cause of **autoimmune hepatitis** is scarring of the liver.
3. _____ Intravenous drug users and people who share needles are not at risk for **hepatitis B,** a serious liver infection.
4. _____ One cause of damage to the liver is **alcoholic cirrhosis.**
5. _____ The noun form of **hepatic** is hepatitis.
6. _____ **Hepatitis B** is transmitted through food.
7. _____ **Cirrhosis** of the liver is caused by alcohol only.
8. _____ **Hepatitis A** is transmitted through blood and bodily fluids.
9. _____ **Autoimmune hepatitis** is caused by years of alcohol abuse.
10. _____ The noun form of **toxin** is toxic.
11. _____ Contaminated needles used in body piercing and body tattooing are one cause of **hepatitis C.**
12. _____ Cirrhosis makes it difficult for blood to flow through the liver to detoxify harmful substances and to purify the blood.
13. _____ Immune disorders such as diabetes, ulcerative colitis, and Sjögren's syndrome can be found in people with **autoimmune hepatitis.**
14. _____ **Hepatitis B** can be transmitted through sexual contact, needle sharing, accidental needle sticks, and from mother to child.
15. _____ The word **contagion** is an adjective.

Multiple Choice Questions

Choose the correct answer from a, b, and c.

1. _____ Causes of **cirrhosis** include:
   a. hepatitis A and hepatitis B
   b. chronic hepatitis B and hepatitis C, alcoholism, and autoimmune hepatitis
   c. alcoholism only

2. _____ A risk factor for contracting **hepatitis B** is:
   a. having unprotected sex with more than one partner
   b. eating contaminated food
   c. alcohol consumption

3. _____ Complications of **cirrhosis** include:

a. bleeding and bruising, edema in the abdomen and legs, and hypertension in the vein from the liver

b. bleeding and bruising only

c. edema in the legs only

4. _____ People exhibiting symptoms such as yellowing of the whites of the eyes and the skin and abdominal swelling should be tested for:

a. hepatitis A

b. autoimmune hepatitis

c. contaminated body piercings

5. _____ Another term for fluid in and swelling of the abdomen is:

a. edema

b. encephalopathy

c. ascites

6. _____ Liver cancer can be caused by:

a. hepatitis A, hepatitis B, and cirrhosis

b. cirrhosis only

c. hepatitis B, hepatitis C, and cirrhosis

7. _____ A complication of **cirrhosis** is:

a. jaundice

b. dark urine

c. hepatic encephalopathy

8. _____ **Hepatitis B** is transmitted through:

a. contact with blood and bodily fluids of an infected person

b. body piercing and illegal drug use

c. contaminated blood

9. _____ The word contaminated is:

a. a verb

b. a verb and an adjective

c. an adjective

10. _____ The expression **"What am I, chopped liver?"** means the person:

a. likes liver

b. feels frustrated and ignored

c. has liver disease

How did you do? Check your answers in the Answer Key online.

MEDICAL VOCABULARY

A good understanding of vocabulary words in pharmacy is very important for communication with professors, fellow students, patients, and coworkers. Knowledge and understanding of vocabulary leads to successful communication and success as a pharmacy student, as a pharmacy technician, and as a practicing pharmacist. You may already know many of the vocabulary words in this chapter, but for words that are unfamiliar, pay careful attention to them and make every effort to know their correct spelling, meaning, and pronunciation. It is a good idea to keep a list of new words and to look up these new words in a bilingual dictionary or dictionary in your first language. A good command of pharmacy-related vocabulary and good pronunciation of vocabulary will help to prevent embarrassing mistakes and increase effective verbal communication skills.

Hepatic System Vocabulary

alcoholism
ascites
bile duct
cirrhosis
contagious
contamination
edema
hemochromatosis
hemolytic anemia

hepatic encephalopathy
hepatitis
immune globulin
immunization
inoperable
jaundice
liver transplant
outbreaks
pernicious anemia

platelets
portal hypertension
scarring
spider angioma
toxin
vaccination
varices
viral hepatitis

PARTS OF SPEECH

A good understanding of parts of speech, such as verbs, nouns, adjectives, and adverbs, is important for successful communication when speaking or writing. It is equally important to know the various forms of words and to use them appropriately.

Word Forms

The table below lists the main forms of some terms that you will likely encounter in pharmacy practice. Review the table and then do the exercises that follow to assess your understanding.

Noun (n)	Infinitive/Verb (v) —Past Tense	Adjective (adj)	Adverb (adv)
alcoholism; alcoholic		alcoholic	
ascites		ascitic	
cirrhosis		cirrhotic	
contagion; contagiousness		contagious	contagiously
contamination; contaminant	to contaminate; contaminated	contaminated	
duct		ductal; ductless	
encephalopathy		encephalopathic	
hemolysis		hemolytic	
hepatitis; hepatectomy		hepatic	
immunization	to immunize; immunized	immune; immunized	
inoperability		inoperable	inoperably
toxic; toxicity		toxic	toxically
transplant; transplanter; transplantation	to transplant; transplanted	transplantable	
vaccine; vaccination	to vaccinate; vaccinated		
virus		viral	virally

Word Forms Exercise

Read the following sentences carefully. Then indicate the word form of the bolded word(s), choosing from v, n, adj, or adv.

1. Symptoms of **cirrhosis** include **swelling** in the legs, **fluid** in the abdomen, **intense itching,** fatigue, and nausea.

   cirrhosis _____   swelling _____   fluid _____   intense _____   itching _____

2. **Autoimmune hepatitis,** a disease of the **liver** in which the body **attacks** itself, may be caused by other diseases, **toxins,** and certain **medications.**

   autoimmune hepatitis _____   liver _____   attacks _____   toxins _____   medications _____

3. **Chronic hepatitis B** is caused by the hepatitis B **virus** and can lead to scarring of the liver, also known as **cirrhosis,** liver cancer, and liver **failure.**

   chronic _____   hepatitis B _____   virus _____   cirrhosis _____   failure _____

4. **Contaminated** food or water can **cause hepatitis A,** a **contagious** liver **infection** that does not lead to chronic hepatitis or cirrhosis.

   contaminated _____   cause _____   hepatitis A _____   contagious _____   infection _____

5. Fatigue, anemia, **itching** (also known as **pruritus**), **jaundice,** which is yellowing of the white of the eyes and the skin, and **discomfort** in the **abdomen** are symptoms of autoimmune hepatitis.

   itching _____   pruritus _____   jaundice _____   discomfort _____   abdomen _____

6. It is **critical** for anyone with cirrhosis to avoid **alcohol,** which is broken down by the liver into highly **toxic** chemicals that **trigger inflammation** that **destroys** liver cells.

   critical _____   alcohol _____   toxic _____   trigger _____   inflammation _____   destroy _____

7. Hepatitis C is **contracted** by coming in contact with blood, needles used to **inject** drugs, and **needles** used in **tattooing** and body piercing that are **contaminated** with the hepatitis C virus.

   contracted _____   inject _____   needles _____   tattooing _____   contaminated _____

8. Hepatitis B, one strain of **viral** hepatitis, can i**nfect** a person who has **unprotected** sex with an **infected** person; a person who uses or shares needles and syringes **contaminated** with infected blood; a person, such as a health care worker, who accidentally comes in contact with infected human blood; and a baby whose infected mother has **transmitted** the virus during pregnancy.

   viral _____   infect _____   unprotected _____   infected _____   contaminated _____
   transmitted _____

9. Autoimmune hepatitis, which can be **triggered** after being **infected** with hepatitis A, hepatitis B, Epstein-Barr virus, or measles, can **lead** to other health **complications** such as pernicious **anemia** and hemolytic anemia.

   triggered _____   infected _____   lead _____   complications _____   anemia _____

10. Because hepatitis A is highly **contagious,** it is important for the **infected** person to **wash** his or her hands after using the bathroom, **avoid** oral, anal, and digital **sexual contact,** and not prepare food for others or share utensils.

    contagious _____   infected _____   wash _____   avoid _____   sexual _____   contact _____

11. A person suffering from **alcoholic** cirrhosis will most likely be **malnourished** and require a nutrition program that will help to **regenerate** the **damaged** liver.

    alcoholic _____   malnourished _____   regenerate _____   damaged _____

12. Jaundice, **loss** of appetite, **abdomina**l pain around the liver, **joint** pain, and dark **urine** are **symptomatic** of hepatitis B.

    loss _____   abdominal _____   joint _____   urine _____   symptomatic _____

13. People **diagnosed** with hepatitis B need to avoid alcohol, avoid **certain** prescription and **over-the-counter** drugs such as acetaminophen that can cause damage to the liver, and should not **share** toothbrushes and **razors** with others.

diagnosed _____   certain _____   over-the-counter _____   share _____   razors _____

14. Autoimmune hepatitis can cause cirrhosis of the liver, which can lead to **complications** such as **enlarged** veins, known as **varices,** and **portal hypertension,** which is **increased** blood pressure in the vein from the liver.

complications _____   enlarged _____   varices _____   portal hypertension _____   increased _____

15. Symptoms of hepatitis A include **low-grade** fever, **vomiting,** nausea, **loss** of appetite, and **discomfort** in the **abdominal** area.

low-grade _____   vomiting _____   loss _____   discomfort _____   abdominal _____

How did you do? Check your answers against the Answer Key online.

Typical Medical Conditions and Patient Complaints

The sentences below contain vocabulary that describes and explains typical medical conditions, diseases, symptoms, and patient complaints that a pharmacist encounters. Read the sentences carefully. Then indicate the word form of the bolded word(s), choosing from v, n, adj, or adv. Look up words you do not know in your bilingual or first-language dictionary.

1. Hepatitis A can be spread by **contaminated** foods, such as shellfish, **uncooked** vegetables, and **raw** fruit that cannot be peeled, and by **ice** and tap water.

contaminated _____   uncooked _____   raw _____   ice _____

2. Some people **infected** with hepatitis B **virus** and most people infected with hepatitis C virus will develop **chronic hepatitis,** which can lead to cirrhosis and **liver cancer.**

infected _____   virus _____   chronic _____   hepatitis _____   liver cancer _____

3. It is important to **wash** one's hands with soap and **warm** water to **guard** against **contracting** hepatitis A, a highly **contagious** disease.

wash _____   warm _____   guard _____   contracting _____   contagious _____

4. **Alternative** medicines such as herb milk thistle, which is believed to **heal** and **rebuild** the liver, and omega-3 fatty acids, which can help to **protect** the liver, are recommended alternative **therapies** for patients suffering from cirrhosis.

alternative _____   heal _____   rebuild _____   protect _____   therapies _____

5. Hepatitis B cannot be **contracted** by **casual contact** such as shaking hands, sharing a phone, sitting on a toilet seat, or coming in contact with the tears or **sweat** of an **infected** person.

contracted _____   casual _____   contact _____   sweat _____   infected _____

6. **Autoimmune** hepatitis can lead to other **diseases** such as **ulcerative** colitis, Hashimoto's thyroiditis, **rheumatoid** arthritis, and **type I** diabetes.

autoimmune _____   diseases _____   ulcerative _____   rheumatoid _____   type I _____

7. Hepatitis A, which is most **contagious** before **signs** and symptoms appear, is **transmitted** through water and food **contaminated** with **feces.**

contagious _____   signs _____   transmitted _____   contaminated _____   feces _____

8. Coming in **contact** with blood, semen, **vaginal** secretions, or **saliva** that is **infected** with the hepatitis B virus and that **enters** the body will cause a person to **contract** hepatitis B.

contact _____   vaginal _____   saliva _____   infected _____   enters _____

contract _____

9. Symptoms such as sleeping during the day instead of at night, the inability to concentrate, and memory loss are typical of **hepatic** encephalopathy, which is **impairment** of the brain as a result of **toxic** substances that have **accumulated** in the blood caused by cirrhosis.

   hepatic _____   impairment _____   toxic _____   accumulated _____

10. Although there is a **vaccine** for hepatitis A and hepatitis B, there is no vaccine for hepatitis C, a **virus** that **silently attacks** the liver without the person having any **symptoms.**

    vaccine _____   virus _____   silently _____   attacks _____   symptoms _____

11. The many causes of cirrhosis include alcohol abuse, **chronic viral** hepatitis, autoimmune hepatitis, **inherited** disorders such as hemochromatosis, which is an **abnormal** accumulation of iron, **toxins,** and certain medications.

    chronic _____   viral _____   inherited _____   abnormal _____   toxins _____

12. Receiving the **immune globulin** or hepatitis vaccine can protect a person from **contracting** hepatitis A, as can **washing** one's hands after **using** the toilet, washing all fruits and vegetables before consuming, and drinking **bottled** water, especially in countries where hepatitis A is common.

    immune globulin _____   contracting _____   washing _____   using _____   bottled _____

How did you do? Check your answers against the Answer Key online.

Medical Vocabulary Comprehension

Now that you have read sentences 1 through 12 describing language regarding the hepatic system, assess your understanding by doing the exercises below.

Multiple Choice Questions

Choose the answer that correctly completes each sentence below.

1. _____ A liver disease that causes the body to attack itself is:
   a. cirrhosis
   b. autoimmune hepatitis
   c. hepatitis C

2. _____ **Jaundice** is yellowing of:
   a. the whites of the eyes
   b. the liver
   c. the skin and the whites of the eye

3. _____ Contaminated water or food can cause:
   a. hepatitis C
   b. hepatitis A
   c. cirrhosis

4. _____ One cause of **cirrhosis** is:
   a. alcohol abuse
   b. hepatitis A
   c. contaminated food

5. _____ Complications of **autoimmune hepatitis** include:
   a. hepatitis B
   b. Epstein-Barr virus
   c. pernicious anemia and hemolytic anemia

6. _____ Symptoms of **hepatitis B** include:

a. jaundice, abdominal pain, and dark urine

b. sleeping during the day

c. increased blood pressure in the vein leading to the liver

7. _____ **Chronic hepatitis** can develop in people who have:

a. hepatitis A

b. hepatitis B and hepatitis C

c. cirrhosis

8. _____ To reduce the risk of contracting **hepatitis A,** it is important to:

a. drink plenty of water

b. wash one's hands with soap and water

c. stop drinking alcohol

9. _____ **Hepatitis C** is contracted by:

a. coming in contact with blood, intravenous needles, and tattooing and body piercing needles that are contaminated with the virus

b. coming in contact with feces

c. having unprotected sex

10. _____ **Hemochromatosis** is a disorder that produces:

a. toxins in the blood

b. toxins in the brain

c. an abnormal accumulation of iron

11. _____ Avoiding acetaminophen and the sharing of razors and toothbrushes with others needs to be practiced by people who have been diagnosed with:

a. cirrhosis

b. hepatitis B

c. autoimmune hepatitis

12. _____ A complication of **autoimmune hepatitis** is:

a. enlarged veins

b. impairment of the brain

c. hemochromatosis

13. _____ There is no vaccine for:

a. hepatitis A and hepatitis C

b. hepatitis B

c. hepatitis C

14. _____ Symptoms of **hepatic encephalopathy** include:

a. sleeping during the day instead of at night and the inability to concentrate

b. sleeping during the day instead of at night only

c. sleeping during the day instead of at night, the inability to concentrate, and memory loss

15. _____ Another term for **cirrhosis** is:

a. scarring of the portal vein

b. scarring of the liver

c. alcoholism

True/False Questions

Indicate whether each sentence below is true (T) or false (F).

1. _____ Hepatitis C is contracted through feces.

2. _____ Cirrhosis is a disease of the liver in which the body attacks itself.

3. _____ Fatigue, anemia, itching, jaundice, and yellowing of the whites of the eyes and the skin are symptoms of autoimmune hepatitis.

4. _____ Hepatitis B can be contracted through casual contact such as shaking hands and coming in contact with the tears and sweat of an infected person.

5. _____ Hepatitis A is not a contagious disease but can be contracted through contaminated water and food.

6. _____ The word "encephalopathic" is a noun.

7. _____ There is no vaccine for hepatitis C, a virus that silently attacks the liver.

8. _____ Swelling of the legs, fluid in the abdomen, itching, nausea, and fatigue are symptoms of cirrhosis.

9. _____ Hepatitis B can be spread through unprotected sex, shared needles, tattooing, and body piercing.

10. _____ A person infected with hepatitis A should avoid oral, anal, and digital sexual contact, as well as wash their hands after using the bathroom.

How did you do? Check your answers against the Answer Key online.

Writing Exercise

An important part of communication is the ability to write about what you read, to write correctly, and to spell correctly. In the exercises below, write your understanding of the meaning of the bolded words.

1. Describe in writing what **hepatitis A, hepatitis B,** and **hepatitis C** are.

_____

_____

_____

_____

2. Describe in writing what **cirrhosis** is.

_____

_____

_____

_____

3. Describe in writing what **autoimmune hepatitis** is.

_____

_____

_____

_____

Check what you have written with acceptable answers that appear in the Answer Key online.

LISTENING AND PRONUNCIATION

The ability to listen and understand what is being said and heard, and the ability to pronounce words clearly, is extremely important. A word misheard and a word mispronounced will lead to poor communication and can seriously put both the pharmacist and patient in danger. Therefore, it is very

3. _____ The patient's doctor's name is:

a. Dr. Sorenson

b. Dr. Sorrysen

c. Dr. Soringsun

4. _____ The patient's medical condition is:

a. cirrhosis, and he has been prescribed Actonel

b. liver failure, and he has been prescribed Aldactone

c. cirrhosis, and he has been prescribed Aldactone

5. _____ The prescribed medication is a:

a. diuretic that will help remove fluid from the patient's body

b. liquid that will help remove fluid from the patient's body

c. diuretic that will help the patient to retain fluid in his body

6. _____ The patient tells the pharmacist that he:

a. has fluid in his legs

b. has an abdomen full of water

c. has a lot of fluid in his abdomen and that his legs are swollen

7. _____ The pharmacist tells the patient that:

a. alcohol is not a toxin that is processed through the liver and that it does not do damage to the liver

b. alcohol is a toxin that is processed through the liver and that it does damage to the liver

c. alcohol does not damage the liver

8. _____ The doctor has prescribed the patient to take:

a. two 25-mg tablets once a day in the morning

b. two 25-mg tablets a day: one in the morning and one in the early evening

c. one 25-mg tablet in the evening

9. _____ The patient tells the pharmacist that:

a. he is also taking rifampin to relieve the itching caused by cirrhosis

b. he used to take rifampin to relieve the itching caused by cirrhosis

c. he used to take rifampin to relive the water retention in his body

10. _____ A common side effect of Aldactone is:

a. impotence, and rare side effects include breast enlargement and drowsiness

b. drowsiness, and rare side effects include impotence and breast enlargement

c. breast enlargement, and rare side effects include impotence and drowsiness

11. ____ The pharmacist tells the patient he:

a. should not take rifampin and Aldactone together

b. can take rifampin and Aldactone together

c. should take rifampin in the morning and Aldactone in the evening

12. ____ The patient is allergic to:

a. wasps and bees

b. sulfa and iodine

c. wasps, bees, shellfish, sulfa, and iodine

13. ____The pharmacist tells the patient that people with cirrhosis should avoid:

a. uncooked shellfish, because it contains mercury

b. uncooked shellfish, because it is not always free of bacteria, which is extremely dangerous to people with cirrhosis

c. cooked shellfish

14. ____ The patient tells the pharmacist that he:

a. drinks two cans of beer a week, and the pharmacist tells the patient that that is acceptable

b. has stopped drinking entirely

c. drinks two cans of beer a week and does not drink hard liquor, and the pharmacist tells the patient that he must stop drinking alcohol entirely because his damaged liver can lead to liver disease, a liver transplant, or death

15. ____ The pharmacist tells the patient, who is:

a. 43 years old, to eat a healthy diet, restrict salt intake, not to take Aleve or Motrin, and to stay away from sick people because he is not able to fight infection like healthy people can

b. 28 years old, to eat a healthy diet, restrict intake, and not to take Aleve or Motrin

c. 43 years old, to get the hepatitis A and hepatitis B vaccine

Check your answers in the Answer Key online. How did you do? Are there new words you do not know? Take the time now to look them up in your bilingual or first-language dictionary.

 Dialogue #2

Listen to Dialogue #2, stop, listen again and take notes. Listen to the dialogue as many times as you need or until you feel you have written sufficient notes and feel confident. You can use your notes to answer the multiple choice questions at the end of the dialogue.

Notes _____

_____

_____

_____

_____

Answer the questions below by selecting the answer that correctly completes each sentence.

1. ____ The patient's name is:

a. Mustafa Pasdar, and the pharmacist's name is Samantha Duffy

b. Samantha Pasdar, and the pharmacist's name is Mustafa Duffy

c. Samantha Duffy, and the pharmacist's name is Mustafa Pasdar

2. ____ The patient is in a:

a. hospital

b. clinic

c. retail pharmacy

3. ____ The patient is:

a. 25 and her date of birth is May 14, 1982

b. 25 and her date of birth is May 14, 1992

c. 25 and her date of birth is May 4, 1982

4. ____ The patient's has been diagnosed with:

a. hepatitis B

b. chronic hepatitis

c. hepatitis C

5. ____ The patient's doctor is:

a. Dr. Len Whitman, and he has prescribed Hepsera

b. Dr. Ben Winman, and he has prescribed Hepsera

c. Dr. Ben Whitman, and he has prescribed Hepsera

6. _____ The medication prescribed to the patient will:

a. cure the virus

b. slow down the virus

c. slow down the virus and eventually cure it

7. _____ The patient contracted the virus through:

a. sharing of contaminated needles

b. protected sex

c. unprotected sex with an infected person

8. _____ The patient's symptoms included:

a. pain around the abdomen, dark urine, and yellowing of the skin and whites of the eyes

b. jaundice

c. pain around the abdomen, dark urine, yellowing of the skin and whites of the eyes, and itchy skin

9. _____ The doctor prescribed that the patient take the medication:

a. once a day with food

b. twice a day with or without food

c. once a day with or without food

10. _____ The pharmacist tells the patient that:

a. her condition cannot be spread to others

b. she needs to prevent spreading the infection to others

c. she will infect only some people

11. _____ The pharmacist tells the patient that:

a. discontinuing the medication will not make her condition worse and that side effects of the medication include headaches, fever, weakness, and diarrhea

b. discontinuing the medication could make her condition worse but that the medication has no serious side effects

c. discontinuing the medication could make her condition worse, that side effects of the medication include headaches, fever, weakness, and diarrhea, and that serious side effects include rash, swelling, and a change in urine amount

12. _____ The pharmacist tells the patient that it is:

a. important that she keep her doctor's appointments, and that if the infection lasts more than 6 months, she has acute hepatitis and that the infection will not clear up

b. important that she keep her doctor's appointments, and that if the infection lasts more than 6 months, she has chronic hepatitis B and that her body will not be able fight the infection

c. not important that she keep her doctor's appointments if her infection lasts less than 6 months

13. _____ When the patient says, "This just boggles the mind," she means that:

a. what the pharmacist is telling her is confusing

b. the infection has made her confused

c. she finds her condition confusing and difficult to accept

14. _____ The pharmacist tells the patient:

a. that it is very important to protect her partners from the virus and to protect them from exposure to blood, saliva, and vaginal secretions, and that her partners wear a condom for vaginal and anal sex and that both partners wear dental condoms for oral sex

b. that it is very important to protect her partners from the virus by avoiding blood contact

c. to stop having sexual intercourse for 6 months

15. _____ The pharmacist tells the patient:

a. not to share syringes and needles, to eat a healthy diet of whole grains, protein, fruits, and vegetables, and that not taking care of her infection can lead to cirrhosis of the liver, liver damage, and liver cancer

b. not to share syringes and needles, to eat a healthy diet of whole grains, protein, fruits, and vegetables, and that not taking care of her infection can lead to hepatitis A and hepatitis C

c. not to share syringes and needles and that not eating a healthy diet of whole grains, proteins, fruits, and vegetables can lead to autoimmune hepatitis

Check your answers in the Answer Key online. How did you do? Are there new words you do not know? Take the time now to look them up in your bilingual or first-language dictionary.

IDIOMATIC EXPRESSIONS

Idioms and idiomatic expressions are made up of a group of words that have a different meaning from the original meaning of each individual word. Native speakers of the English language use such expressions comfortably and naturally. However, individuals who are new speakers of English or who have studied English for many years may still not be able to use idioms and idiomatic expressions as comfortably or naturally as native speakers. As pharmacy students, pharmacy technicians, and practicing pharmacists, you will hear many different idiomatic expressions. Some of you will understand and know how to use these expressions correctly. At times, however, you may not understand what your professors, colleagues, and patients are saying. This of course can lead to miscommunication, embarrassment, and possibly dangerous mistakes.

Unlike the previous chapters that contain idioms and expressions with words related to the chapter theme, there are no idioms or expressions that contain words related to the hepatic system. However, there is one idiomatic expression using the word "liver." For example, "What am I, chopped liver?" means "Why are you ignoring me?" or "Don't ignore me." The term "chopped liver" also has a second meaning and refers to a food made of cooked chicken liver that is chopped up and mixed with chopped eggs and onions.

POST-ASSESSMENT

True/False Questions

Indicate whether each sentence below is true (T) or false (F).

1. _____ **Hepatitis A** is contracted through contaminated needles.

2. _____ The adjective of **cirrhosis** is cirrhotic.

3. _____ **Hepatitis C** is a viral infection in which the body attacks itself.

4. _____ The words **transplant** and **transplantation** are nouns.

5. _____ Yellowing of the whites of the eyes and skin, anemia, and itching are symptoms of **hepatitis B.**

6. _____ **Chronic hepatitis B** is caused by cirrhosis.

7. _____ One way to contract **hepatitis C** is through contaminated tattooing and body piercing needles.

8. _____ Another term for scarring of the liver is **autoimmune hepatitis.**

9. _____ Dark urine, jaundice, loss of appetite, vomiting, and abdominal pain are symptoms of **hepatitis A.**

10. _____ A low-grade fever, loss of appetite, vomiting, and abdominal pain are symptoms of **hepatitis A.**

11. _____ Another term for enlarged veins is **varices.**

12. _____ People infected with **autoimmune hepatitis** cannot share razors and toothbrushes.

13. _____ **Autoimmune hepatitis** can lead to hepatitis B.

14. _____ **Hepatitis B** can be contracted through casual contact such as hand shaking.

15. _____ **Hepatic encephalopathy** is caused by hepatitis A.

Multiple Choice Questions

Choose the correct answer from a, b, and c.

1. _____ The word **alcoholic** is:

a. a noun

b. an adjective and a noun

c. a verb

2. _____ A person suffering from **hepatitis B** should:

a. drink plenty of water

b. not share toothbrushes and razors with others

c. avoid casual contact with others

3. _____ Pernicious anemia and hemolytic anemia can be triggered by:

a. autoimmune hepatitis

b. hepatitis A

c. hepatitis B and hepatitis C

4. _____ Alternative medicines such as herb milk thistle are believed to heal:

a. autoimmune hepatitis

b. the liver of people suffering from cirrhosis

c. the liver of people suffering from hepatitis A

5. _____ In this sentence, "Hepatitis A is most contagious before signs and symptoms appear," the word **contagious** is:

a. a verb and a noun

b. an adjective

c. a noun

6. _____ Hepsera is used to:

a. cure the hepatitis B virus

b. slow down the hepatitis A virus

c. slow down the hepatitis B virus

7. _____ Aldactone is used to:

a. treat water retention caused by cirrhosis

b. treat water retention caused by the hepatitis B virus

c. slow down the hepatitis B virus

8. _____ Impairment of the brain as a result of toxic substances that accumulate in the blood is caused by:

a. autoimmune hepatitis

b. hepatic encephalopathy

c. cirrhosis

9. _____ The word **toxicity** is a:

a. verb and a noun

b. verb only

c. noun only

10. _____ In the sentence, "Alcohol and chronic viral hepatitis are two causes of cirrhosis," the word **chronic** is:

a. an adjective and viral is a noun

b. an adjective and viral is an adjective

c. a noun and viral is a noun

11. _____ **Hepatitis A** is contracted through:

a. unprotected sex

b. contaminated food, water, and feces

c. accidental needlesticks

12. _____ A person with **cirrhosis:**

a. can drink alcohol in moderation

b. should constantly wash his or her hands

c. should not drink alcohol

13. _____ **Autoimmune hepatitis** can lead to:

a. hepatitis B

b. diseases such as type II diabetes and Hashimoto's thyroiditis

c. hepatitis C

14. _____ The word **contaminant** is:

a. a verb and the word contamination is a noun

b. a noun and the word contamination is a noun

b. an adjective and the word contamination is a noun

15. _____ In the sentence, "It's very important for people infected with hepatitis A, which is very contagious, to wash their hands," the word **contagious** is:

a. an adjective

b. a past tense verb

c. a noun

Listening and Comprehension Exercises

Dialogue #1

Listen to Dialogue #1, stop, listen again and take notes. Listen to the dialogue as many times as you need or until you feel you have written sufficient notes and feel confident. You can use your notes to answer the multiple choice questions at the end of the dialogue.

Notes _____

_____

_____

_____

_____

Answer the questions below by selecting the answer that correctly completes each sentence.

1. _____ The pharmacist's name is:

a. James Arroyo, and the patient's name is Fela Richter

b. Fela Arroyo, and the patient's name is James Richter

c. Fela Arroyo, and the patient's name is James Rickter

Noun (n)	Infinitive/Verb (v)— Past Tense	Adjective (adj)	Adverb (adv)
sex		sexual	sexually
syndrome		syndromic	
syphilis		syphilitic	
testicle		testicular	
transmission	to transmit; transmitted		
uterus		uterine	
vagina; vaginitis		vaginal	vaginally
yeast; yeastiness		yeasty	yeastily

Word Forms Exercise

Read the following sentences carefully. Then indicate the word form of the bolded word(s), choosing from v, n, adj, or adv.

1. **Untreated pelvic** inflammatory disease (PID), which is caused by sexually transmitted diseases such as gonorrhea and chlamydia, can damage **reproductive** organs as a result of infected fluid that collects in the **fallopian tubes** and **scarring.**

   untreated _____ pelvic _____ reproductive _____ fallopian tubes _____ scarring _____

2. Many **females** will experience a **yeast infection,** a type of **vaginitis,** which is caused **naturally** by *Candida*, a **fungus.**

   females _____ yeast infection _____ vaginitis _____ naturally _____ fungus _____

3. Men who suffer from **erectile dysfunction,** also known as **impotence,** may experience the **inability** to occasionally achieve an **erection,** the inability to have a **full** erection, or the inability to maintain an erection during intercourse.

   erectile dysfunction _____ impotence _____ inability _____ erection _____ full _____

4. Symptoms of **gonorrhea,** also known as "the clap," a highly contagious **sexually** transmitted disease or **STD** that affects both men and women, include a thick **vaginal** or **penile discharge** and a burning sensation when urinating.

   gonorrhea _____ sexually _____ STD _____ vaginal _____ penile _____ discharge _____

5. An uncomfortable and embarrassing symptom of **menopause** is **hot flashes,** which are characterized by a **flushed, blotchy,** red face and skin, a feeling of **warmth** through the upper body and face, and **sweat** on the upper body.

   menopause _____ hot flashes _____ flushed _____ blotchy _____ warmth _____
   sweat _____

6. Some mothers who are **lactating,** or breast-feeding their babies, will develop **mastitis,** which is inflammation of the **breast** tissue caused by bacteria that enters the breast tissue through a **crack** in the skin of the **nipple** or through the **milk duct.**

   lactating _____ mastitis _____ breast _____ crack _____ nipple _____ milk duct _____

7. Primary **amenorrhea refers** to lack of **menstruation** by the age of 16, and **secondary** amenorrhea refers to **lack** of menstruation for more than 6 months.

   amenorrhea _____ refers _____ menstruation _____ secondary _____ lack _____

8. Signs of an **ectopic** pregnancy, in which the **fertilized** egg **implants** itself outside the uterus, are abnormal **vaginal** bleeding, **pelvic** pain in the lower part of the **pelvis,** and feeling faint and dizzy.

   ectopic _____ fertilized _____ implants _____ vaginal _____ pelvic _____ pelvis _____

9. **Dysmenorrhea** is the term that refers to painful **menstrual cramps,** which are characterized by **painful** lower **abdominal** pain accompanied by nausea, vomiting, and loose **stool.**

   dysmenorrhea _____   menstrual _____   cramps _____   painful _____   abdominal _____
   stool _____

10. Most women in **perimenopause,** which is the years leading to menopause, will experience a variety symptoms that include **irregular** periods, heavy **bleeding** during periods, hot flashes, mood changes, **vaginal** dryness, and **urinary** incontinence.

    perimenopause _____   irregular _____   bleeding _____   vaginal _____   urinary _____

11. Causes of male **infertility** include, but are not limited to, **impaired** shape and impaired movement of the **sperm,** a low sperm **count, testosterone** deficiency, and sexually transmitted diseases such as gonorrhea and **chlamydia.**

    infertility _____   impaired _____   sperm _____   count _____   testosterone _____
    chlamydia _____

12. The use of latex **condoms** during **sexual** intercourse reduces the risk of **contracting sexually** transmitted infections such as gonorrhea and chlamydia and preventing the transmission of the HIV virus by **blocking** the **exchange** of bodily fluids.

    condoms _____   sexual _____   contracting _____   sexually _____   blocking _____
    exchange _____

13. Symptoms of **polycystic** ovary syndrome, a **hormonal** disorder, include no **menstruation** or **irregular** menstruation, **excessive** hair growth on the face, chest, and other parts of the body, and **multiple** cysts on the ovaries.

    polycystic _____   hormonal _____   menstruation _____   irregular _____
    excessive _____   multiple _____

14. The morning-after pill, also referred to as emergency **contraception,** is a **birth control** pill taken to **prevent** pregnancy after **unprotected** or **unwanted** sex has occurred.

    contraception _____   birth control _____   prevent _____   unprotected _____
    unwanted _____

15. Women whose **cervical** cancer has **progressed** will experience **pelvic** pain and pain during intercourse, have **vaginal** bleeding between periods and during menopause, and have a **foul,** bloody vaginal **discharge.**

    cervical _____   progressed _____   pelvic _____   vaginal _____   foul _____
    discharge _____

How did you do? Check your answers against the Answer Key online.

Typical Medical Conditions and Patient Complaints

The sentences below contain vocabulary that describes and explains typical medical conditions, diseases, symptoms, and patient complaints that a pharmacist encounters. Read the sentences carefully. Then indicate the word form of the bolded word(s), choosing from v, n, adj, or adv. Look up words you do not know in your bilingual or first-language dictionary.

1. Symptoms of **testicular** cancer, which is highly **treatable** when **diagnosed** early, include discomfort or pain in the **testicle** or **scrotum,** a lump or **enlargement** in either testicle, and fatigue.

   testicular _____   treatable _____   diagnosed _____   testicle _____   scrotum _____
   enlargement _____

2. Complications of **untreated** pelvic inflammatory disease—whose symptoms include pelvic pain, heavy vaginal discharge with a foul odor, and pain during intercourse—include **infertility, ectopic** pregnancy, which can cause life-threatening **bleeding,** and **chronic** pelvic pain.

   untreated _____   infertility _____   ectopic _____   bleeding _____   chronic _____

3. **Endometriosis,** a painful **reproductive** disease in which tissue that normally lines the inside of the **uterus** implants itself in the **fallopian** tubes, ovaries, and in the tissue lining of the **pelvis,** can interfere with conception and lead to impaired **fertility.**

endometriosis _____   reproductive _____   uterus _____   fallopian _____   pelvis _____
fertility _____

4. Substance **abuse,** certain **medical** conditions such as heart disease and diabetes, certain **medications,** and stress and anxiety are **risk factors** for developing **erectile** dysfunction, or ED.

abuse _____   medical _____   medications _____   risk factors _____   erectile _____

5. After menopause, some women may develop **atrophic vaginitis,** a condition that is caused by **low estrogen levels** and characterized by **vaginal** burning, itching, or pain.

atrophic _____   vaginitis _____   low estrogen _____   levels _____   vaginal _____

6. **Cervicitis** is inflammation of the **cervix** caused by viruses and bacteria transmitted by **STDs** such as gonorrhea, chlamydia, **genital** herpes, and genital **warts** and can lead to **pelvic** inflammatory disease (PID).

cervicitis _____   cervix _____   STDs _____   genital _____   warts _____   pelvic _____

7. **Hormonal** imbalance, stress, too much **exercise,** low body **weight,** certain medications, a thyroid condition, **contraceptives,** and pregnancy can cause **amenorrhea.**

hormonal _____   exercise _____   weight _____   contraceptives _____   amenorrhea _____

8. Symptoms of **menopause,** which occurs when a woman has not had a **period** for 12 months, include **night sweats,** irregular periods, decreased **fertility, vaginal** dryness, urinary incontinence, irritability, and weight gain.

menopause _____   period _____   night sweats _____   fertility _____   vaginal _____

9. Women who experience **adenomyosis** during menstruation will experience **prolonged** and heavy bleeding, severe and **sharp cramps,** and **pass blood clots.**

adenomyosis _____   prolonged _____   sharp _____   cramps _____   pass _____
blood clots _____

10. In men, **gonorrhea** can lead to **infertility;** in women, it can lead to PID and other complications such as **ectopic** pregnancy, **transmission** to the child during pregnancy, and infertility; and in both men and women gonorrhea can spread to the **anal** area, the mouth and throat, and eyes.

gonorrhea _____   infertility _____   ectopic _____   transmission _____   anal _____

11. While **tender** breasts, **mood swings,** food cravings, and irritability a few days before a woman gets her period are typical symptoms of **premenstrual** syndrome (**PMS**), more **persistent** sadness, depression, anger, anxiety, loss of control, and overeating or lack of appetite are typical symptoms of premenstrual dysphoric disorder (**PMDD**), which is a more severe form of PMS.

tender _____   mood swings _____   premenstrual _____   PMS _____   persistent _____
PMDD _____

12. **HPV,** or human papillomavirus, infection is transmitted through sexual contact, and symptoms of sexually contracted HPV in females are **genital warts** that can **appear** in the vulva, cervix, vagina, and near the anus; and in males the warts can appear in the scrotum, **penis,** and around the anus.

HPV _____   genital _____   warts _____   appear _____   penis _____

13. A **hysterectomy** might be a good option for women who suffer from **cervical** or **uterine** cancer, endometriosis, uterine fibroids that cause heavy **bleeding,** and who suffer from persistent bleeding during periods when **non-surgical** methods have not been successful.

hysterectomy _____   cervical _____   uterine _____   bleeding _____
non-surgical _____

14. **Premature ovarian failure,** which is used to refer to a woman's **ovaries' inability** to function before age 40, can lead to infertility, osteoporosis, and depression.

premature _____ ovarian _____ failure _____ ovaries' _____ inability _____

15. Signs of **endometrial** cancer, also known as **uterine** cancer, include prolonged periods, bleeding between periods, a **watery,** pink **vaginal** discharge, and more **frequent** spotting during the perimenopause years.

endometrial _____ uterine _____ watery _____ vaginal _____ frequent _____

16. A woman with an **ovarian** cyst may experience **irregular** periods, pelvic pain, pain during **intercourse,** breast **tenderness** as though she were **pregnant, fullness** in the abdomen, pressure in the bladder and rectum, nausea, and vomiting.

ovarian _____ irregular _____ intercourse _____ tenderness _____ pregnant _____ fullness _____

17. The symptoms of **genital herpes,** also known as herpes simplex virus 2, a highly **contagious** STD that has no **cure,** include **itching** around the **genital** area and buttocks, and small red bumps and **blisters** in the genital area.

genital herpes _____ contagious _____ cure _____ itching _____ genital _____ blisters _____

18. A **complication** of prolonged and heavy **menstrual** bleeding, known as **menorrhagia,** is **anemia,** which results from iron **deficiency.**

complication _____ menstrual _____ menorrhagia _____ anemia _____ deficiency _____

19. Signs of **ovarian** cancer, which mimic symptoms of bladder and **digestive** disorders, include **bloating, urinary** urgency, nausea and gas, diarrhea, constipation, lack of appetite, pain during sexual intercourse, and **increased waist** size.

ovarian _____ digestive _____ bloating _____ urinary _____ increased _____ waist _____

20. To help increase the performance of **sperm,** men should **watch** their weight, **exercise,** and avoid tobacco, alcohol, **recreational** drugs, steroids, and testosterone **supplements.**

sperm _____ watch _____ exercise _____ recreational _____ supplements _____

How did you do? Check your answers against the Answer Key online.

Medical Vocabulary Comprehension

Now that you have read sentences 1 through 20 describing language regarding the reproductive system, assess your understanding by doing the exercises below.

Multiple Choice Questions

Choose the answer that correctly completes each sentence below.

1. _____ A disease that if left untreated can damage the fallopian tubes is:
a. vaginitis
b. pelvic inflammatory disease
c. cervicitis

2. _____ **Menorrhagia** is:
a. absence of menstruation
b. prolonged and heavy bleeding during menstruation
c. painful intercourse

3. _____ Human papillomavirus (HPV) infects:
a. the penis and scrotum only

b. the vagina and anus only

c. the cervix, vulva, vagina, penis, scrotum, and anal area

4. _____ Persistent sadness, depression, anger and anxiety, loss of control, and overeating or lack of appetite are typical symptoms of:

a. premenstrual syndrome (PMS)

b. hot flashes

c. premenstrual dysphoric disorder (PMDD)

5. _____ Risk factors for **erectile dysfunction** include:

a. stress and certain medical conditions such as heart disease and diabetes

b. impotence

c. penile discharge

6. _____ **Cervicitis** is caused by:

a. viruses and bacteria transmitted by STDs

b. infertility

c. a hormonal disorder

7. _____ Characteristics of **perimenopause** include:

a. regular periods and normal bleeding

b. irregular periods, heavy bleeding, and hot flashes

c. premature ovarian failure

8. _____ **Genital herpes** is:

a. a highly contagious STD that has a cure

b. a highly contagious disease with no cure that causes itching and red bumps and blisters around the genital area of men only

c. a highly contagious disease with no cure that causes itching and red bumps and blisters around the genital area of both men and women

9. _____ **Amenorrhea** refers to:

a. absence of menstruation

b. painful cramps during menstruation

c. pain during sexual intercourse

10. _____ Avoiding tobacco, alcohol, recreational drugs, steroids, and testosterone supplements can help a man:

a. avoid STDs

b. increase sperm performance

c. treat genital warts

11. _____ Bloating, increased waist size, and urinary urgency are symptoms of:

a. PMS

b. PID

c. ovarian cancer

12. _____ A complication of **menorrhagia** is:

a. absence of periods

b. anemia

c. infertility

13. _____ Irregular periods, breast tenderness, pain during intercourse, and pressure in the bladder and rectum are some symptoms of:

a. ovarian cyst

b. cervicitis

c. endometriosis

14. _____ The condition in which women experience prolonged and heavy bleeding, severe and sharp cramps, and pass blood clots is called:

a. dyspareunia

b. menorrhagia

c. adenomyosis

15. _____ Another term for **gonorrhea** is:

a. the snap

b. the clap

c. scabies

True/False Questions

Indicate whether each sentence below is true (T) or false (F).

1. _____ **Genital herpes** is a highly contagious STD that has a cure.

2. _____ A **hysterectomy** might be a good option for women who suffer from uterine fibroids that cause heavy bleeding, from cervical and uterine cancer, and from endometriosis.

3. _____ **Premature ovarian failure** can lead to pelvic inflammatory disease.

4. _____ **Erectile dysfunction** can lead to testicular cancer.

5. _____ **Atrophic vaginitis** is a condition that is by caused by low estrogen levels and characterized by vaginal burning, itching, or pain.

6. _____ The word **"menopausal"** is a noun.

7. _____ **Endometriosis** does not interfere with conception and does not lead to infertility.

8. _____ Another term for emergency contraception is the **morning-after pill.**

9. _____ A **yeast infection** is a type of STD that is caused by the *Candida* fungus.

10. _____ Discomfort or pain in the testicle or scrotum, a lump or enlargement in either testicle, and fatigue are signs of **testicular cancer.**

How did you do? Check your answers against the Answer Key online.

Writing Exercise

An important part of communication is the ability to write about what you read, to write correctly, and to spell correctly. In the exercises below, write your understanding of the meaning of the bolded words.

1. Describe in writing what **pelvic inflammatory disease** is.

_____

_____

_____

_____

2. Describe in writing what **erectile dysfunction** is.

_____

_____

_____

_____

3. Describe in writing what **amenorrhea, menorrhagia, dysmenorrhea, and adenomyosis** are.

_____

_____

_____

_____

4. Describe in writing what **perimenopause** and **menopause** are.

_____

_____

_____

_____

5. Describe in writing what **gonorrhea, genital herpes,** and **human papillomavirus** are.

_____

_____

_____

_____

Check what you have written with acceptable answers that appear in the Answer Key online.

LISTENING AND PRONUNCIATION

The ability to listen and understand what is being said and heard, and the ability to pronounce words clearly, is extremely important. A word misheard and a word mispronounced will lead to poor communication and can seriously put both the pharmacist and patient in danger. Therefore, it is very important that one hear clearly what another person has said, and that one speak clearly with correct pronunciation.

Listen carefully to the pharmacy-related words presented in the audio files found in Chapter 12 on thePoint (thePoint.lww.com/diaz-gilbert), and then pronounce them as accurately as you can. Listen and then repeat. You will listen to each word once and then you will repeat it. You will do this twice for each word. Listening and pronunciation practice will increase your listening and speaking confidence. Many languages do not produce or emphasize certain sounds produced and emphasized in English, so pay careful attention to the pronunciation of each word.

Pronunciation Exercise

Listen to the audio files found in Chapter 12 on thePoint (thePoint.lww.com/diaz-gilbert). Listen and repeat the words. Then say the words aloud for additional practice.

1. adenomyosis   ăd′n-ō-mī-ō′sĭs
2. amenorrhea   ā-mĕn′ə-rē′ə
3. atrophic vaginitis   ā-trŏf′ĭk văj′ə-nī′tĭs
4. bacterial vaginosis   băk-tîr′ē-əl văj′ə-nō′sĭs
5. birth control   bûrth kən-trōl′
6. bloated   blō′tĭd
7. breast lump   brĕst lŭmp
8. cervix   sûr′vĭks
9. condom   kŏn′dəm
10. contraceptive   kŏn′trə-sĕp′tĭv
11. cramps   krămps
12. cyst   sĭst
13. diaphragm   dī′ə-frăm
14. douche   dōōsh
15. dysmenorrhea   dĭs-mĕn′ə-rē′ə
16. dyspareunia   dĭspĕru niēə
17. early menarche   ûr′lē mə-när′kē
18. ectopic pregnancy   ĕk-tō′p′ĭk prĕg′nən-sē
19. ejaculation   ĭ-jăk′yə-lā′shən
20. endometriosis   ĕn′dō-mē′trē-ō′sĭs

21. erectile dysfunction   ĭ-rĕk′tǝl, -tīl′ dĭs-fŭngk′shǝn
22. fallopian tube   fǝ-lō′pē-ǝn to͞ob
23. fertile   fûr′tl
24. fibrocystic breasts   fī′brō-sĭs′tĭk brĕsts
25. fibroids   fī′broids′
26. foul odor   foul ō′dǝr
27. frothy discharge   frô′thē dĭs-chärj
28. gonorrhea   gŏn′ǝ-rē′ǝ
29. hormone   hôr′mōn
30. hot flash   hŏt flăsh
31. hysterectomy   hĭs′tǝ-rĕk′tǝ-mē
32. infertility   ĭn′fǝr-tĭl′ĭ-tē
33. inseminate   ĭn-sĕm′ǝ-nāt
34. intercourse   ĭn′tǝr-kôrs
35. intrauterine device   ĭn′trǝ-yo͞o′tǝr-ĭn dĭ-vīs
36. lactation   lăk-tā′shǝn
37. lumpectomy   lŭm-pĕk′tǝ-mē
38. mastectomy   mă-stĕk′tǝ-mē
39. mastitis   mă-stī′tĭs
40. menopause   mĕn′ǝ-pôz
41. menorrhagia   mĕn′ǝ-rā′jē-ǝ
42. menses   mĕn′sēz
43. menstruation   mĕn′stro͞o-ā′shǝn
44. miscarriage   mĭs′kăr′ĭj
45. mittelschmerz   mĭtl ʃmɛǝrts
46. nipple   nĭp′ǝl
47. ovary   ō′vǝ-rē
48. ovulate   ō′vyǝ-lāt
49. Pap smear   păp smîr
50. pelvic inflammatory disease   pĕl′vĭk ĭn-flăm′ǝ-tôr′ē dĭ-zēz
51. pelvis   pĕl′vĭs
52. penis   pē′nĭs
53. perimenopause   pîr′ēmĕn′ǝ-pôz
54. polycystic ovarian syndrome   pŏl′ē-sĭs′tĭk ō-vâr′ē-ǝn sĭn′drōm
55. postpartum   pōst-pär′tǝm
56. premenstrual syndrome   prē-mĕn′stro͞o-ǝl sĭn′drōm′
57. progesterone   prō-jĕs′tǝ-rōn′
58. scabies   skā′bēz
59. scrotum   skrō′tǝm
60. semen   sē′mǝn
61. seminal fluid   sĕm′ǝ-nǝl flo͞o′ĭd
62. sexually transmitted disease   sĕk′sho͞o-ǝllē trăns-mĭtĕd dĭ-zēz′
63. sexually transmitted infection   sĕk′sho͞o-ǝllē trăns-mĭtĕd ĭn-fĕk′shǝn
64. sperm   spûrm
65. spermicide   spûr′mĭ-sīd
66. syphilis   sĭf′ǝ-lĭs
67. testicle   tĕs′tĭ-kǝl
68. testosterone   tĕs-tŏs′tǝ-rōn
69. toxic shock syndrome   tŏk′sĭk shŏk sĭn′drōm
70. uterine fibroid   yo͞o′tǝr-ĭn fī′broid
71. vaginitis   văj′ǝ-nī′tĭs

72. venereal disease   və-nîr′ē-əl dĭ-zēz

73. yeast infection   yēst ĭn-fĕk′shən

Which words are easy to pronounce? Which are difficult to pronounce? Use the space below to write in the words that you find difficult to pronounce. These are words you should practice saying often.

_____

_____

_____

_____

_____

_____

_____

Listen to the audio files found in Chapter 12 on thePoint (thePoint.lww.com/diaz-gilbert) as many times as you need to increase your pronunciation ability of the difficult words. Pronounce these words with a friend or a colleague who speaks English.

English Sounds That Are Difficult for Speakers of Other Languages to Pronounce

Spanish

In Spanish there is no English "v" sound, but the "v" consonant in Spanish is pronounced like the English "b." The vowel "i" is pronounced like a long "e." Pay careful attention to the "v" sound in English when pronouncing words that begin with "v." Also pay careful attention to English words that begin with "s;" do not use the Spanish "es" sound when pronouncing English words that begin with "s."

For example, in English,

pelvis is not pronounced pelbees

Vietnamese

In Vietnamese, the "t" consonant is pronounced "s," but in English the "t" is pronounced "t" and "s" is pronounced "s." Be careful with English words that begin with "t." In Vietnamese, the "b" consonant is pronounced "p," but in English "p" is pronounced "p" and "b" is pronounced "b."

In Vietnamese, words do not end in "b," "ch," "f," "d," "j," "l," "p," "r," "s," "sh," "v," and "z." In English, words end in these letters. Pay special attention to pronouncing these English sounds. In Vietnamese, there is no "dzh" or "zh" sound, so English words like "judge" (dzh) and "rupture" (zh) will be hard for Vietnamese speakers to pronounce.

For example, in English,

birth control is not pronounced pir contoh

Gujarati

In Gujarati, "v" is pronounced "w," "f" is pronounced "p," "p" is pronounced "f," and "z" is pronounced "j." Short "i" is pronounced long "e," "x" is pronounced "ch," and "th" is pronounced "s." In English, "v" is pronounced "v," "f" is pronounced "f," "z" is pronounced "z" or "s," "j" is pronounced "j," and "x" is pronounced "x." Pay careful attention when pronouncing these sounds.

For example, in English,

fertile is not pronounced pertile

(continued)

Korean

In Korean, the "v" consonant is pronounced "b" and the "f" consonant is pronounced "p." In English, the "v" is pronounced "v," the "f" is pronounced "f," and the "p" is pronounced "p." Pay special attention when pronouncing these sounds.

For example, in English,

vaginitis is not pronounced baginitis

Chinese

In Chinese, the "r" consonant is pronounced "l" or "w," and "b," "d," "g," and "ng" are not pronounced at all. Pay careful attention to English words that begin with "r" because the "r" is not pronounced "l" or "w," and "b," "d," "g," and "ng" are pronounced in English.

For example, in English,

pregnancy is not pronounced prehnehcee

Russian

The "w" consonant is pronounced like a "v" and the "v" sound like a "w." Pay careful attention to the English "th." It is not pronounced "s."

For example, in English,

vaginitis is not pronounced waginitis

DICTATION

Listening/Spelling Exercise: Word and Word Pairs

Listen to the words or word pairs on the audio files found in Chapter 12 on thePoint (thePoint.lww.com/diaz-gilbert) and then write them down on the lines below.

1. _____
2. _____
3. _____
4. _____
5. _____
6. _____
7. _____
8. _____
9. _____
10. _____
11. _____
12. _____
13. _____
14. _____
15. _____

Listening/Spelling Exercise: Sentences

Listen to the sentences on the audio files found in Chapter 12 on thePoint (thePoint.lww.com/diaz-gilbert) and then write them down on the lines below.

become familiar with these different models. These types of documentation seek a variety of information, such as personal patient information, medical history, medication history, allergies and adverse drug reactions, social and family history, and much more. In this chapter, you will also have the opportunity to practice interpreting abbreviations and to read and write pharmacy documentation.

Appropriate pharmacy documentation is very important and critical for obvious reasons. First, you want to provide the best possible care to your patients. Second, you want to prevent potential lawsuits that can result from poor documentation, poor patient care, and errors. Third, you will need to communicate patient information to individuals such as fellow students, professors, pharmacists, other health care professionals, insurance companies, and drug companies.

It is important to be knowledgeable of the various terms, vocabulary words, and abbreviations used in written pharmacy documentation of patient complaints and health and medication concerns. The documentation forms are interrelated. For example, SOAP notes help you to obtain valuable information from a patient who is being assessed and are helpful in making a pharmaceutical care plan for the patient. The pharmaceutical care plan will help the pharmacist to write and document important information, plan treatment goals, monitor outcomes, and record any intervention made. The patient case presentation or patient medical and physical database will help pharmacy students and pharmacists to share knowledge about their patients, to get advice about a patient from pharmacy students and pharmacists, and help pharmacy students to present patient cases to their professors and other pharmacists.

A good command of pharmacy documentation vocabulary and abbreviations is absolutely necessary because pharmacy documentation of patient complaint, history, assessment, patient care, and more is mandatory. As pharmacy students and pharmacists you will be advising and counseling patients. You will assess their general health, their medical and medication history, and the goals, problems with, and outcomes of their drug therapy. You will inform and instruct your patients about their medical conditions and how to use medications properly. You will determine whether the patient will need to change, continue, or discontinue a certain medication.

You may already know many of the vocabulary words and abbreviations in this chapter, but if some words and abbreviations are new to you, pay careful attention to them and make every effort to know their correct spelling, meaning, and pronunciation. It is a good idea to keep a list of new words and abbreviations and to look up these new words in a bilingual dictionary, in a dictionary in your first language, in an English language dictionary, and in a dictionary of abbreviations and acronyms.

Pharmacy Documentation Abbreviations

Patient Information—Personal and Physical

ADR	adverse drug reaction
All	allergies
A&O	alert and oriented
A&O × 1	alert and oriented to person
A&O × 2	alert and oriented to person and place
A&O × 3	alert and oriented to person, place, and time
BF	black female
BM	black male
BMF	black married female
BMM	black married male
BP	blood pressure
BPM, bpm	beats per minute
CC	chief complaint
C/O	complains of
CV	cardiovascular
DD	demographic data
DH	drug history
DOB	date of birth
Dx	diagnosis

ETHO	alcohol
Ext	extremities
F	female
FH	family history
F/U	follow-up
Gen	general appearance
Genit/Rectal	genital/rectal
HO	history of
HPI	history of present illness
Hx	history
ID	identification
Kg	kilogram
Labs	laboratory tests and results
lb	pound
LMP	last menstrual period
M	male
MAR	medication administration record
Meds	medications
MedHx	medication history
MS	musculoskeletal
NKA	no known allergies
NKDA	no known drug allergies
NL	normal
OTC	over the counter
P	pulse, pressure, plan
PE	physical examination
PMD	private medical doctor
PMH	past medical history
PMI	past medical illness
PP	patient profile
PPD	packs per day
PSH	past surgical history
Pt.	patient
R/O	rule out
ROS	review of system
RR	respiration rate
SH	social history
S/P	status post
S/S	signs/symptoms
SQ	subcutaneous
Sx	symptom
T, Temp	temperature
TPR	temperature, pulse, respiration

Tx	treatment
UNK	unknown
VS	vital signs
VSS	vital signs stable
WD	well developed
WDM	white divorced male
WDWN-BF	well-developed, well-nourished black female
WDWN-BM	well-developed, well-nourished black male
WDWN–WF	well-developed, well-nourished white female
WDWN–WM	well-developed, well-nourished white male
WF	white female
WM	white male
WMF	white married female
WMM	white married male
WN	well-nourished
WNL	within normal limits
Wt.	weight
yo	year old

Body Parts

Abd	abdomen
AD	right ear
AS	left ear
AU	each ear
CNS	central nervous system
Cx	cervix
EENT	eyes, ears, nose, throat
HEENT	head, eyes, ears, nose, throat
HR	heart rate
OD	right eye
OS	left eye
OU	both eyes

Symptoms/Signs/Side Effects

CFNS	chills, fever, and night sweats
Cig	cigarettes
CP	chest pain
DOE	dyspnea on exertion
FUO	fever of unknown origin
HA	headache
LBP	lower back pain
NSR	normal sinus rhythm

N&V	nausea and vomiting
N/V/D	nausea/vomiting/diarrhea
PND	paroxysmal nocturnal dyspnea
SOB	shortness of breath

Diseases/Medical Conditions

AD	Alzheimer's disease
AIH	autoimmune hepatitis
ALD	alcoholic liver disease
ALL	acute lymphocytic leukemia
ALS	amyotrophic lateral sclerosis (Lou Gehrig's disease)
AMI	acute myocardial infarction
ANLL	acute non-lymphocytic leukemia
AOM	acute otitis media (middle ear infection)
CA	cancer
CAD	coronary artery disease
CF	cystic fibrosis
CHD	coronary heart disease
CHF	coronary heart failure
COPD	chronic obstructive pulmonary disease
CP	chest pain, cerebral palsy
CV	cardiovascular
CVA	cerebrovascular accident
DI	diabetes insipidus
DJD	degenerative joint disease
DM	diabetes mellitus
DVT	deep venous thrombosis
ED	erectile dysfunction
Fx.	fracture
GE	gastroesophageal/gastroenterology
GERD	gastroesophageal reflux disease
GI	gastrointestinal
GU	gastric ulcer, genitourinary
HAV	hepatitis A virus
HBV	hepatitis B virus
HCV	hepatitis C virus
HD	Hodgkin's disease
HH	hiatal hernia
HPV	human papilloma virus
HSV	herpes simplex virus
HTN	hypertension
IBD	inflammatory bowel disease
IBS	irritable bowel syndrome
IDDM	insulin-dependent diabetes mellitus
IM	infectious mononucleosis

MI	myocardial infarction
MS	multiple sclerosis
NHL	non-Hodgkin's lymphoma
NIDDM	non-insulin-dependent diabetes mellitus
OA	osteoarthritis
PE	pulmonary embolism
PID	pelvic inflammatory disease
PMDD	postmenopausal dysphoric disorder
PMS	premenstrual syndrome
PUD	peptic ulcer disease
PVD	peripheral vascular disease
RA	rheumatoid arthritis
STD	sexually transmitted disease
TB	tuberculosis
TIA	transient ischemic attack
TSS	toxic shock syndrome
UC	ulcerative colitis
URI	upper respiratory infection
UTI	urinary tract infection

Medication

APAP	acetaminophen
ASA	aspirin
ATB	antibiotic
BCP	birth control pill
Nitro	nitroglycerin
NSAID	nonsteroidal anti-inflammatory drug
OC	oral contraceptive
PCN	penicillin
Tyl	Tylenol

Diagnostic Tests

BC	blood culture
Bx	biopsy
CBC	complete blood count
Cx	culture
CXR	chest x-ray
Endo	endoscopy, endotracheal
INR	international normalization ratio

| UA | urinalysis |
| XR | x-ray |

Dosage/Dosage Method

aa	of each
AC	before meals
BID	twice daily
Cap	capsule
Crm	cream
D	day
Gt	drop
H	hour
Hrly	hourly
Hrs	hours
HS	at bedtime
IM	intramuscular
Inj	injection
INH	inhalation
IV	intravenous
mcg	micrograms
mg	milligrams
mos	month
NPO	nothing by mouth
oint	ointment
PC	after meals
pil	pill
po	by mouth
pr	per rectum
prn	as needed
pulv	powder
PV	per vagina
Q	every
q1d	every day
q1w	every week
q4h	every 4 hours
q6h	every 6 hours
QAM	every morning
QPM	every evening
QD	once daily, every day
QH	every hour
QHS	every night at bedtime
QID	four times daily
QM	every morning

QOD	this is no longer an acceptable abbreviation for every other day; you must spell out "every other day"
Qs	up to
qwk	once a week
Rx	prescription
SID	once a day
SC, SQ	subcutaneous
SL	sublingual (beneath the tongue)
Ss	one half
tab	tablet
tsp	teaspoon
TID	three times daily
ud	as directed
ung	ointment
wk	week
×	period of time (e.g., "for five days" = × 5 days)
yr	year

Recommendations

BR	bed rest
D/C	discontinue; discharge
F/U	follow-up

Pharmacy Documentation Abbreviations Exercise

Provide the appropriate abbreviation or definition for the terms below.

1. The abbreviation for **four times daily** is: _____

2. The abbreviation for **every night at bedtime** is: _____

3. The abbreviation for **once a week** is: _____

4. **HPI** means: _____

5. **A&O** means: _____

6. **bpm** means: _____

7. The abbreviation for **musculoskeletal** and **multiple sclerosis** is: _____

8. **VSS** means: _____

9. The abbreviation **WD** means: _____

10. **SID** is the abbreviation for: _____

11. **TPR** is the abbreviation for: _____

12. The abbreviation for **antibiotic** is: _____

13. **AU** is the abbreviation for: _____

14. **PE** is an abbreviation for: _____

15. The abbreviation for **of each** is: _____

Multiple Choice Questions

Choose the correct answer from a, b, and c.

1. _____ The abbreviated sentence, "The Pt.'s DH includes OTC medications and ASA BID," means:

a. The patient's demographic history includes over-the-counter medications and Tylenol twice daily

b. The patient's drug history includes over-the-counter medications and aspirin twice daily

c. The patient's drug history includes over-the-counter medications and two aspirins twice daily

2. _____ The abbreviated sentence, "The Pt. was Dx with DM and instructed how to administer her medication SQ q1d" means:

a. The patient was diagnosed with dementia and instructed how to administer her medication subcutaneously daily

b. The patient was diagnosed with diabetes mellitus and instructed how to administer her medication subcutaneously weekly

c. The patient was diagnosed with diabetes mellitus and instructed how to administer her medication subcutaneously daily

3. _____ The abbreviated sentence, "The WDWN-BF C/O of CFNS" means:

a. The well-developed and well-nourished black female was complaining of chills, fever, and night sweats

b. The well-developed and divorced black female was complaining of chills, fever, and nervousness

c. The well-developed and undernourished black female was complaining of chills, fever, and night sweats

4. _____ The abbreviated sentence, "The 64 yo WM's CC was CP and SOB" means:

a. The 64-year-old white male's chief complaint was chest pain and shortness of breath

b. The 64-year-old white male's cardiology complaint was chest pain and shortness of breath

c. The 64-year-old white male's chief complaint was cerebral palsy and shortness of breath

5. _____ The abbreviated sentence, "Pt.'s MedHx includes 2 puffs of his inhaler for COPD and ADR to iodine" means:

a. the patient's medical history includes 2 puffs of his inhaler for chronic obstructive pulmonary disease and an adverse drug reaction to iodine

b. the patient's medication history includes 2 puffs of his inhaler for chronic obstructive pulmonary disease and an adverse drug reaction to iodine

c. the patient's medication history includes 2 puffs of his inhaler for chronic bronchitis and an adverse drug reaction to iodine

6. _____ The abbreviated sentence, "The Pt. was instructed to F/U in 2 wks to monitor CP, ADR to Nitro-Dur patch, and storage of SL nitro" means:

a. The patient was instructed to follow-up for a period of 2 weeks to monitor chest pain, adverse drug reaction to sublingual nitroglycerin, and to check proper storage of the Nitro-Dur patch

b. The patient was instructed to follow-up in 2 weeks to monitor chest pains, adverse drug reaction to sublingual nitroglycerin, and to check proper storage of the Nitro-Dur patch

c. The patient was instructed to follow-up in 2 weeks to monitor chest pain, adverse drug reaction to the Nitro-Dur patch, and to check proper storage of sublingual nitroglycerin

7. _____ The abbreviated sentence, "The 37 yo WF's C/C of PMS and Sx of abd pain and HA, and she treated it with ibuprofen 400 mg TID" means:

a. The 37-year-old white female's chief complaint of postmenstrual syndrome and symptoms of abdominal pain and hiatal hernia was treated with 400 milligrams of ibuprofen three times daily

b. The 37-year-old white female's chief complaint of premenstrual syndrome and symptoms of abdominal pain and headache was treated with 400 milligrams of ibuprofen three times daily

c. The 37-year-old white female's chief complaint of premenstrual syndrome and symptoms of abdominal pain and headache was treated with 40 milligrams of ibuprofen four times daily

8. _____ The abbreviated sentence, "The 21 yo WDWN-WM with HO GERD and asthma C/O pain in AS and was taking Tyl po prn" means:

a. The 21-year-old well-developed, well-nourished white male with a history of gastrointestinal reflux disease and asthma complained of pain in his left ear and was taking Tylenol by mouth as needed

b. The 21-year-old white, divorced, well-nourished male with a history of gastrointestinal reflux disease and asthma complained of pain in his right ear and was taking Tylenol by mouth as needed

c. The 21-year-old well-developed, well-nourished white male with a history of gastrointestinal reflux disease and asthma complained of pain in both ears and was taking Tylenol by mouth as needed

9. _____ The abbreviated sentence, "The Pt.'s MedHx includes Flexeril 10 mg TID for LBP and muscle spasms, and Captopril 25mg BID for HTN" means:

a. The patient's medication history includes 10 milligrams of Flexeril three times daily for lower back pain and muscle spasms, and 20 milligrams Captopril twice daily for hypertension

b. The patient's medication history includes 25 milligrams of Flexeril three times daily for lower back pain and muscle spasms, and 10 milligrams Captopril twice daily for hypertension

c. The patient's medical history includes 10 milligrams of Flexeril twice daily for lower back pain and muscle spasms, and 20 milligrams Captopril three times daily for hypertension

10. _____ The abbreviated sentence, "The 69 yo WF has Hx glaucoma OU and cataracts OD, and was Dx with OA 5 days ago after XR revealed left hip Fx." means:

a. The 69-year-old white female has a history of right eye glaucoma and cataracts in both eyes and was diagnosed with osteoarthritis 5 days ago after x-ray revealed a left hip fracture

b. The 69-year-old white female with a history of glaucoma in both eyes and right eye cataracts was diagnosed with osteoarthritis for a period of 5 days after x-ray revealed a left hip fracture

c. The 69-year-old white female with a history of glaucoma in both eyes and right eye cataracts was diagnosed with osteoarthritis 5 days ago after x-ray revealed a left hip fracture

How did you do? Check your answers against the Answer Key online.

Pharmacy and Medical Abbreviations Exercise

Read the following sentences carefully. Then write in the abbreviation of the bolded words on the lines provided.

1. The 41-**year-old female** patient is **complaining** that she is feeling fatigued, tired, and cold all the time. She began taking 50 mcg of Levoxyl **once a day** three weeks ago. She is currently on **birth control pills.**

   year-old _____   female _____   complaining _____   once a day _____   birth control pills _____

2. A 26-year-old **male patient** complains of heartburn and feeling dizzy. He states he has **tuberculosis** and is taking rifampin capsules 2 hours **before meals.** He has **no known allergies to drugs** but is **allergic** to latex.

   male _____   patient _____   tuberculosis _____   before meals _____   no known allergies to drugs _____   allergic _____

3. The patient has a **history of hypertension** and chronic bronchitis. Her **chief complaint** today is **chest pain** and **shortness of breath.**

   history of _____   hypertension _____   chief complaint _____   chest pain _____   shortness of breath _____

4. A 54-year-old man complains of dizziness and frequent urination at night. He is currently taking 40 **milligrams** of valsartan **twice daily by mouth** to treat **congestive heart failure** and 20 milligrams of Lasix **once daily** by mouth to treat edema in his legs.

   milligrams _____   twice daily _____   by mouth _____   congestive heart failure _____   once daily _____

5. A 35-year-old woman has a **history of pelvic inflammatory disease.** Her **chief complaint** today is severe cramping, fainting, and dizziness after taking tegaserod **twice daily before meals** for 2 days to treat her **irritable bowel syndrome.**

history of _____   pelvic inflammatory disease _____   chief complaint _____
twice daily _____   before meals _____   irritable bowel syndrome _____

6. The patient is **complaining of** mouth sores, a persistent cough, and black stools. These **symptoms** could be the side effects of Rheumatrex. He was recently **diagnosed** with ankylosing spondylitis. The patient also suffers from **chronic obstructive pulmonary disease** and chronic bronchitis. He has an Atrovent inhaler and takes two to four **inhalations every day twice a day.**

complaining of _____   symptoms _____   diagnosed _____   chronic obstructive
pulmonary disease _____   inhalations _____   every day twice a day _____

7. A **16-year-old girl** recently diagnosed with epilepsy and grand mal seizures **complains of nausea, vomiting, diarrhea,** and fatigue. She is presently taking **one Dulcolax tablet daily. Allergies** include Ceclor and cats.

16-year-old girl _____   complains of _____   nausea, vomiting, and diarrhea _____
one Dulcolax tablet daily _____   allergies _____

8. A 60-year-old man is **complaining of** constipation. He has a **history of** constipation and takes Metamucil, but the Metamucil is not working as effectively as he would like. He suffers from Parkinson's disease and is currently taking a **5-milligram capsule of Eldepryl twice a day, one with breakfast and one with lunch.**

complaining of _____   history of _____   5-milligram capsule of Eldepryl twice a day,
one with breakfast and one with lunch _____

9. An 18-year-old woman is complaining of a rash on her legs and arms. She states she woke up this morning with the rash. She has **no known drug allergies,** but is allergic to tomatoes. She began taking Macrodantin 7 days ago to treat her first **urinary tract infection.** She was taking one **100-milligram Macrodantin capsule four times a day,** one capsule **every 6 hours.** She has a **history of** exercise-induced asthma but has not had an asthma attack in a long time and is not taking an asthma medication.

no known drug allergies _____   urinary tract infection _____   100-milligram Macrodantin capsule four times a day _____   every 6 hours _____   history of _____

10. The patient is complaining that he has been having **lower back pain** for about a week. He has also been feeling dizzy and having some diarrhea. He has a **history of** depression and took Zoloft **once a day for 6 weeks** about 4 months ago. He is no longer taking Zoloft and he can't remember the dosage. He was recently diagnosed with **erectile dysfunction** and is currently taking one **50-milligram Viagra tablet about twice a week** before sexual activity.

lower back pain _____   history of _____   once a day for 6 weeks _____   erectile dysfunction _____   50-milligram Viagra table about twice a week _____

11. The 56-year-old female patient was **diagnosed** with **autoimmune hepatitis** 2 months ago. A **biopsy** for cirrhosis of the liver was negative. She is currently taking **two 20-milligram prednisone tablets daily.** She has also been taking Fosamax for osteoporosis for 2 years. Her **chief complaint** today is fatigue and discomfort in her **abdomen.**

diagnosed _____   autoimmune hepatitis _____   biopsy _____   two 20-milligram
prednisone tablets daily _____   chief complaint _____   abdomen _____

12. The patient has **history of** hepatitis B. His **chief complaint** today is diarrhea and abdominal pain. He was **diagnosed** with gonorrhea and chlamydia 7 days ago. He was taking **doxycycline twice a day, once in the morning and once in the evening, and taking azithromycin once a day, both for 5 days.** Both medication dosages are unknown. He has **no known drug allergies.**

history of _____   chief complaint _____   diagnosed _____   doxycycline twice a day,
once in the morning and once in the evening, and taking azithromycin once a day, both for
5 days _____   no known drug allergies _____

13. A **23-year-old female** with a history of vaginal yeast infections and menorrhagia **complains of** waking up with a body rash. She is currently being treated for cystitis. Her doctor prescribed **one tablet of Bactrim be taken in the morning and one tablet in the evening for 15 days**. Today is day 6. Her **allergies** include Ceclor, iodine, and peanut butter.

    23-year-old female _____ complains of _____ one tablet of Bactrim be taken in the morning and one tablet in the evening for 15 days _____ allergies _____

14. A 60-year-old man was **diagnosed** with glaucoma 2 weeks ago and prescribed **1 drop of Isopto Carpine in each eye four times a day** by his **private medical doctor**. Patient is **complaining of** cloudy vision, spasms of the eyelids, and blurred vision. He has a **hiatal hernia** and has a **history of gastroesophageal reflux disease.**

    diagnosed _____ 1 drop of Isopto Carpine in each eye four times a day _____ private medical doctor _____ complaining of _____ hiatal hernia _____ history of gastroesophageal reflex disease _____

15. A 47-year-old man is complaining of severe abdominal pain, bloody diarrhea, and flu-like **symptoms.** He was diagnosed with colitis 2 weeks ago. He went to the doctor after bleeding from his rectum and complaining of diarrhea. His doctor prescribed **one Asacol pill daily, but patient does not know the dosage.** Patient states he is not getting better. Patient has a **history of** fungal infection in his groin area and was prescribed Nizoral. The fungal infection cleared up and he is no longer taking Nizoral. Patient's **known drug allergies** include **penicillin.**

    symptoms _____ one Asacol pill daily, but patient does not know dosage _____ history of _____ known drug allergies _____ penicillin _____

How did you do? Check your answers against the Answer Key online.

Abbreviations Writing Exercise

Read the following sentences written with abbreviations and rewrite them as complete sentences.

1. A 47 yo WM recently Dx with ED is C/O feeling dizzy, flushed, and LBP. He has taken one Viagra 50-mg tab po 6 different times about 1 hr before sexual activity.

    _____
    _____
    _____
    _____

2. A 29 yo WF with HO Hep B is C/O a thick Vag D/C that looks like cottage cheese. Her MedHx includes Hepsera to Tx Hep B and Nasonex for nasal congestion.

    _____
    _____
    _____
    _____

3. A 33 yo WMD with HPI cirrhosis is C/O of n/v/d and drowsiness. He is currently taking one Aldactone 25-mg tab po AM, po PM SID, to Tx water retention in abd and legs. He has NKDA.

    _____
    _____
    _____
    _____

4. A 56 yo BF with HTN × 5 yrs is C/O a rapid heart beat. All include sulfa. She is currently smoking 1 ppd cig and has been smoking for 36 yrs. Current MedHx includes Captopril 25-mg po TID × 5 yrs and digoxin 5-mg po SID.

_____

_____

_____

_____

5. The pt. is C/O abd pain and worsening bloody diarrhea. He states he feels like he has the flu. He was Dx with UC 3 wks ago. He has been taking Asacol po SID (dosage UNK). All include PCN.

_____

_____

_____

_____

6. The 43 yo WF is C/O abd pain and a foul vag D/C. Her LMP was 2 mos ago. She is on BCP and denies she is pregnant. She has MS and is currently taking Betaseron Inj SID.

_____

_____

_____

_____

7. The 61 yo Pt.'s CC is a gout flare-up in his right toe. He states it's tender to the touch and very red and hot. The flare-up started 3 days ago. He's been taking 2 Tyl tab prn. He wants to get a cortisone Inj and an Rx for probenecid, which he received the last time he had a gout attack 2 years ago.

_____

_____

_____

_____

8. The 21 yo WF's CC is nausea, loss of appetite, dizziness, and HAs. She began taking Macrodantin cap po SID × 5 days to Tx UTI. Pt has NKDA but other All include wasps, bees, and iodine. She is on BCP and has been taking Aleve 1 tab prn for her HAs.

_____

_____

_____

_____

9. The 30 yo BM is C/O painful and burning urination, and penile discharge for about 1 wk. He has NKDA but is allergic to latex. Pt. had HO TB 5 yrs ago and was prescribed rifampin. Pt. also has history of STDs—gonorrhea and chlamydia. He was Dx 2 yrs ago and was prescribed doxycycline and azithromycin. Pt does not remember dosage. Pt. does not always use condoms or practice safe sex.

_____

_____

_____

_____

10. The 26 yo WF's CC is hair loss, trembling, and shaking. Pt. was recently Dx with hypothyroidism and is currently taking Levoxyl 50 mcg po SID. Pt. has been taking Levoxyl $\times$ 2 wks. Her LMP was 3 wks ago. She is not on BCP. Pt. takes Tyl prn for HAs. She states she cut her finger yesterday and has applied Neosporin on the cut. All include sulfa, iodine, and dog dander.

_____

_____

_____

_____

11. The Pt. was brought in by her husband. He stated she was experiencing terrible pain in her sternum and in her back and heartburn. Pt. was A&O. She had Endo 4 days ago and was Dx with HH, GERD, and an inflamed esophagus. Her PMD prescribed ranitidine 1 tsp AM and 1 tsp PM SID. PSH includes appendectomy and rt. knee surgery. All include Bactrim and cats.

_____

_____

_____

_____

12. The 5 yo WNF Pt. was brought in by her mother. Her mother states her daughter is tugging at her AS, that her OD is pink and watery, and that she is crying a lot. Her mother has been giving her daughter children's Tyl.1 tsp po prn. Mother states her daughter has Hx of ear infections and has had one episode of croup. Their PMD has prescribed amoxicillin to Tx her ear infections. The Pt.'s VS are NL. Pt.'s SH includes parents who each smoke 1–2 ppd cigs.

_____

_____

_____

_____

13. The 32 yo BM is C/O constipation $\times$ 2 wks. He is taking Metamucil BID. The Pt.'s other current medications include Lipitor 20 mg po QHS to treat cholesterol and 2 glyburide 5 mg tab po BID for DM type II.

_____

_____

_____

14. The 56 yo WF had liver Bx 1 wk ago and was Dx with cirrhosis of the liver. The Pt.'s C/C is anxiety and depression. The Pt. has Hx of COPD. Current medications include albuterol, 2 puffs prn for SOB $\times$ 7 yrs. She has 25 yr smoking Hx, but quit 1 year ago, and has 20 yr Hx of ETHO consumption. Pt. denies drinking ETHO after cirrhosis Dx.

_____

_____

_____

15. The 69 yo BM is C/O of weakness and aching pain in both legs around the calf area for a long time. He can't walk as far as he used to. Pt. has Hx of CAD, angina, and high cholesterol. His Meds include Atenol 50-mg tab po SID, Mevacor 20-mg tab po daily, and ASA 325-mg tab po SID.

_____

_____

_____

_____

Check what you have written with acceptable answers that appear in the Answer Key online.

Pharmacy Documentation Abbreviations Comprehension

Now that you have been introduced to written pharmacy documentation abbreviations and have read and completed sentences 1 through 15 using language regarding patient information and pharmacy documentation, assess your understanding by doing the exercises below.

Multiple Choice Questions

Choose the answer that correctly completes each sentence below.

1. _____ The abbreviation for **chief complaint** is:

a. CCO

b. C/O

c. CC

2. _____ The abbreviation for **"doxycycline twice a day, once in the morning and once in the evening"** is:

a. BID doxycycline AM/PM

b. doxycycline po AM BID, po PM BID

c. BID doxycycline AM and BID doxycycline PM

3. _____ The abbreviation for **"every 6 hours"** is:

a. HQ6

b. hq6

c. q6h

4. _____ The sentence: "Patient is complaining of chest pain and shortness of breath" can be abbreviated as:

a. Pt. C/O CP and SOB

b. Pt. CC of Ch Pn and SOB

c. Patient CC of CP and SOB

5. _____ The sentence: "The patient has been taking Dulcolax twice daily before meals for a period of 2 days to treat her irritable bowel syndrome" can be abbreviated as:

a. Pt. is taking Dulcolax po BID AC to treat IBS × 2 days

b. Pt. is taking Dulcolax po TID PC × 2 days to treat IBS

c. Pt. is taking Dulcolax po BID PC to treat IBS

6. _____ The abbreviation for **"one 50-milligram Viagra tablet approximately twice a week"** is:

a. Viagra 50-mg tab qwk

b. Viagra 50-mg tab po appr. biwk

c. Viagra 50-mcg tab po qwk

7. _____ **HPI** is the abbreviation for:

a. history of present illness

b. history of past illness

c. history of present and past illness

8. _____ **"The patient's VS are NL"** means:

a. The patient's vital signs are normal

b. The patient's vaginal symptoms are normal

c. The patient's vascular symptoms are normal

9. _____ **"Pt. takes Tyl prn for HAs"** means:

a. the patient takes Tylenol intravenously for headaches

b. the physical therapist only takes Tylenol when he has a headache

c. the patient takes Tylenol as needed for headaches

10. _____ **PV** is the abbreviation for:

a. pelvic virus

b. per vagina

c. powder

11. _____ The sentence: "The Pt. has been taking Macrodantin cap po QID × 5 days to Tx UTI" means:

a. The patient has been taking a Macrodantin capsule by mouth four times a day for a period of 5 days to treat urinary tract infection

b. The patient takes 5 Macrodantin capsules a day to urinary tract infection

c. The patient took a Macrodantin capsule by mouth once a day for only 5 days to treat urinary tract infection

12. _____ **ADR** is the abbreviation for:

a. attention deficit recurrence

b. Alzheimer's disease relapse

c. adverse drug reaction

13. _____ The sentence: "He suffers from Parkinson's disease and is currently taking a 5-milligram capsule of Eldepryl twice a day, one with breakfast and one with lunch" means:

a. He suffers from Parkinson's disease and is taking 5 Eldepryl capsules with breakfast and 5 Eldepryl capsules with lunch

b. He suffers from Parkinson's disease and takes Eldepryl 5-mg cap po BID, one AM/one PM

c. He suffers from Parkinson's disease and takes Eldepryl 5-mg cap po SID, one AM/one PM

14. _____ **TPR** is the abbreviation for:

a. treatment, pulse, and respiration

b. temperature, pulse, and respiration

c. treatment, pain, respiration

15. _____ The sentence: "He has been taking Asacol po SID (dosage UNK)" means:

a. He has been taking Asacol injections daily but dosage is not known

b. He has been taking Asacol by mouth daily and the patient knows the dosage

c. He has been taking Asacol by mouth daily but the dosage is unknown

True/False Questions

Indicate whether each sentence below is true (T) or false (F).

1. _____ **DOB** is the abbreviation for diagnosis of biopsy.

2. _____ **Hx** of **PID** is the abbreviation for history of peptic inflammatory disease.

3. _____ "Patient has **KDA** but is allergic to peanuts" means the patient has no known drug allergies and is not allergic to peanuts.

4. _____ **BID AC** means twice daily after meals.

5. _____ "Current **MedHx** includes Captopril **25 mg po TID × 5 years**" means current medication history includes taking a 25-mg Captopril by mouth three times for a period of 5 years.

6. _____ The abbreviation **DD** means demographic data and the abbreviation **DH** means drug history.

7. _____ "Her **PMD** prescribed Isopto **1 Gt OD QID**" means her private medical doctor prescribed 1 drop of Isopto Carpine in her right eye four times daily.

8. _____ The abbreviation for acetaminophen is **ASA.**

9. _____ "She is taking Levoxyl **50 mcg po SID**" means she is taking 50 milligrams of Levoxyl daily.

10. _____ **QHS** is the abbreviation for every night at bedtime.

How did you do? Check your answers against the Answer Key online.

PHARMACY DOCUMENTATION AND STANDARDIZED PATIENT FORMS

A common method used to document a patient's pharmaceutical care is the SOAP note. SOAP is the acronym for subjective (S), objective (O), assessment (A), and plan (P). Subjective information includes information the patient shares with the pharmacy student and pharmacist during the patient interview, observations that the pharmacist and pharmacy student make about the patient, and information about the symptoms the patient is experiencing. Objective information is data that is obtained from the results of laboratory and diagnostic tests. An assessment of the patient is made by the pharmacy student and the pharmacist and is based on subjective and objective information. The plan in the SOAP note includes information about how to treat the patient, whether to discontinue medication and prescribe a new medication, whether to adjust dosage, and whether to order additional diagnostic tests.

The patient case presentation or patient workup is another method to document a patient's pharmaceutical care. The case presentation is also a way for pharmacy students to learn how to manage a patient's disease state. Practicing pharmacists use case presentations to discuss a patient's care with colleagues and other pharmacists who will also be taking care of the patient. The case presentation form includes a lot of information and can include up to 22 sections to be completed. Some of these sections are chief complaint, history of present illness, family and social history, medications, physical examination, and laboratory tests and results. An example of a case presentation or patient workup is the Patient History and Physical Database form. Pharmacotherapy Workup Notes are another way to document a patient's pharmaceutical care, and include three sections: assessment, care plan, and evaluation. Pharmacotherapy Workup Notes also provide a case presentation form.

The SOAP note, the Patient History and Physical Database, and the Pharmacotherapy Workup Notes require that the patient's record be clear and concise and that the data collected by the pharmacy student and the pharmacist be organized and logical. The information that is written in these types of pharmacy documentation forms contains abbreviations, acronyms, and short/incomplete sentences as well as complete sentences. Familiarity with and complete knowledge of abbreviations and acronyms and their meanings, and a good command of written English, is therefore essential.

In this section, you will be introduced to the SOAP note format and the Patient History and Physical Database (Patient H&P Database), and you will learn how to complete them. You also will be introduced to a sample of the Pharmacotherapy Workup Notes format that appears in Appendix B.

SOAP Notes Model

Figure 13-1 shows a model of a SOAP note. The purpose of this model is to introduce you to and familiarize you with the language and abbreviations used on this form. The SOAP note format is used to communicate patient information in writing. The information for a SOAP note is obtained from the patient interview, from pharmacy students' and pharmacists' assessments, and from lab and test results. There are variations of the SOAP form, but the important thing to remember is that you need to document certain information to be able to treat a patient and to be able to share patient information in writing with professors, pharmacists, fellow students, medical doctors, and other health care professionals involved in the treatment and pharmaceutical care of the patient.

SOAP Notes Form

Patient's name: _____ DOB: _____

S: (Subject)
In this section, you write and document subjective information shared with you by the patient. This information includes:

1) the patient's chief complaint
2) the patient's history of their present illness
3) the patient's past medical history
4) the patient's family history
5) the patient's social history
6) the patient's review of system, which is the patient's summary of their health

O: (Objective)
In this section, you document objective information. This information includes:
1) the patient's current medications
2) the patient's allergies
3) the patient's vital signs
4) the patient's physical exam
5) the results of any tests such as X-rays, blood tests, etc.

A: (Assessment)
In this section, you document:

1) your interpretation of the patient's complaint(s) and adherence to the medication regimen, as well as the diagnosis based on the patient's medical condition(s), current medication condition, and the results of any tests that may have been ordered
2) the need for instructions and education to the patient about medications, dosage, and treatment

P: (Plan)
In this section, you document:

1) how you will address the concerns and issues found in the assessment
2) suggestions and recommendations for treatment, medications, dosage
3) any referrals or other suggestions for the patient
4) instructions to the patient to self-check and self-monitor

FIGURE 13-1 Model of a SOAP note

Completing a SOAP Note Exercise

Read the following patient scenario carefully. After reading it thoroughly, complete the blank SOAP note form below. Put the information that you have read into the appropriate sections. Use abbreviations and pay careful attention to spelling. Based on the patient scenario presented, not every section of the SOAP note will be completed.

Patient Scenario

MC is a 68-year-old white woman who is brought to the clinic by her son, who lives with her. Her son states that his mother is not feeling well and has been coughing a lot. She did not sleep well last night because the cough kept waking her up. MC has also been coughing up phlegm and sputum. Her son also states that his mother is not eating as much. MC has had chronic bronchitis since she was 22 and has been smoking since she was 15 years old. She developed chronic obstructive pulmonary disease 10 years ago. She has had an Atrovent inhaler and is supposed to take four to six inhalations four times a day, but she doesn't always do so.

MC has had hypertension for 8 years and is taking 20 milligrams of Lisinopril once a day. MC also takes 10 milligrams of Fosamax daily in the morning for osteoporosis. She also had a complete hysterectomy when she was 42 as a result of fibroids and severe menstrual bleeding. MC has also had two benign breast nodules removed. She had a negative right breast biopsy in 1999 and a negative left breast biopsy in 2005. The son states there is no history of breast cancer in the family, but that MC's sister died from ovarian cancer at the age of 45 fifteen years ago. There is no history of diabetes or CAD in her family.

MC is allergic to iodine and sulfa. She is also allergic to cats. MC lives with her son and his wife and two grandchildren ages 6 and 8. She worked until age 64 as a supermarket cashier. She has been a widow 18 years. Her husband died of colon cancer. She smokes a pack of cigarettes a week. She has tried to quit and wore the patch but with no success. She doesn't drink alcohol. MC is tired, experiencing labored breathing, but is cooperative.

Her blood pressure is 137/82. Her pulse is 84. She weighs 135 pounds and measures 66 inches tall. Her temperature is 98 degrees. There is no nasal discharge. Labs and x-ray have been ordered and results are pending.

Patient: _____

S:

CC: _____
_____
_____
_____

HPI: _____
_____
_____
_____

PMH: _____
_____
_____
_____

FH: _____
_____
_____
_____

SH: _____
_____
_____
_____

O:

Meds: _____

_____

_____

_____

Allergies: _____

_____

_____

_____

PE: _____

_____

_____

_____

Labs: _____

_____

_____

_____

A: _____

_____

_____

_____

P: _____

_____

_____

_____

How did you do? Check your answers against the Answer Key online.

SOAP Notes Comprehension Exercise

Now that you have completed a written SOAP related to the patient scenario, assess your understanding of the patient's information in the SOAP note by doing the exercises below.

Multiple Choice Questions

Choose the correct answer from a, b, and c.

1. _____ The patient's chief complaint is:
   a. she has been a widow for 18 years
   b. she is not feeling well and coughing a lot
   c. she is allergic to sulfa and iodine

2. _____ The patient's husband's death of colon cancer and the patient's sister's death of ovarian cancer documents:

a. PMH

b. FH

c. SH

3. _____ The patient's allergies are documented in the:

a. assessment section of the SOAP note

b. subjective section of the SOAP note

c. objective section of the SOAP note

4. _____ The patient:

a. works as a supermarket cashier and lives with her son and his family

b. is retired and lives alone

c. is retired and lives with her son and his family

5. _____ The patient's medication information includes:

a. medications to treat DM, CAD, and OA and is documented in the objective section of the SOAP note

b. medications for HTN, chronic bronchitis, and COP and is documented in the assessment section of the SOAP note

c. medications for HTN, chronic bronchitis, COPD, and osteoporosis and is documented in the objective section of the SOAP note

6. _____ The patient's VS and pending lab results are recorded in the:

a. objective section of the SOAP note

b. assessment section of the SOAP note

c. PE section of the SOAP note

7. _____ The medication the patient does not take every day like she is supposed to is:

a. Fosamax

b. Atrovent inhaler

c. Lisinopril

8. _____ According to the plan section of the SOAP note:

a. the patient's Lisinopril dosage will be increased

b. the patient has been referred to a smoking cessation program

c. a plan cannot be developed because the assessment is incomplete

9. _____ The patient is:

a. anxious and uncooperative, and continues to smoke a pack of cigarettes a day

b. tired, has labored breathing, but is cooperative, and smokes a pack of cigarettes a week

c. experiencing SOB, is cooperative, and no longer smokes

10. _____ The patient's medical history includes:

a. a complete hysterectomy, negative breast biopsies on each breast, and benign breast nodules

b. partial hysterectomy, negative breast biopsies, and benign breast nodules

c. a complete hysterectomy, negative left breast biopsy, and a malignant breast nodule on her right breast

How did you do? Check your answers in the Answer Key online.

Patient History and Physical Database Model

Below is a model of a Patient History and Physical (H&P) Database form. The purpose of the H&P Database form is to obtain patient information and to communicate and share the patient information with pharmacy students, pharmacists, and other health care professionals in writing and verbally. Information obtained in the H&P Database form comes from the patient interview and from lab and test results. There are variations of the H&P Database form, but the important thing to remember is that you need to document certain information to be able to treat a patient and to be able to share patient information in writing with professors, pharmacists, fellow students, medical doctors, and other health-care professionals involved in the treatment and pharmaceutical care of the patient.

Completing a Patient H&P Database Form Exercise

Read the following patient scenario carefully. After reading it thoroughly, complete the appropriate sections of the guided Patient H&P Database form below. Use abbreviations and pay careful attention to spelling. Based on the patient scenario presented, not every section of the Patient H&P Database form will be completed.

ID: In this section, you identify the patient by age, race, and sex.

CC: In this section, you document the patient's chief complaint.

HPI: In this section, you document the patient's history of present illness.

PMH: In the section, you document the patient's past medical history.

DH: In this section, you document the patient's drug history.

Allergies: In this section, you document the patient's allergies.

FH: In this section, you document the patient's family medical history.

SH: In this section, you document the patient's social history.

ROS: In this section, you document the patient's own summary of their health status.

PE: In this section, you document the patient's vital signs during the physical examination.

Labs: In this section, you document any lab results.

Recommendation: In this section, you make recommendations based on lab and test results, and you instruct and educate patient.

Monitoring Plan: In this section, you plan for the patient to return, to self-monitor, and to self-check.

Patient Scenario[a]

Scenario: You are a pharmacy student at a community pharmacy. Mr. Smith, a 68-year-old gentleman who has been a patient this pharmacy for several years, enters the store and presents a prescription for Coumadin 2 mg #30, i po SID. You have available to you Mr. Smith, his pharmacy profile, and a sheet of his laboratory values, which your preceptor has trained him to bring every time he comes to the pharmacy. The following information is the history and physical data you are able to obtain, your assessment of Mr. Smith's situation, and your chart note.

Read the information that appears in the patient's profile below:

The patient is a 68-year-old man whose chief complaint is that he needs to increase his warfarin dose due to decreased efficacy in his past dose. The patient takes warfarin daily to prevent deep vein thrombosis. Because today his international normalization ratio is 1.5, his doctor has increased his warfarin dosage from 5 milligrams by mouth every day to 7 milligrams by mouth every day. The patient was diagnosed with deep vein thrombosis. He had hip replacement surgery 3 months ago. He had a single episode of atrial fibrillation 4 years ago and is currently in normal sinus rhythm. He was diagnosed with congestive heart failure 7 years ago and with chronic obstructive pulmonary disease 5 years ago. He had an anterior myocardial infarction 14 years ago and is not currently experiencing

[a]Adapted with permission from O'Sullivan T, Boh L. *Pharmacy Practice Manual: A Guide to the Clinical Experience.* Baltimore: Lippincott Williams & Wilkins; 2001:600,603–604. Example of a case workup.

chest pain. He has been taking 5 milligrams of warfarin by mouth once daily for 2 months for deep vein thrombosis. It is the same dose since he was discharged from the hospital 2 months ago. He's been taking .25 milligrams of digoxin by mouth daily for a period of 7 years for congestive heart failure, 2 puffs of ipratropium four times daily for a period of 9 years for chronic obstructive pulmonary disease, and 2 puffs of albuterol four times daily for a period of 9 years for chronic obstructive pulmonary disease.

His over-the-counter medications include one multivitamin with iron and minerals by mouth daily for his general health for a period of 7 months. For constipation he has been taking one scoop of psyllium in a glass of water daily for a period of 4 years. He takes four tablespoonfuls of bismuth salicylate as needed for diarrhea. He states he took one dose twice in the past year for stomach flu. He's also been taking two to three alfalfa tablets daily for health. His friend recommended this to him about a month ago. The patient's medication refill history indicates that he obtains his refills on time. He obtains all prescription and over-the-counter medications from this pharmacy, but he buys the alfalfa tablets at the health food store. His recreational drug use includes a 40-packs-a-year smoking history. He quit 2 years ago. He drinks one to two drinks per week, and there has been no recent change in that amount. He denies any history of medication or environmental allergies. His father died at age 54 from acute myocardial infarction.

The patient is retired and lives with his wife, who helps him with medication management at home. He denies any changes in ingesting foods that contain vitamin K. A summary of the patient's own health status indicates he has no current complaints. His sputum is clear, he has had no coughing spells recently, and he denies shortness of breath, dyspnea on exertion, and paroxysmal nocturnal dyspnea. The patient states he sleeps with one pillow and that he is comfortable walking short distances and there has been no change in 3 months. He denies any chest pain and bleeding or bruising on his skin. He states his urine is clear and yellow with no blood and that his stools are dark brown.

The patient weighs 80 kilograms, which is his usual weight, and he stands 5 feet 10 inches tall. His heart rate is 85 with regular rhythm. His blood pressure is 135/82. His rate and rhythm is 20 and his temperature is 37.2. His lab results indicate that today his international normalization ratio is 1.5. Two weeks ago it was 1.9; 4 weeks ago it was 2.4; 6 weeks ago it was 2.6; and 8 weeks ago at discharge from the hospital it was 2.3 and his albumin was 4.5. The recommendation is to treat anticoagulation by having the patient discontinue taking alfalfa tablets and to start taking 80 milligrams of enoxaparin subcutaneously every 12 hours but to discontinue enoxaparin when his international normalization ratio is greater than or equal to 2.0. The patient will be instructed in how to self-administer the medication subcutaneously. The recommendation also includes continuing warfarin at the current dose.

To treat myocardial infarction prophylaxis, it is recommended the patient take 81 milligrams of aspirin by mouth daily. Patient has been instructed to return for an international normalization ratio check in 5 days and to self-monitor for signs/symptoms of deep vein thrombosis, which include calf warmth, tenderness, or pain, and to call his doctor immediately if he experiences chest pain or shortness of breath. The patient has been instructed to also check for signs/symptoms of major bleeding in the gums, urine, stool, skin bruising, and epistaxis and to come back for a stool guaiac test in 3 months.

Patient H&P Database Form Comprehension Exercise

ID: _____

CC: _____

_____

HPI: _____

_____

_____

PMH: _____

_____

_____

_____

_____

DH: _____

_____

_____

_____

_____

OTC MEDS: _____

_____

_____

_____

_____

Allergies: _____

_____

FH: _____

_____

SH: _____

_____

ROS: _____

_____

_____

_____

PE: _____
_____
_____
_____
_____

Pertinent Labs:

Today	2 weeks ago	4 weeks ago	6 weeks ago	8 weeks ago (at discharge)
INR:	INR:	INR:	INR:	INR: Alb:

Current Medical Problems	Goal of Therapy	Measurable End-Point

Current Drug-Related Problems	Justification	Therapeutic Alternatives

Recommendation	Monitoring Plan

How did you do? Compare your written answers with the completed sample Patient H&P Database form in the Answer Key online.

Completing SOAP Note from Patient H&P Database Form

Complete the SOAP note below using patient information from the Patient H&P Database above.

S: _____
_____
_____
_____

O: _____
_____
_____
_____

A: _____

_____

_____

_____

P: _____

_____

_____

_____

How did you do? Compare your written answers with the completed sample SOAP note related to the patient scenario in the Answer Key online.

Pharmacy Documentation Forms Comprehension: Patient H&P Database Form and SOAP Note

Now that you have read the patient scenario and have completed the Patient H&P Database form and SOAP note, assess your understanding by doing the exercises below.

True/False Questions

Indicate whether each sentence below is true (T) or false (F).

1. _____ The patient is an 86-year-old man.
2. _____ The patient has a prescription for Coumadin 2 mcg #20, i po SID.
3. _____ The patient's chief complaint is that he wants his digoxin medication increased.
4. _____ The patient was diagnosed with DVT 2 years ago.
5. _____ The patient's OTC medications include alfalfa tablets, multivitamins with iron and minerals, psyllium, and bismuth salicylate.
6. _____ The patient lives with his daughter.
7. _____ The patient's father died of COPD at age 54.
8. _____ The patient smokes and drinks regularly.
9. _____ The lab results indicate the patient needs to discontinue taking alfalfa tablets.
10. _____ The lab results indicate the patient should continue with the current warfarin dose.

Multiple Choice Questions

Choose the correct answer from a, b, and c.

1. _____ The patient is a (an):
a. 68-year-old woman
b. 68-year-old man
c. 86-year-old man

2. _____ The patient's prescription is for:
a. Coumadin 2 mg #30, i po SID
b. Coumadin 2 mg #30 i po BID
c. Coumadin 2 mcg #20, i po SID

3. _____ The patient's complaint is that he needs his:
a. warfarin dosage increased
b. digoxin dosage increased
c. warfarin dosage decreased

4. _____ The patient was diagnosed with:

a. CHF 2 months ago

b. COPD 2 months ago

c. DVT 2 months ago

5. _____ The patient's OTC medications include:

a. alfalfa tablets and multivitamins with iron and minerals

b. alfalfa tablets, multivitamins with iron and minerals, psyllium, and bismuth salicylate

c. psyllium, bismuth salicylate, and alfalfa tablets

6. _____ The patient:

a. lives with his spouse

b. is a widow

c. lives with his daughter

7. _____ The patient's:

a. mother died of AMI at age 54

b. father died of AMI at age 54

c. father died of COPD at age 54

8. _____ The patient:

a. tried to quit smoking 2 years ago, but continues to smoke

b. smokes a pack of cigarettes per week

c. quit smoking 2 years ago

9. _____ The lab results indicate the patient needs to:

a. continue taking alfalfa tablets

b. discontinue taking alfalfa tablets

c. take alfalfa tablets as needed

10. _____ The patient will:

a. continue with warfarin at current dose to treat DVT

b. discontinue current dose

c. continue with increased warfarin dosage to treat DVT

11. _____ The patient information, "DVT, 2 mos ago" and "1–2 drinks/week" is indicated in the:

a. objective section of the SOAP note

b. SH section of the Patient H&P Database form

c. subjective part of the SOAP note

12. _____ The recommendation to discontinue alfalfa tablets should be included in the:

a. plan section of the SOAP note and in the monitoring plan section of the Patient H&P Database

b. labs section of the Patient H&P Database

c. DH section of the Patient H&P Database

13. _____ The patient's PE data should be included in the:

a. objective section of the SOAP note and in the PE section of the Patient H&P Database

b. assessment section of the SOAP note

c. subjective section of the SOAP note and in the PE section of the Patient H&P Database

14. _____ The history of the patient's INR lab results should be documented in the:

a. assessment section of the SOAP note and in the Labs section of the Patient H&P Database

b. labs section of the Patient H&P Database and in the objective section of the SOAP notes

c. subjective section of the Patient H&P Database

15. _____ The patient's new medications, patient education, and patient instructions should be documented in the:

   a. assessment section of the SOAP note

   b. recommendation and plan section of the Patient H&P Database and in the assessment section of the SOAP note

   c. plan section of the SOAP note and in the recommendation and plan section of the Patient H&P Database

How did you do? Check your answers against the Answer Key online.

POST-ASSESSMENT

True/False Questions

Indicate whether each sentence below is true (T) or false (F).

1. _____ **Tx** is the abbreviation for treat/treatment.
2. _____ The patient's PMH and PHI is documented in the objective section of the SOAP note.
3. _____ **TID × 5** yrs means "taken three times daily for a period of 5 years."
4. _____ Vital signs and current medications are documented in the objective section of the SOAP note, and the patient's allergies are documented in the subjective section of the SOAP note.
5. _____ The abbreviation for **nitroglycerin** in nigly.
6. _____ The Patient H&P Database includes only information about the patient's current health and physical data.
7. _____ **MedHx** is the abbreviation for medical history.
8. _____ The recommendation section of the Patient H&P Database is used to make recommendations based on lab and tests results, and to instruct and educate patients about medication use.
9. _____ The abbreviation for cancer is **Cx.**
10. _____ The patient's smoking and recreational drug use history is documented in the subjective section of the SOAP note and in the DH section of the Patient H&P Database.
11. _____ **ABT** is the abbreviation for antibiotic.
12. _____ Objective information in a SOAP note is obtained through lab tests and diagnostics tests.
13. _____ The abbreviation for **allergy** is All.
14. _____ **CFNS** is the abbreviation for cold, fatigue, and night sweats.
15. _____ There is only one form that is used to document patient pharmacy documentation.
16. _____ **cig** is the abbreviation for cigarettes.
17. _____ Knowledge of pharmacy and medical abbreviations is not needed to read and write pharmacy documentation.
18. _____ **PND** is the abbreviation for paroxysmal nocturnal dyspnea.
19. _____ Pharmacy documentation is shared with patients only.
20. _____ The abbreviation **WN** means well nourished.

Multiple Choice Questions

Choose the correct answer from a, b, and c.

1. _____ The abbreviated sentence: "The 26 yo WF's CC of NVD" means:

   a. The 26-year-old female widow is complaining of nausea, vertigo, and dizziness

   b. The 26-year-old white female's chief complaint of nausea, vomiting, and diarrhea

   c. The 26-year-old well female is complaining of nausea, vomiting, and diarrhea

2. _____ The abbreviated form of the sentence, "The patient is taking 50 micrograms of Levoxyl by mouth once a day," is:

a. The Pt. is taking Levoxyl 50 mcg po SID

b. The Pt. is taking Levoxyl 50 mg po SID

c. The Pt. is taking Levoxyl 50 mcg SQ SID

3. _____ The abbreviated form of the sentence, "Her private medical doctor prescribed one teaspoon of ranitidine in the morning and one tsp in the evening daily," is:

a. Her PMD prescribed ranitidine 1 tsp AM and 1 tsp PM QD

b. Her PMD prescribed ranitidine 2 tsp BID

c. Her PMD prescribed ranitidine 2 tsp AM and 2 tsp PM QD

4. _____ The abbreviated sentence, "Pt.'s SH includes parents who each smoke 1–2 ppd cigs," means:

a. Patient's smoking history includes parents who each smoke one to two packs of cigarettes per day

b. Patient's social history includes parents who each smoke one to two packs of cigarettes per week

c. Patient's social history includes parents who each smoke one to two packs of cigarettes per day

5. _____ The abbreviated sentence, "The 32 yo BM is C/O constipation $\times$ 2 wks and is taking Metamucil BID," means:

a. The 32-year-old black male is complaining that he had constipation 2 weeks ago and is taking Metamucil twice daily

b. The 32-year-old black male is complaining that he has had constipation for a period of 2 weeks and is taking Metamucil twice daily

c. The 32-year-old black male is complaining of constipation for at least 2 weeks and has been taking Metamucil twice weekly

6. _____ The abbreviated form of the sentence, "The patient has chronic obstructive pulmonary disease, chronic bronchitis, and is taking two to four inhalations of Atrovent every day twice a day," is:

a. The Pt. has COPD and chronic bronchitis and is taking 2–4 IHN Atrovent BID SID

b. The Pt. has COPD and chronic bronchitis and is taking 2–4 IHN Atrovent SID

c. The Pt. has COPD and chronic bronchitis and is taking 2–4 INH Atrovent BID

7. _____ The abbreviated form of the sentence, "He is currently taking one 25-milligram tablet of Aldactone by mouth in the morning and one in the evening daily to treat water retention in the abdomen and legs," is:

a. He is currently taking 1 Aldactone 25-mcg tab po AM, po PM BID to Tx water retention in abd and legs

b. He is currently taking 1 Aldactone 25-mg tab po AM, po PM QD to Tx water retention in abd and legs

c. He is currently taking 2 Aldactone 25-mg tab po AM, PM QD to Tx water retention in abd and legs

8. _____ The abbreviated sentence, "A 47 year WDWN–WF came to the ED C/O of CFNS and LBP" means:

a. A 47-year-old well-developed, well-nourished white female came to the emergency department complaining of chills, fatigue, nausea, sweating, and lower back pain

b. A 47-year-old white divorced and well-nourished female came to the emergency department complaining of chills, fever, night sweats, and lower blood pressure

c. A 47-year-old well-developed, well-nourished white female came to the emergency department complaining of chills, fever, night sweats, and lower back pain

Mini Dialogue #3

Person A: Have you met the new pharmacist? What do you think of her?
Person B: She's only been here 1 week and she's already getting under my skin.

Mini Dialogue #4

Person A: It's really quiet today—not too many patients coming in with prescriptions.
Person B: I'm not complaining. It's nice not to have patients getting in my hair.

Mini Dialogue #5

Person A: I can't believe I have to work tonight and study for my pharmacy exam, which is tomorrow morning.
Person B: I would be tearing my hair out if I were you.

Mini Dialogue #6

Person A: How's your new boss?
Person B: He's like my old boss, who was friendly and kind, but he's also tough as nails.

Chapter 1 Post-Assessment

Dialogue #1

Patient: Hi. Can I speak with the pharmacist?
Pharmacist: I am the pharmacist on duty today. What can I help you with?
Patient: When I woke up yesterday, I noticed that my arm was a reddish-brown color and was swollen. It is painful and itchy. It seems to be getting worse today. Is there a cream that I can buy that will reduce the swelling and relieve the itchiness?
Pharmacist: Let's take a look at the arm. You're right. It is a brown color and it is swollen. Let me ask you a couple of questions. Were you bitten by an insect or did you hit your arm?
Patient: Not that I remember. But I was camping during the Labor Day weekend 2 days ago. Maybe I was bitten by an insect and did not notice it.
Pharmacist: OK. That seems possible, as I can see a possible bite mark. Has the swelling spread in the last 2 days?
Patient: Yes. At first, the brown color and swelling was only around my wrist. Today, they nearly reach my elbow!
Pharmacist: Have you noticed any pus?
Patient: Yes. As I was scratching my arm this morning, I noticed a small amount of clear fluid discharge.
Pharmacist: OK. It looks like you may have what is called impetigo, which is a mild skin condition that can be caused by an insect bite. I really think you should see a doctor today since the infection in your arm is pretty big and spreading.
Patient: Really?
Pharmacist: It looks like you're going to need a prescription for an antibiotic. But in the meantime, you may take Benadryl for the itching so you don't continue to scratch and spread the infection.
Patient: Benadryl? I've never taken Benadryl.
Pharmacist: You need to be careful. Benadryl can make you drowsy, so don't drive or operate heavy machinery right after you take it. To relieve the pain, I recommend you take Tylenol or Motrin unless you have any kidney or liver problems.
Patient: Actually, I take Tylenol a lot when I have a headache and I don't have any kidney problems.
Pharmacist: Good. You can find both Benadryl and Tylenol in aisle 4. And I know it's hard not to, but try not to scratch. The infection can spread and make things worse.
Patient: Thanks for all your help. I will call my doctor as soon as I get home. Thank you for your help.
Pharmacist: Sure, glad to be of help.

Dialogue #2

Patient: Hi, can I speak with the pharmacist?

Pharmacist: Hi, I am Mrs. Smith, the pharmacist on duty. What can I help you with today?

Patient: My feet are burning and itching, and the skin is peeling off. I'm starting to tear my hair out! How can I make the burning and itching stop?

Pharmacist: Do you mind if I examine your feet?

Patient: Not at all.

Pharmacist: OK, you said that both feet are burning and itching?

Patient: Yes!

Pharmacist: OK, I am going to remove your socks and shoes. Let's take a look at your feet.

Patient: Do I have athlete's foot?

Pharmacist: Yes, the skin is scaly between your toes and on the soles of your feet. This scaliness, in combination with the burning and itching, is characteristic of a fungal infection called athlete's foot.

Patient: What should I do?

Pharmacist: I recommend that you apply Lamisil cream twice a day to the affected area. You will use this cream for 2 weeks.

Patient: Can I stop using it if the burning sensation and itchiness go away?

Pharmacist: It is important that you continue to use the cream for the entire 2 weeks, even if the burning and itching stop before then. If you don't use the cream for 2 weeks, the infection may return. Do you have any questions?

Patient: Do I need to do anything to my feet before I put the cream on?

Pharmacist: You should wash and completely dry your feet, even between the toes, before applying the cream. In addition, you should change your socks daily and should consider wearing different shoes, as the fungus may possibly be living in your shoes if they are old or if they are constantly worn.

Patient: Where can I find the Lamisil?

Pharmacist: Follow me. I'll show you where we keep it.

Dialogue #3

Patient: Hi, are you the pharmacist?

Pharmacist: Yes, I am. What can I help you with?

Patient: I feel a little embarrassed. But, well, I have a bad habit of biting my nails when I am nervous. I was biting my nails yesterday, and a very thin piece of my nail was ripped from the side of the nail. Today the side of my index finger is red, swollen, and very painful. I was wondering what I should do for the finger?

Pharmacist: I see. Have you noticed any pus or discharge from the nail?

Patient: Yes. There was yellow pus from the nail this morning when I pressed on the finger.

Pharmacist: Well, it looks like you have an ingrown fingernail. There is a small infection in the finger, which is the reason for the redness, inflammation, pus, and pain. I recommend that you soak the finger twice a day in an Epsom salts soak. You can also apply peroxide to the finger. In addition, you should apply Neosporin to the finger during the day and cover it with a Band-Aid. You may take Motrin for the pain until the infection heals. The infection should be gone in several days. Do you have any questions?

Patient: Not at this time. Can you show me where the Epsom salts and the Neosporin are?

Pharmacist: Sure. Follow me.

CHAPTER 2

Pharmacist/Patient Dialogues

Dialogue #1

Patient: Hi, I need help. I woke up this morning with my right eye crusted and shut tight. I washed my face, and the eye was red. And it's gotten worse throughout the day. Now it's itchy, swollen, and really red.

Pharmacist: It looks like you have conjunctivitis, or what we call pink eye.

Patient: I don't think I've ever had pink eye. I've had a stye, but not pink eye.

Pharmacist: Pink eye is very contagious. That's probably how you got it. Do your eyes also feel itchy?

Patient: Yeah, it feels like there is something in my eye, but I can't get it out. Anyway, I have a prescription to treat it. I have a big presentation in 2 days and I don't want to look like this. Here's the prescription.

Pharmacist: OK. It's a prescription for tobramycin ophthalmic solution. They're eyedrops. Do you wear contacts?

Patient: Yeah, but I didn't put them in this morning. As you can see, I'm wearing my glasses.

Pharmacist: Good. Don't wear your contacts while using eyedrops and until your eye clears up.

Patient: That's it. Will it clear up in 2 days?

Pharmacist: Your doctor has prescribed that you use the eyedrops for 5 days. Put one drop in your eye every 4 hours. It should relieve the redness, inflammation, and itchiness. And even if you see that your eye has cleared up before the 5 days, continue using the drops.

Patient: OK. I just hope my eye gets better before my presentation.

Pharmacist: I hope so too. And don't be surprised if you experience a burning or stinging sensation. These are just some of the side effects. Make sure you read the instructions carefully. And good luck with your presentation.

Patient: Thanks.

Dialogue #2

Patient's mother: Hi. Could you fill this prescription quickly? We just got back from the pediatrician's office and my daughter has an ear infection. She's been crying non-stop. Here's the prescription.

Pharmacist: The prescription is for amoxicillin, an antibiotic. Has she had amoxicillin before?

Patient's mother: No. I don't think so. This is her first ear infection.

Pharmacist: How old is she?

Patient's mother: She's almost 3...34 months old.

Pharmacist: Is she allergic to penicillin?

Patient's mother: No. I don't think so.

Pharmacist: OK. The doctor has ordered the amoxicillin in suspension form, liquid form. I suggest that you also buy a dose-measuring spoon if you don't have one so that you can measure the dosage as precisely as possible.

Patient's mother: I have one.

Pharmacist: Good.

Patient's mother: How about the side effects? Is there anything I should look for?

Pharmacist: Yes. Keep your eyes open for any side effects such as watery diarrhea. And if she gets a rash or starts itching or wheezing, call your doctor immediately.

Patient's mother: Can she eat with the medicine?

Pharmacist: Sure. And make sure she drinks plenty of water when you give her her dosage.

Patient's mother: OK. I'll follow the directions on the bottle.

Pharmacist: Oh, one more thing. Make sure you refrigerate the medicine and make sure she finishes the entire amount, even if she begins to feel better.

Patient's mother: Sure. Thank you so much.

Dialogue #3

Pharmacist: Hello. Can I help you?

Patient: I hope so. My eye doctor tells me I have glaucoma and he gave me this prescription. What's it for?

Pharmacist: Well, it's a prescription for Isopto Carpine. It will help treat your glaucoma. Did your doctor explain how to use this medicine?

Patient: He did. But I was so upset when he told me I have glaucoma that I didn't really listen. He told me that he would put me on this medicine. What did you say the name of the medicine is and what does it do?

Pharmacist: Well, it will help to reduce the high pressure in your eyes. By lowering the pressure, it will help to prevent problems with your vision.

Patient: Yeah, I don't see well, especially at night. And yeah, I do feel some pressure. So what kind of medicine is it?

Pharmacist: Well, Isopto Carpine is an eyedrop. Do you wear contact lenses?

Patient: No, no.

Pharmacist: OK, before applying the drops, make sure your hands are clean and don't touch the eye dropper with your hands or let it touch your eyes.

Patient: Yeah, I know. I've used Visine eyedrops in the past for red eye. I know how to use eyedrops.

Pharmacist: Good, but you need to be careful with these eyedrops. Pull your lower eyelid to make a pouch and then squirt one eyedrop in the eyelid pouch. Then close your eye and place your index finger in the corner of your eye by your nose and put pressure on it for about a minute. And try not to blink. When you've done this with one eye, do the same to the other eye. Do you have any questions?

Patient: Not right now. The medication box will have the label to tell me how many times I should put the eyedrops in my eye.

Pharmacist: That's right. And, of course, if you have any questions, call your doctor.

Patient: Yeah, if I can get through.

Pharmacist: I know what you mean. In the meantime, I need to get some information. Have you been here before?

Patient: Are you kidding me? I've been here for all kinds of ailments. I should be in your fancy computer. My name is Aldo Mancini—A-L-D-O M-A-N-C-I-N-I—and I'm 62 years young.

Pharmacist: OK, but I need your birth date.

Patient: I was born on April 5, 1944.

Pharmacist: OK, here you are. You still live at the same address and you still have the same insurance? And you have no allergies?

Patient: That's right. Hey, I do have a question. Are there any, you know, side effects from this medicine?

Pharmacist: Good question. It's very common to feel a little irritation, burning, or stinging. You might temporarily experience blurred vision. But of course, if these side effects persist, call your doctor. And call your doctor immediately if you experience a rash, itching, dizziness, or difficulty breathing. These are rare, but just in case.

Patient: Can I call you, if I can't get through at the doctor's office?

Pharmacist: Myself or another pharmacist will be happy to help you. Our phone number appears on your prescription label.

Patient: By the way, how do you spell the name of the eyedrops?

Pharmacist: That's I-S-O-P-T-O and C-A-R-P-I-N-E. Isopto Carpine.

Patient: All those letters for small eyedrops. Thank you so much. What's your name?

Pharmacist: I'm Eman Hussain. My name is on the label, too.

Patient: You've been wonderful. Thank you so much.

Pharmacist: You're very welcome, Mr. Mancini.

Mini Dialogue Listening Exercises

Mini Dialogue #1

Person A: Why are you smiling from ear to ear?

Person B: I just passed my pharmacy licensing exam and I have three job offers, but I don't know which one to accept.

Mini Dialogue #2

Person A: Did you see the World Cup soccer championship game between Italy and Brazil? It was such a great game.

Person B: Are you kidding me? My eyes were glued to the TV and I didn't go to work.

Mini Dialogue #3

Person A: Have you met the new head pharmacist? What do you think of him?

Person B: Poor guy. He's only been here 4 days and he's already up to his ears in work.

Mini Dialogue #4

Person A: It's really quiet today—not too many patients coming in with prescriptions.
Person B: I'm not complaining. It's nice not to have patients bend your ear about all their health problems.

Mini Dialogue # 5

Person A: I can't believe I have to work tonight by myself. I feel I shouldn't work alone because I'm still green behind the ears.
Person B: Your boss has a lot of confidence in your ability.

Mini Dialogue #6

Person A: How's your new boss?
Person B: He's like my old boss, who was friendly and kind, but he has eyes like a hawk.

Mini Dialogue #7

Person A: It's amazing how much customers and patients will try to steal batteries for their hearing aids.
Person B: I know. The batteries are so small. That's why we need to have eyes in the back of our head at all times to be able to stop them.

Chapter 2 Post-Assessment

Dialogue #1

Patient: Hi. I need a prescription filled. I have swimmer's ear and the doctor gave me a prescription for an antibiotic.
Pharmacist: Sure. It's for Cortisporin Otic solution. Have you had swimmer's ear before?
Patient: Yeah, a couple of times. Usually I just put a little bit of diluted vinegar in my ears and take Tylenol for the pain and it usually clears it up. But this time the infection is pretty bad and I'm in more pain than usual.
Pharmacist: Do you swim a lot?
Patient: Actually, I do triathlons, so I spend a lot of time in the pool or in Cooper River training.
Pharmacist: That's probably how you got the infection.
Patient: I know, and I have a triathlon coming up in a month.
Pharmacist: Wow. I can barely walk a block without running out of breath. OK, let me fill this prescription for you. Have you been here before?
Patient: No. Do you need my insurance card?
Pharmacist: Sure, I'll take that, but I'll need to ask you a couple of questions. What's your full name? And what's your date of birth?
Patient: Michael P. Francis and my birth date is February 2, 1960.
Pharmacist: Is Francis with an "i" or and "e"?
Patient: With an "i" as in F-R-A-N-C-I-S.
Pharmacist: OK. And your address?
Patient: 21 Chester Lane, apartment three "s" in Wayne. The zip is 11920.
Pharmacist: Thanks. Your co-pay for the prescription is $10.00.
Patient: OK. You think this antibiotic will get rid of this infection soon?
Pharmacist: Well, it should. It will help to stop the growth of bacteria in your ears. And it will reduce the swelling and inflammation that is causing the pain. You should start feeling better in 3 to 5 days, but make sure you use the medication regularly.
Patient: How many times a day should I put drops in?
Pharmacist: Your doctor has prescribed three to four times a day. You need to finish the entire prescription even if you're feeling better.
Patient: OK. I guess I'll read the directions and instructions in the package.

Pharmacist: That's a good idea, and pay attention to possible side effects such as stinging or burning that won't go away after you apply the drops. Call the doctor if you experience this, and call the doctor if you feel that you are experiencing some hearing loss.

Patient: Thanks. I'll read the label carefully.

Pharmacist: Good. And good luck in your triathlon.

Dialogue #2

Patient: Hi, can I speak with the pharmacist?

Pharmacist: Hi, I am Dr. Newmark, the pharmacist on duty. What can I help you with today?

Patient: I just had cataract surgery on my right eye and the doctor told me I should get this medicine. He said it will help with inflammation.

Pharmacist: OK. It's a prescription for Lotemax eyedrops. Have you been here before?

Patient: Oh, yeah. Many times, for this and that.

Pharmacist: What is your name?

Patient: Ethel Burns, honey. That's B-U-R-N-S, not B-Y-R-N-E-S.

Pharmacist: Mrs. Burns, what's your date of birth?

Patient: Do you really need to know? I'm just kidding. My birth date is December 4, 1938. I'm 68 and now I have cataracts. Can you believe it?

Pharmacist: Actually, they're quite common. Mrs. Burns, are you allergic to any medication?

Patient: Yes, penicillin.

Pharmacist: Are you taking any other medications?

Patient: No, not right now. I consider myself pretty healthy. I walk 2 miles every day, except in bad weather. I don't want to fall and break my hip.

Pharmacist: That's wise. OK, let me explain how to use the eyedrops. Make sure you shake the bottle well. Gently pull the lower eyelid and then squirt the eyedrop. Close your eyes for a couple of minutes and try not to blink.

Patient: It sounds easy, but will it hurt?

Pharmacist: Well, it's not unusual to feel some stinging or burning and some temporary vision loss. In rare cases, some people experience dizziness, rash, itching, and trouble breathing. If you do, please call your doctor immediately.

Patient: Are you serious? If I'd known that, I would have kept my cataract. One eyedrop can cause all of that?

Pharmacist: I'm glad you have a good sense of humor about it, but please call your doctor if you experience any of these side effects. Do you have any other questions?

Patient: Well, now I'll know what to expect if I get a cataract on my left eye.

Pharmacist: I hope not, but if you do, we're here.

Patient: Thanks, hon. It's nice to be young.

Pharmacist: You're welcome. Enjoy your walks.

Dialogue #3

Patient: Hi, are you the pharmacist?

Pharmacist: Yes, I am. What can I help you with?

Patient: Well, I got into a brawl. I got punched in my left ear a few times. I went to the emergency room a couple of days later after the pain wouldn't go away and it looks like I have a ruptured eardrum. It hurts a bit. The doctor said it should heal in a couple of months, but in the meantime to prevent an infection he gave me this prescription.

Pharmacist: I see. What's your name?

Patient: Thomas Miller.

Pharmacist: Mr. Miller, have you been here before?

Patient: No, and I don't have any insurance. I'll charge it on my credit card.

Pharmacist: OK, Mr. Miller. The prescription is for Cortisporin Otic. Do you have any allergies?

Patient: I'm allergic to cats. Is the medicine going to get rid of the pain? It's getting a little intense.

Pharmacist: Well, the medicine contains antibiotics to help stop bacteria from growing, as well as hydrocortisone to help reduce the ear swelling and the discomfort you're having. Mr. Miller, what's your date of birth and what's your address?

Patient: I have Best Health Insurance. Here's my card. It also has my home address on it.

Pharmacist: What's your home number?

Patient: 555-0171.

Pharmacist: Thanks. While your prescription is being filled, and it won't be long, let me explain to you how to use amoxicillin. Have you ever taken amoxicillin?

Patient: No. I've never had sinusitis before.

Pharmacy: OK. Make sure to take the dosage prescribed by your doctor. It's on the medicine bottle label.

Patient: Is it OK to stop taking it if I start to feel better?

Pharmacist: No. It's very important to take all the amoxicillin. Even if you start feeling better, your sinus infection may not be completely treated. And don't break open the capsules. Swallow them whole.

Patient: Can I take it with food?

Pharmacist: You can, and you can also take it on an empty stomach, but make sure you drink a full glass of water with the capsules.

Patient: Will they make me feel different or sick?

Pharmacist: Actually, since this is your first time with amoxicillin, read the computer printout we will give you of the side effects. These side effects could include some nausea, vomiting, and diarrhea. But if you experience shortness of breath, or you feel that your throat is closing up, or you get hives and swelling, stop taking it and get medical help immediately. I don't want you to panic, but just be mindful of these possible side effects.

Patient: Wow. Getting a sinus infection is no fun. I just want to feel better soon.

Pharmacist: You will. And call your doctor if you have other concerns.

Patient: Thank you so much. You've been so helpful.

CHAPTER 4

Pharmacist/Patient Dialogues

Dialogue #1

Pharmacist: Hello, are you here to pick up a prescription or to get one filled?

Patient: Actually, I'm here to get a prescription filled.

Pharmacist: I see. It's a prescription for Levoxyl. Have you been here before?

Patient: Yeah. I was here last year for a sinus infection. I was on ampicillin.

Pharmacist: What's your name?

Patient: Linda Anderson. My birth date is 1/2/69. I was wondering . . . could you hurry up? I'm really cold. It's so cold in here.

Pharmacist: I'll try. OK, I see you are in our system. You still live on Sunset Road?

Patient: No, I moved. I live on 32 Harvard Road, but same town. And I have the same phone number.

Pharmacist: OK. Thanks for the update. Now, I need to ask you a couple of questions. Are you taking any medication?

Patient: Well, I take vitamins. And I cut my finger 2 days ago, so I've been taking Tylenol and putting Neosporin on the cut.

Pharmacist: Have you been on Levoxyl before?

Patient: No, this is my first time. I have hypo . . . something to do with my thyroid. It's so confusing. All I know is that I'm always cold and really super tired and I forget things and I can't concentrate. And I've gained weight but I'm not eating more.

Pharmacist: Your doctor has given you a prescription for Levoxyl because you have hypothyroidism or an underactive thyroid. Levoxyl is a synthetic thyroid hormone that will replace the hormone that is normally produced by your thyroid gland.

Patient: How often do I take it?

Pharmacist: Your doctor has prescribed 50 mcg once a day. It's a good idea to take it in the morning on an empty stomach about a half hour before breakfast. Your doctor will monitor you.

Patient: Are there any strange side effects?

Pharmacist: Well, not all people react in the same way. But let your doctor know if you begin experiencing headaches, nervousness, trembling, or sweating. There's a list of possible side effects on the computer printout you will receive with the medication. In very rare cases, some people might experience some hair loss until their bodies adjust to the medication. Let your doctor know.

Patient: Will it make me sleepy?

Pharmacist: Well, no, but it may cause insomnia.

Patient: Great. Just what I need.

Pharmacist: You can always call us or your doctor if you have any concerns.

Patient: I know. Thanks. Here is my insurance card. I think I only have a $5 co-pay.

Dialogue #2

Patient: Hi. I'm here to pick up my insulin medicine.

Pharmacist: What is your name?

Patient: Sean Smith.

Pharmacist: Sean, have you been here before?

Patient: No.

Pharmacist: OK, I need to ask you a few questions. Sean, how do you spell your first name?

Patient: S-E-A-N.

Pharmacist: What's your birth date?

Patient: March 18, 1980.

Pharmacist: Your home address?

Patient: 88 Marlboro Lane in Waine.

Pharmacist: Is that W-A-Y-N-E?

Patient: No, it's W-A-I-N-E.

Pharmacist: And the phone number where you can be reached?

Patient: My cell number is best. It's 818-0818.

Pharmacist: Can you confirm your doctor's name?

Patient: Dr. Harwicke, with an "e" at the end.

Pharmacist: And your insurance?

Patient: I have Optimal Health. Here's my card.

Pharmacist: OK, now I have all the information I need. Oh, one more thing. Any allergies?

Patient: I'm allergic to peanuts and peanut butter.

Pharmacist: OK. Now here's your prescription. This is NovoLog.

Patient: Novo what?

Pharmacist: NovoLog. It's spelled N-O-V-O-L-O-G. This is insulin that you inject to treat your diabetes.

Patient: Yeah, my doctor said it's the kind I inject.

Pharmacist: That's right. Has your doctor taught you how to inject it?

Patient: Yeah. And I've watched my mother inject herself many times. She has diabetes, too.

Pharmacist: Some important things to remember. Don't inject cold insulin, so keep the insulin at room temperature. Clean the area you want to inject like the back of your arm, your thigh, or your abdomen with rubbing alcohol. Make sure you inject the correct amount as prescribed by your doctor.

Patient: Do I inject the insulin before or after I eat?

Pharmacist: Inject it 5 to 10 minutes before you eat. And pay attention to some possible side effects. Too much insulin can cause low blood sugar, or hypoglycemia, and you might experience chills, dizziness, sweating, and hunger. Too little insulin can cause hyperglycemia, or high blood sugar, and you might feel very thirsty, urinate a lot, and feel a little confused and drowsy. Call your doctor immediately. I know it's a lot to remember. Do you have any questions?

Patient: No, I'll be all right. My doctor has explained a lot to me and I can always ask my mother.

Pharmacist: OK, Sean. Here you go. There's more information about the insulin on the package. Take care. And feel free to call us any time.

Dialogue #3

Pharmacist: Good morning. How can I help you today?

Patient: My doctor called in a prescription for Sofran. I think that's what it's called.

Pharmacist: What are you having treated?

Patient: For my nausea. I have leukemia.

Pharmacist: OK. You mean Zofran with a "z". It's spelled Z-O-F-R-A-N. That's OK. So many medications sound identical. Anyway, would you like to sit down while you wait?

Patient: No, I'm OK.

Pharmacist: OK. What's your name?

Patient: My last name is Morales. My first name is Martin.

Pharmacist: Could you spell your last name for me?

Patient: M-O-R-A-L-E-S.

Pharmacist: Is your date of birth July 27, 1966?

Patient: Yeah.

Pharmacist: OK. Here we are. You still live at the same address?

Patient: Yeah. And I still have the same phone number.

Pharmacist: Is your doctor Dr. Thomas Miller?

Patient: Yeah.

Pharmacist: Have you used Zofran before?

Patient: No. But after a few rounds of chemotherapy I started to have more nausea and more vomiting.

Pharmacist: That's not uncommon. Hopefully, the Zofran will help alleviate both.

Patient: I hope so. Am I going to feel any other side effects?

Pharmacist: Well, you might experience some lightheadedness, headaches, drowsiness, and even constipation. Some people experience muscle stiffness and vision problems.

Patient: How about any allergic reactions? I'm allergic to iodine.

Pharmacist: Well, as indicated in the packaging, some rare allergic reactions include severe rash, difficulty breathing, and swelling. Of course, please seek medical attention immediately if any of these occur.

Patient: Wow, all of that just to make my nausea and vomiting go away.

Pharmacist: You said you're receiving chemotherapy?

Patient: Yeah.

Pharmacist: OK. Your doctor has prescribed that you need to take one tablet about 30 minutes before your treatment, and your doctor has probably told you not to eat before your treatment. Let your doctor know if the medication is not working for you.

Patient: OK, I will. I have another round of chemotherapy tomorrow morning.

Pharmacist: Good luck and I hope you get well soon.

Patient: Thanks a lot. Here's my insurance card.

Mini Dialogue Listening Exercises

Mini Dialogue #1

Person A: I hate when patients yell at me when their prescription is not ready in time. Don't they know how busy we are?

Person B: Oh, don't let them make your blood boil. Just do your job with a smile on your face.

Mini Dialogue #2

Person A: Have you seen the movies "Saw" and "Saw II?" I can't wait to see "Saw III."

Person B: No way. Those types of movies make my blood run cold.

Mini Dialogue #3

Person A: No, I'm not the only pharmacist in my family. My grandmother was a pharmacist; so was my mother and my older brother.

Person B: Wow. Pharmacy really runs in your blood.

Mini Dialogue #4

Person A: Your sister called while you were out. She said she needs to borrow money from you.

Person B: I'm never going to lend her money again. The last time I loaned her money, she paid me in pennies. It was like getting blood from a stone.

Mini Dialogue #5

Person A: My brother and I had a big fight last night. I don't like his fiancé and I don't think he should marry her. And I don't want to be in their wedding.

Person B: Well, whether you like her or not or don't want to be in their wedding, he's still your brother. And you know what they say—blood is thicker than water.

Chapter 4 Post-Assessment

Dialogue #1

Pharmacist: Hello. How can I help you today?

Patient: Well, I need to get my prescription for my diabetes filled.

Pharmacist: OK. Do you have the prescription?

Patient: Yeah. Here it is. My doctor, Dr. Menken, wants me to try a new pill to control my diabetes. I also have to follow a new diet and exercise more.

Pharmacist: Is that M-E-N-K-E-N or M-E-N-K-I-N?

Patient: With an "e".

Pharmacist: He has ordered Amaryl in 2-mg tablets.

Patient: Yeah, he said they would be pills and not the insulin I've been injecting. By the way, how do you spell that? It sounds like a girl's name.

Pharmacist: It's spelled A-M-A-R-Y-L. You look familiar. Have you been here before?

Patient: For my insulin. My name is Ann Marie Jones. No "e" in Ann and they're two separate names.

Pharmacist: So that's capital A-N-N and capital M-A-R-I-E. And Jones is J-O-N-E-S.

Patient: That's right.

Pharmacist: Is your birth date January 20, 1977?

Patient: Yep.

Pharmacist: Is your insurance still Healthy Living?

Patient: No. I have a new job and a new insurance plan. It's Health Now Plan. Here's my card.

Pharmacist: Thanks. Is your address still 64 Robin Circle in Haddonfield?

Patient: No. I've moved. My new address is 17 Princeton Road in Maple Shade.

Pharmacist: And your phone?

Patient: Also new. It's 632-1129.

Pharmacist: Thanks. Now, do you have any questions about the new medication?

Patient: I didn't have any problems with my old insulin injection, but I used to get red where I injected myself and felt a little pain for a little while, but that's about it.

Pharmacist: Well, you won't experience that with the tablet, but keep your eyes open for other side effects such as yellowing of your eyes or skin, dark urine, or stomach pains. These are rare, but not to be ignored. Of course, if you have difficulty breathing, swelling, or a rash, seek medical attention immediately.

Patient: I will. I will read the pamphlet and the instructions in the box. And the nurse at the doctor's office also explained to me what to look for.

Pharmacist: That's good. And remember you can always call us if you have any questions.

Patient: I know. Thanks.

Pharmacist: Sure. It will be just a few minutes

Patient: Oh, yeah. I just remembered, how often do I take the tablet?

Pharmacist: Your doctor wants you to take one tablet once a day with breakfast. Try to take it regularly and of course monitor and check your glucose levels and let your doctor know if your glucose levels are elevated.

Dialogue #2

Pharmacist: Hello. How can I help you today?

Patient: I'm here to pick up my prescription. Dr. Schneider called it in this morning.

Pharmacist: Sure. What's your name?

Patient: Ilene, I-L-E-N-E. Last name Willis, W-I-L-L-I-S.

Pharmacist: Is that a prescription for propylthiouracil?

Patient: Yeah, I think so. Dr. Schneider said it's also called PTU. I have Graves disease, a hyperactive thyroid.

Pharmacist: Did your doctor explain how to use it?

Patient: Well, I think he said I have to take one tablet three times a day.

Pharmacist: That's what he prescribed. Did he explain to you some of the side effects that you might have?

Patient: No, but will I feel drowsy?

Pharmacist: Well, that's one side effect. You might also experience joint pain, nausea, upset stomach, and some tingling and burning sensation on your hands and feet. You can read more about the side effects in the computer printout stapled to the prescription bag. But I need to get additional information.

Patient: Sure.

Pharmacist: Do you have any allergies?

Patient: No medicines, but I'm allergic to onions, bees, and wasps.

Pharmacist: What's your birth date?

Patient: April 22, 1952.

Pharmacist: I see you're in our computer. Is your address still 2733 Phoenix Avenue?

Patient: Yes.

Pharmacist: And your insurance?

Patient: Mutual Health and Life.

Pharmacist: OK, you're all set. You don't have a co-pay. Don't hesitate to call us or your doctor if you have any concerns.

Patient: I will. Thank you.

Dialogue #3

Customer: Hi, I'm here to pick up my wife's prescription. The last name is Graham.

Pharmacist: Can you spell it for me?

Customer: G-R-A-H-A-M. Her first name is Christina with an "h".

Pharmacist: OK. Here it is. Did the doctor explain to your wife or to you how Aranesp is used?

Customer: Well, Dr. Patel told us it's an injection to help her with the anemia she has as a result of her chemotherapy.

Pharmacist: Which doctor Patel?

Customer: Amit Patel. A-M-I-T.

Pharmacist: OK. I'll explain how to use it and the possible side effects as soon as I confirm some information. Has Christina been here before?

Customer: Many, many times. Her birth date is February 12, 1955. We live on 4601 Westmont Road.

Pharmacist: OK. I see this information in our system. Insurance is the same?

Customer: Yeah. And I don't have a co-pay.

Pharmacist: That's right. Aranesp is a colorless vial. Your doctor has ordered two vials that you can refill. She needs to inject it under her skin. If she's too weak, you can do it. Needles don't make you queasy, do they?

Customer: I've been a diabetic for years and have experience injecting my insulin.

Pharmacist: OK then. Her doctor wants her to use it once a week. It usually takes 2 to 6 weeks before she'll start feeling better. You can read the patient information pamphlet regarding preparation and usage instructions.

Customer: I will. Any side effects?

Pharmacist: It's possible to experience a headache, body aches, and diarrhea. In rare cases, the medication can cause blood clots, so keep an eye out for swelling, redness, and weakness of arms and legs. Call the doctor immediately. And of course, if you or your wife have any questions, please call us.

Customer: Sure. We will. Thanks.

CHAPTER 5

Pharmacist/Patient Dialogues

Dialogue #1

Pharmacist: Hello. Can I help you?

Patient's mother: I hope so. I have a prescription for my daughter. She's home with bronchitis.

Pharmacist: OK. It's for Entex. Has your daughter been taking any other medication?

Patient's mother: Well, she was taking Robitussin, but her cough and congestion got worse. And now she has a lot of mucus in her lungs.

Pharmacist: How old is your daughter?

Patient's mother: She's 16.

Pharmacist: What's your daughter's name?

Patient's mother: Aurea Cuevas.

Pharmacist: Can you please spell her name for me?

Patient's mother: Aurea is A-U-R-E-A and Cuevas is C-U-E-V-A-S.

Pharmacist: Thanks. And what's her date of birth?

Patient's mother: August 19, 1990.

Pharmacist: I see from the computer she's been here before.

Patient's mother: Yeah. For ear infections when she was younger.

Pharmacist: Is she allergic to any medications?

Patient's mother: She broke out into a rash the first time she took Bactrim for some kind of infection.

Pharmacist: Is your address still 11 Morningside Terrace?

Patient's mother: Yeah.

Pharmacist: Is the phone number the same?

Patient's mother: Yes.

Pharmacist: And the doctor is Dr. Swee?

Patient's mother: Yep.

Pharmacist: Well, the medication should start to make her feel better. The medication will help to loosen the mucus in her lungs and clear the congestion. She'll start to breathe easier.

Patient's mother: Will it make her drowsy?

Pharmacist: It might, so don't let her drive while she's taking it. She might also experience some nausea and upset stomach. It's rare, but keep your eyes out for other side effects such as . . .

Patient's mother: I'll just read the insert in the box. I read everything.

Pharmacist: That's a good idea. How will you be paying for this?

Patient's mother: I'll pay cash. By the way, is it pills or liquid?

Pharmacist: Her doctor prescribed capsules. And make sure she drinks plenty of fluids when she takes the capsules. Do you have any other questions?

Patient's mother: No, but how much is it?

Pharmacist: That'll be $33.99.

Patient's mother: OK.

Dialogue #2

Patient: Hi, I need to get this prescription filled. I have asthma.

Pharmacist: Your doctor has given you a prescription for the albuterol oral inhaler.

Patient: What do you mean? It's not a pill I can take?

Pharmacist: No. Your doctor ordered the inhaler instead.

Patient: How do I use it? This is the first time I've had asthma. She told me I have exercise-induced asthma and wheezing.

Pharmacist: Do you play sports?

Patient: Yeah, I play field hockey, basketball, and softball.

Pharmacist: Good for you. Now, it's important to read the leaflet in the package, but I'll show you how to use it. First, shake the inhaler and spray-test it. Then put the mouthpiece near your mouth and exhale. Next, place the mouthpiece in your mouth and press the inhaler as you inhale deeply. Make sure you hold your breath for at least 10 seconds so that the medication gets absorbed.

Patient: How often do I do that?

Pharmacist: Well, your doctor has prescribed that you inhale two to three puffs 15 to 30 minutes before exercise or physical activity to help you with exercise-induced wheezing. Make sure you don't take more puffs than prescribed by your doctor.

Patient: So this will help me get rid of my wheezing and the shortness of breath I get when I run?

Pharmacist: It should, but if you find that it's not helping, please see your doctor. And keep you eyes out for any possible side effects such as headache and nausea. And if you begin to feel dizzy, get medical help.

Pharmacist: Can you tell me your name so I can get your chart and take a look at it?

Patient: Margaret Peters.

Pharmacist: Here it is. Give me a minute to take a quick look at it. OK. According to your chart, you were prescribed captopril. Do you have the bottle with you?

Patient: Yeah. It's in my purse. Here it is.

Pharmacist: Thank you. I just need to update your chart before I give you the refill. Do you have a few minutes?

Patient: Sure.

Pharmacist: I see from your chart that you have been on other medications. Are you still taking Lipitor for your cholesterol?

Patient: No. I stopped after I had the heart attack.

Pharmacist: Did the doctor tell you to stop?

Patient: No.

Pharmacist: Mrs. Peters, you need to take the medical advice of your doctor.

Patient: Medicine is so expensive, even with insurance.

Pharmacist: I understand. Speak to your doctor about reduced-cost medications, OK? And before you leave I'll give you a list of reduced-cost cholesterol medicines for your doctor to review.

Patient: OK. I will. And thanks for the list.

Pharmacist: I see that you take over-the-counter multivitamins with iron and minerals. Are you still taking them?

Patient: Yes.

Pharmacist: Now, do you feel that the captopril is working for you?

Patient: I think so.

Pharmacist: Have you had any side effects?

Patient: Well, I noticed I felt a little dizzy and lightheaded when I first took it, but then it went away. I'm feeling fine now.

Pharmacist: Good. Have you experienced a fast heartbeat?

Patient: No.

Pharmacist: How about a cough?

Patient: No.

Pharmacist: Change in your urine?

Patient: No.

Pharmacist: Any other side effects that you can think of?

Patient: No. Actually, I think the medicine is making me feel better. That's why I'm here for a refill. I want to continue to feel good.

Pharmacist: That's a wise idea. Give me a few minutes while I get you the refill. Remember, you need to take one pill three times a day and an hour before you eat. And avoid any potassium supplements or salt substitutes.

Patient: I know.

Dialogue #2

Pharmacist: Good morning, Mr. Jackson. How are you today? Do you remember me?

Patient: I think so. Were you the pharmacist the last time I was here?

Pharmacist: Yes, I'm Linda Riley.

Patient: Linda. Now I remember.

Pharmacist: So how are you doing? How are you feeling?

Patient: OK.

Pharmacist: I remember that you started to see us after you were diagnosed with congestive heart failure. Are you taking your meds?

Patient: Yes.

Pharmacist: Can you tell me what you're taking?

Patient: Well, let me get my bottles out. I'm taking val . . . sar . . . tan. I'm taking La . . . six. And 2 weeks ago I had a cataract removed, so I'm taking drops. I think they're called Lo . . . te . . . max. Here you go.

Pharmacist: Thank you. Can you tell me what you're taking valsartan for?

Patient: For my heart.

Pharmacist: Can you tell me why you're taking the Lasix?

Patient: Doctor told me it stops me from having too much water in my lungs and helps with the swelling in my legs.

Pharmacist: And how about the Lotemax?

Patient: After she took out my cataract from my left eye, she told me to put the drops in so I don't get inflammation. My eye is fine. I'm gonna see her next week for a checkup.

Pharmacist: Are you able to see better?

Patient: Yes, very much.

Pharmacist: Good. Mr. Jackson, you've done a good job of bringing in all your meds. Are you taking your medications as directed by your doctor and as on the medication labels?

Patient: Yes.

Pharmacist: Are any of the medicines giving you any trouble?

Patient: Well, sometimes when I get up from sitting, I feel a little dizzy. And I'm going to the bathroom a lot.

Pharmacist: Well, the Lasix helps to remove the extra fluid, or what we call edema, in your body and your legs. That explains why you're urinating more. The dizziness is a common side effect of valsartan and Lasix. Try to get up slowly. Can you tell me when you're taking your valsartan?

Patient: Well, I really try to take the val . . . sar . . . tan with food, but the doctor said I don't need to take it with food.

Pharmacist: How about the Lasix?

Patient: The doctor told me to take it around eight in the morning every day so I don't have to wake up so much in the night to urinate. So I try not to take my pills at night.

Pharmacist: That's a good idea. I see from your chart you have smoked in the past. Are you smoking now?

Patient: No. I wish I could.

Pharmacist: According to your chart, part of your treatment includes some exercise. What kind of physical activity do you do?

Patient: Well, I have been going out for walks in the evenings and on weekends if the weather is nice. But I didn't walk for almost 2 weeks when I had the eye patch over my eye.

Pharmacist: Well, I'm glad you are walking as much as you can. It's important. Mr. Jackson, do you have any questions for me?

Patient: No, I'm OK. Thank you so much, dear.

Dialogue #3

Pharmacist: Good morning. My name is Larry Brand. I'm your pharmacist today. Are you Mrs. Eva Gonzalez?

Patient: Yes.

Pharmacist: I understand that you are being discharged from the hospital today, so I just want to go over with you what you need to know about your medication to help you treat your stroke. I see from your chart that you are 51.

Patient: Yes.

Pharmacist: I also see from you chart that you have type I diabetes.

Patient: Yes.

Pharmacist: Are you still taking NovoLog?

Patient: Yes.

Pharmacist: Have you had any problems with NovoLog?

Patient: No.

Pharmacist: I see from your chart that this is your first stroke. Your doctor has prescribed Aggrenox.

Patient: What?

Pharmacist: Here, I'll spell it for you. A-G-G-R-E-N-O-X. I'm going to explain to you what it is and how it will help decrease your chances of having another stroke. I know it's difficult to talk, but you can stop me to ask questions.

Patient: OK.

Pharmacist: Is a family member going to pick you up?

Patient: Yes.

Pharmacist: I'll try to come back and explain things to your family member.

Patient: OK.

Pharmacist: This medication comes in a capsule. It contains aspirin and another medication with a long name. It's spelled d-i-p-y-r-i-d-a-m-o-l-e. The capsule will help to stop blood clots in the brain. The doctor wants you to take one capsule in the morning and one capsule in the evening. You can take it with food or without food. It's important that you swallow the capsule whole. Don't crush or chew the capsule. Do you understand me so far?

Patient: Yes.

Pharmacist: Good. Also, drink eight ounces of water.

Patient: OK.

Pharmacist: OK. Now I'm going to explain some possible side effects, some problems that the medication may give you. These side effects include nausea, dizziness, heartburn, diarrhea, and sleepiness. Understand?

Patient: Yes.

Pharmacist: But if you have bruising on your skin or dark and bloody stool when you go to the bathroom, or if you have a severe headache or if you get a rash or have difficulty breathing, call your doctor immediately. I will give you a list of all the side effects for you to take home and read. Also have a family member read them. I'm sorry I have so much information to tell you, but it's important.

Patient: OK.

Pharmacist: According to your chart, you're not currently taking any medication that cannot be taken with the capsules, but remember not to take ibuprofen like Motrin and naproxen like Aleve.

Patient: OK.

Pharmacist: Also, let the doctor that treats you for diabetes know that you've had a stroke and that you're taking Aggrenox. He may want to adjust your diabetes medicine.

Patient: OK.

Pharmacist: Thank you so much for being patient. My name is Larry Brand. I wish you well. If you or your family has any questions, you can call me. Here is my card with my phone number. Or you can call your doctor or your drugstore pharmacist.

Patient: OK.

Mini Dialogue Listening Exercises

Mini Dialogue #1

Person A: I hate when patients yell at me when their prescription is not ready in time. Don't they know how busy we are?

Person B: Jan, we need to have a heart-to-heart talk about your attitude. The patients have complained about you.

Mini Dialogue #2

Person A: I don't know how much longer I can take working here. All Mike does is yell at me.

Person B: I know what you mean. How can a person with a heart of stone be in charge of this pharmacy?

Mini Dialogue #3

Person A: How was your doctor's visit today? What did he say about your test results?

Person B: It's not good. When he told me, my heart sank.

Mini Dialogue #4

Person A: Sometimes I wish I could be more like Norma. She doesn't hide anything.

Person B: I know what you mean, but I don't know if I could always wear my heart on my sleeve.

Mini Dialogue #5

Person A: My sister and I had a big fight last night. I don't like her fiancé. I don't think he's good for her. She's my baby sister and I want her to be happy.

Person B: Well, there's nothing you can do. Your heart's in the right place, but it's her life.

Mini Dialogue #6

Person A: Don't worry. I'll work for you this weekend. I know how important it is to have a big birthday party for your children.

Person B: Thank you so much for switching weekends with me. You have a heart of gold.

Chapter 6 Post-Assessment

Dialogue #1

Pharmacist: Hello. My name is Frederica Collins. I'm a pharmacist and I will be reviewing your prescription with you and answer any questions you may have. Are you Mr. Arthur Jenkins?

Patient: Yes, I am. Nice to meet you. Do you know what drugs the doctor wants me to take?

Pharmacist: Yes, I do. But first I want you to tell me how you're feeling.

Patient: Well, I have felt better, but it's been hard for me to walk. My legs have been hurting. The doctor told me I have bad arteries. He says they're hard.

Pharmacist: You have what is called peripheral artery disease. What that means is that you have fatty material inside your arteries. This fatty material blocks the blood from flowing to your arteries. That's why your legs hurt when you walk. Your legs need more blood when they move, when you walk or go up the stairs.

Patient: Yeah. My legs feel tight and heavy and my calf muscles feel tired. You know, the pain comes and goes.

Pharmacist: Do you have any other discomfort?

Patient: Well, sometimes my butt hurts and sometimes I have numbness and a tingling feeling in my legs, and my feet ache.

Pharmacist: Those are common symptoms. But you should start feeling much better once you begin your medication. Your doctor has prescribed Pletal. Has your doctor talked to you about Pletal?

Patient: He told me the medicine will help me to walk better, and not limp.

Pharmacist: That's right. It will help to reduce the symptoms you're experiencing. Soon you should be able to walk farther distances without so much pain. It will help improve the oxygen and blood flow in your legs. Here's what Pletal looks like. It comes in tablet form. They are white, and as you can see, the name of the drug is imprinted on the tablet.

Patient: Yeah, I see. P-L-E-T-A-L. It is spelled almost like flower petal.

Pharmacist: Yeah, you're right. Now, you will need to take a tablet twice a day. And make sure you take the tablet 30 minutes before breakfast and dinner, or 2 hours after breakfast and dinner.

Patient: I'm confused. Did you say 30 minutes after breakfast or dinner?

Pharmacist: You're right. It can be a bit confusing, but I'll repeat it. Thirty minutes *before* breakfast *and* dinner or 2 hours *after* breakfast *and* dinner.

Patient: How fast will I start feeling better?

Pharmacist: Well, you should see improvement in as soon as 2 to 4 weeks, or longer. It could take as long as 12 weeks before you'll feel the benefits of the medication.

Patient: That long, huh? I hope it's sooner than later. I have a hard time getting to my car, and I'm uncomfortable when I drive.

Pharmacist: Speaking of driving, be careful. The medication can make you dizzy. Be careful when driving, and limit alcohol intake. And keep your eyes out for other possible side effects such as diarrhea. And if your feet and hands start to swell and you start to feel rapid and pounding heartbeats, call your doctor immediately. And avoid grapefruit. You want to avoid a bad interaction.

Patient: No grapefruit? Not even with my breakfast?

Pharmacist: I wouldn't recommend it, but check with your doctor.

Patient: OK.

Pharmacist: OK, Mr. Jenkins, do you have any questions for me?

Patient: Is there anything I shouldn't take?

Pharmacist: Yes. Don't take aspirin or anti-inflammatory over-the-counter drugs like ibuprofen or naproxen. Are there any drugs you're taking, prescribed or over-the-counter?

Patient: Sometimes I take Tylenol. Is that OK?

Pharmacist: Sure. Do you have any other questions for me?

Patient: No, but I do have a lot to remember. Everything you told me will be on the label?

Pharmacist: Yes, and I'll also give you a patient information sheet for you to take home and refer to. And if you have any questions, you can call the clinic, your local pharmacist, or your doctor.

Dialogue #2

Pharmacist: Good afternoon, Mrs. Davis. How are you today?

Patient: I'm pretty good. You can call me Helen.

Pharmacist: Sure, Helen. I'm Brett Long. I'm the clinic pharmacist and I'm here to see how you're doing and to review your prescriptions with you. I see from your chart that you were hospitalized with chest pains, more specifically, angina. This was your first episode?

Patient: Yes, it was. I thought I was having a heart attack and going to die.

Pharmacist: I also see from your chart that you are a smoker and that you have high cholesterol and high blood pressure.

Patient: Yes, I have tried to quit so many times, and I try to eat healthy, but . . .

Pharmacist: How old are you?

Patient: I'm 49.

Pharmacist: OK, Mrs. Davis. Let's talk about your medications. Can you tell me what you're taking for your angina?

Patient: Well, the doctor gave me a patch. It's right here on my chest.

Pharmacist: Can you tell me the name of the patch and how you're using it?

Patient: Isn't it nitroglycerin?

Pharmacist: Yes, but the name of the patch is Nitro-Dur. Can you tell me how you're using it?

Patient: I put it on my chest. My doctor told me to leave it there for about 12 to 14 hours during the day. But sometimes it itches and irritates my skin so I take it off. And sometimes I take it off when I'm in the shower.

Pharmacist: Don't do that. Don't remove it. You need to keep the patch on when showering and even swimming. To avoid irritation, change the location of the patch; for example, if it irritates your skin on your chest, place the next patch on your upper arm. Do you have any allergies?

Patient: Well, I'm allergic to penicillin.

Pharmacist: OK. It's important to keep the patch on for 12 to 14 hours, and then wait about 10 to 12 hours before you put a new patch on.

Patient: OK.

Pharmacist: Now, let's review your cholesterol medication. What are you taking for your cholesterol?

Patient: Zocor.

Pharmacist: Can you tell me how you use Zocor?

Patient: Well, I know I'm supposed to take one tablet at night but sometimes I forget, especially if I'm not home.

Pharmacist: Mrs. Davis, it's very important to take your Zocor on a daily basis. Is it giving you any problems? Does it give you an upset stomach, do your muscles feel weak, does it make you fatigued?

Patient: No, none of that. I have no problems with it. I just don't take it as I should, and I know I should. But I know I'm not supposed to eat grapefruit because I'm on Zocor, which is fine with me because I don't like grapefruit.

Pharmacist: Well, that's good. Not that you don't like grapefruit, but that you know not to eat it with Zocor. And what are you taking for your blood pressure?

Patient: Well, the doctor put me on Diovan, but I don't always take it like I'm supposed to.

Pharmacist: Has it given you problems?

Patient: Yeah. It would make me dizzy and lightheaded so I told the doctor and he changed the prescription so I wouldn't get dizzy and lightheaded and it worked, but still I don't always take it.

Pharmacist: Mrs. Davis, Helen, I can't emphasize enough how important it is to take all your medications. I also see in your chart that your doctor has prescribed physical activity and weight loss. And he also recommended a smoking cessation program.

Patient: I know, I know. I need to lose weight and I need to stop smoking. It's so hard.

Pharmacist: Mrs. Davis, you're very young, but you have developed coronary heart disease. And angina is caused by coronary heart disease. It's becoming more difficult for oxygen and blood to reach your heart muscles. And the cholesterol is making your arteries hard. And smoking and high blood pressure do not help the situation. Are you aware that the number on killer in women is not cancer, but heart disease?

Patient: Really! I didn't know that.

Pharmacist: Yes! You are putting yourself at great risk for a heart attack and heart failure.

Patient: I had no idea. What should I do?

Pharmacist: First, you need to take all your medications and make regular appointments with your doctor. Next, you need to sign up for a smoking cessation class. The hospital here offers classes. The hospital also offers exercise and weight loss classes. Most insurance plans will pay for all of these classes, and, if not, the hospital charges reasonable rates. And finally, you need to watch your diet. Follow the diet plan your doctor gave you. I have a copy of it in your chart. I'll make a copy for you now.

CHAPTER 7

Pharmacist/Patient Dialogues

Dialogue #1

Pharmacist: Good afternoon. I'm Chris Meloni and I'm the pharmacist working with your doctor, Dr. Gary Lubin. Are you Amanda Adams?

Patient: Yes.

Pharmacist: How are you today?

Patient: I'm OK, except for my esophagus and my reflux.

Pharmacist: Yeah. I see from your chart that you have been having problems with GERD. Can you tell me a little bit about what's been going on and the medications you've been taking?

Patient: Well, about 3 months ago I noticed I was having some heartburn even though I wasn't eating any spicy foods, you know, like Mexican and Thai food. So I took some Maalox, Mylanta, Tums. But those didn't work.

Pharmacist: You got no relief?

Patient: Not only didn't I get relief, but I started to choke and gag on my food. One day about 2 weeks ago it was pretty bad. My husband took me to the emergency room and they referred me to a gas-tro-ento-rol-ogist. And he gave me an endo- something, you know, to look down my esophagus.

Pharmacist: You had an endoscopy, and what did the doctor find?

Patient: Well, he told me my esophagus was really inflamed and that I had a hiatal hernia, and that that was causing my choking and my problems swallowing, so he gave me medication. He gave me Zantac, and I told him if that's the generic, that's fine. I refuse to pay for brand names. He told me that Zantac was the brand-name drug and that the generic is ra-NI-ti-deen. I think it's spelled R-A-N-I-T-I-D-I-N-E. He told me it's in liquid form so I don't have to swallow pills.

Pharmacist: That's right. When did you have the endoscopy?

Patient: Three days ago. But I'm just getting my prescription now.

Pharmacist: OK. Are you still having problems swallowing and choking?

Patient: No. I haven't been eating much since my throat feels a little sore. I'm just eating Jell-O and soup and stuff like that. But I'm starting to feel better.

Pharmacist: Good. What did the doctor tell you about ranitidine?

Patient: I really have no idea. I was drowsy and groggy after the endoscopy; I can't remember what he said. He spoke to my husband, but he can't really remember either. Can you tell me?

Pharmacist: Absolutely! Well, like I said earlier, you have GERD. Ranitidine will help to reduce the stomach acid that is causing the problems. Dr. Lubin wants you to take a teaspoon in the morning and a teaspoon in the evening. You can take it with or without food. Try to take it at the same time every day. Are you taking any other medications?

Patient: Well, I did have pink eye about 2 weeks ago and I was taking tobramycin. And it cleared up.

Pharmacist: OK. That's good. Do you have any questions about the ranitidine?

Patient: Yeah. Is it going to make me stop choking and having problems swallowing? It's pretty scary.

Pharmacist: Well, it's going to help prevent too much stomach acid from producing. It will help to reduce the inflammation in your esophagus. But if you continue to have choking episodes, tell your doctor. I want you to be aware that this medication can cause dizziness, headaches, constipation, and diarrhea. Though very unlikely, if you get a rash, have swelling, and have trouble breathing, call your doctor immediately.

Patient: Are you serious? You know, when I was in college I had a CAT scan and I almost died. I stopped breathing, started convulsing. But they gave me Benadryl and I survived. I found out later I was allergic to iodine.

Pharmacist: Wow! Yeah, I see from your chart that you're allergic to iodine. And another thing, avoid alcohol.

Patient: Don't worry. I don't drink and Dr. Lubin told me because of my bad esophagus I can't have alcohol.

Pharmacist: That's right. Do you have any questions?

Patient: I'm starting to get a headache. Can I take my Tylenol when I get a headache while I'm on this medication?

Pharmacist: Yeah, Tylenol is fine, but try to avoid ibuprofen and naproxen.

Patient: What are they again?

Pharmacist: Motrin and Aleve.

Patient: OK.

Dialogue #2

Pharmacist: Hi. Are you Mr. Alex Hardy?

Patient: Yes, I am.

Pharmacist: How are you today? My name is Gerry Wade and I'm the pharmacist on duty in the clinic today. I'm here to talk to you about the medication Dr. Finkel has prescribed. He has prescribed Asacol. Do you know why you need to take Asacol?

Patient: Well, I have colitis. I've been having diarrhea and bleeding from my rectum, and sometimes I can't go to the bathroom even though I feel like I have to go.

Pharmacist: What you have is ulcerative colitis that is causing inflammation in your rectum. That's why you are having a difficult time moving your bowels. Is this the first time you have experienced colitis?

Patient: Yes.

Pharmacist: OK. Before I begin to explain how to use Asacol, I just want to confirm a few things in your patient chart and ask you a few questions.

Patient: Sure.

Pharmacist: Is your birth date December 12, 1961?

Patient: Yes.

Pharmacist: Your chart states that you're allergic to penicillin. Anything else?

Patient: No, I don't think so.

Pharmacist: I also see that you have had problems with a fungal infection. Can you tell me more about that?

Patient: Well, I had these red, dry patches on my arms and my legs near my groin area, like jock itch, and the doctor told me it was a fungal infection and gave me a pill that starts with an "N". I don't remember the name.

Pharmacist: According to your chart it was Nizoral.

Patient: Yeah, that's it.

Pharmacist: Are you still taking Nizoral?

Patient: No, no. My jock itch went away about 3 weeks after I started taking the medicine. That was about 2 weeks ago.

Pharmacist: OK. Good. Now, let's talk about your medicine for your colitis. The doctor wants you to take two tablets three times a day. You don't need to eat food with it. But make sure you take the tablets whole and that you not chew or crush them. You should also know that it's possible that you might see parts of the tablet or the whole tablet in your stool. If this happens tell your doctor. Any questions so far?

Patient: Is it going to give me gas? When I started taking the medicine for my jock itch, I was having more gas than usual.

Pharmacist: Well, it might. That's one of the possible side effects. You might also have flu-like symptoms and abdominal and back pain. I'll give you a complete list of all the possible side effects for you to take with you. But if you get very bad stomach and abdominal pain, worsening bloody diarrhea, or constipation or a fever, call your doctor. And try not to drink alcohol while on this medicine.

Patient: Not even a beer now and then?

Pharmacist: I don't recommend it. Do you have any questions?

Patient: Yeah. What should I do if I forget to take it?

Pharmacist: Well, if you miss a dose, try to take it as soon as you remember. But if you remember right as you're coming to your next dose, skip the dose you forgot. And don't double up to catch up.

Patient: OK. I just hope this medicine cures whatever it is I have.

Pharmacist: Well, Asacol is not going to cure your colitis. It's going to treat it. Asacol is an anti-inflammatory drug that will help to treat your condition. It will decrease some of the symptoms you're having, such as diarrhea and bleeding from your rectum. Of course, if you feel the medication is not alleviating your symptoms and not making you feel better, call your doctor.

Patient: Thanks. I will.

Dialogue #3

Pharmacist: Good afternoon. Are you Lily Soto?

Patient: Yep. That's me.

Pharmacist: Hi. I'm Chaz Oliver, and I'm the pharmacist whose going to review your patient chart and go over your new prescription with you.

Patient: You mean my prescription for my constipation?

Pharmacist: Yes.

Patient: You have no idea what I'm going through. It's terrible, not being able to go. My stomach is all bloated; my pants don't fit. I feel pregnant. I'm really starting to tear my hair out. Have you ever been constipated?

Pharmacist: I'm sure we've all been at one time or another.

Patient: Please help me. I can't take it anymore. I can't remember the last time I had a good bowel movement.

Pharmacist: OK, Lily. Let me look over your chart. I see the last time you were in the clinic was about 4 weeks ago.

Patient: Yeah. I was here to get my blood pressure medication refilled. I'm taking a drug called telmi-something.

Pharmacist: Telmisartan.

Patient: That's it. I've been taking it for about 2 years and I still don't know how to pronounce the name. High blood pressure runs in my family. Here's my prescription for my constipation.

Pharmacist: It's a prescription for Dulcolax.

Patient: Is it a pill or a suppository?

Pharmacist: It's a suppository that will help to stimulate your digestive tract and your intestines. Have you used suppositories before?

Patient: Yeah, when I had hemorrhoids.

Pharmacist: OK, so then you know how to insert them. I would advise that you try not to have a bowel movement 10 to 15 minutes before you insert the suppository.

Patient: OK, I won't. How many do I use?

Pharmacist: Insert one suppository before bedtime or in the morning before breakfast.

Patient: Will it work fast?

Pharmacist: Well, you may feel it start to work after about 30 minutes.

Patient: How long should I use it?

Pharmacist: Your doctor has ordered a box of six suppositories. You shouldn't use them for more than a week. If you don't have a bowel movement after taking the suppositories, see your doctor.

Patient: I can still take my blood pressure medicine, right?

Pharmacist: Sure.

Patient: Are there any side effects with these suppositories?

Pharmacist: You might experience some irritation in your rectal area, and you might experience cramping and diarrhea. But if you experience bleeding or, like I said earlier, you have no bowel movement, contact your doctor immediately.

Patient: OK, I will. Thanks. Hopefully, I'll start feeling better.

Mini Dialogue Listening Exercises
Mini Dialogue #1

Person A: You must be so relieved the exam is over. Now you can relax.
Person B: I couldn't wait for it to be over. I had butterflies in my stomach the entire time I was taking the test.

Mini Dialogue #2

Person A: Can you believe some of these patients?
Person B: To tell you the truth, some days I just can't stomach them.

Mini Dialogue #3

Person A: I really do not like our chemistry professor. He's way too tough.
Person B: I know what you mean. I don't have the stomach for another course with him.

Mini Dialogue #4

Person A: What's wrong? Did something happen?
Person B: I just saw a dead mouse in my office and it really turned my stomach.

Mini Dialogue #5

Person A: Did you hear that John is going to be promoted to manager?
Person B: I heard, and I'm not happy. His promotion is difficult to stomach.

Mini Dialogue #6

Person A: Why is she always late for work? It's so unprofessional.
Person B: I find it hard to stomach people who are tardy and show no consideration for others.

Chapter 7 Post-Assessment
Dialogue #1

Patient: Hi. Are you the pharmacist?
Pharmacist: Yes, I am. How can I help you?
Patient: Well, I'm a little bit embarrassed, but I need something to help me with my constipation.
Pharmacist: Sure. Do you have a prescription from your doctor?
Patient: No. Do I need one?
Pharmacist: No. We have many over-the-counter treatments that can help you. How long have you been constipated?
Patient: Well, almost 3 weeks now. I'm having difficulty going, you know, moving my bowels. I strain, but nothing happens. In fact, I think I also have a hemorrhoid from all the straining.
Pharmacist: Do you have any allergies?
Patient: Not to medicines, but I'm allergic to milk and onions.
Pharmacist: Are you currently on any medication?
Patient: I take birth control pills.
Pharmacist: OK, come with me and I'll show you some products that you can choose from, but I would suggest Sani-Supp. It's a glycerin suppository that you insert into your rectum. Make sure you moisten the suppository with lukewarm water before inserting. The instructions are on the back of the box.
Patient: OK. This is so embarrassing. I've had suppositories before. After I had my first child, I had so many hemorrhoids from pushing so hard during labor that my doctor gave me suppositories to get rid of my hemorrhoids.
Pharmacist: Good. So it shouldn't be difficult. Use the suppositories as needed but try not to use the suppositories for longer than a week. If you're still constipated, I recommend that you see your doctor.

Patient: Is there anything else you can recommend? Being constipated is so uncomfortable and I feel so bloated.

Pharmacist: Well, first make sure you drink plenty of water every day. Four to six glasses is good. Eat a lot of fiber and roughage. I can also recommend Metamucil or Citrucel.

Patient: What's the difference?

Pharmacist: No difference really. They are both fiber laxatives, which help to increase the amount of water in your stool and to soften your stool. Both come in powder, chewable tablets, and wafers. But you need to drink plenty of water with all of them. And make sure you read the label carefully.

Patient: Will it help me with my hemorrhoid?

Pharmacist: It should. Metamucil is also used to treat hemorrhoids. But if you want a topical ointment, you can use Preparation H.

Patient: Yeah. I've used that in the past. I'll get that too. How long should I take the Metamucil?

Pharmacist: No more than 7 days. If you're still constipated, please tell your doctor. Do you have everything you need?

Patient: Yes, I think so. I have the Sani-Supp suppositories, the Metamucil chewable tablets, and Preparation H, and hopefully the end of my constipation. And thank you so much. You've been very patient and helpful.

Pharmacist: My pleasure. Here, I'll take those to the register where you can pay for them.

Dialogue #2

Pharmacist: Good morning, are you Samuel Torres?

Patient: Yeah, that's me.

Pharmacist: I'm Erin Farrell, and I'm the pharmacist who will go over your prescription to treat your peptic ulcer and answer any questions you might have. How are you today?

Patient: I've been better. This ulcer is really bad news.

Pharmacist: Can you tell me more about the discomfort and pain that you're having?

Patient: Like I told my doctor, I'm still having a pain that burns, you know, a burning pain around my belly button and my breastbone.

Pharmacist: Does the pain last a long time?

Patient: It comes and goes, you know. Sometimes it's just for a little while and sometimes I can have the pain for hours. And it really flares up at night, so I have a hard time sleeping.

Pharmacist: Before you saw your doctor, were you taking anything for it?

Patient: I took Maalox and Mylanta and Pepto-Bismol, and nothing would happen. I wouldn't feel better. So I stopped taking them and I went to the doctor.

Pharmacist: Are you taking any other medications?

Patient: Just my vitamins. That's it.

Pharmacist: OK. Do you know what your doctor prescribed?

Patient: No, I don't remember.

Pharmacist: OK, I just need to confirm one thing—are you allergic to penicillin or any kind of antibiotic?

Patient: No.

Pharmacist: OK, according to your chart, Dr. B. J. Lewis has prescribed Prevpac. It's used to treat ulcers caused by a bacterial infection. Prevpac contains medication to help block the acid in your stomach and also contains antibiotics to help stop bacteria from growing.

Patient: That sounds good. How long do I take it?

Pharmacist: You need to take one tablet in the morning and one tablet in the evening. And you're going to do this for 14 days. Do not stop taking it before then even if you feel better. If you stop taking it before the 14 days, you risk the chance of letting the bacteria continue to grow and then you'll have the problem all over again. And you don't want that.

Patient: Yeah, you're right. Do I need to take it with food?

Pharmacist: No, but take it before you eat. And make sure you swallow the tablets whole. Don't chew or crush them. Do you have any questions?

Patient: No.

Pharmacist: OK. You shouldn't experience any side effects other than maybe a headache and maybe a taste in your mouth you wouldn't normally have. However, if you have bad stomach pain, cramps, and persistent diarrhea, let your doctor know. And one more thing—it's important not to drink alcohol when taking Prevpac. It can make you dizzy or drowsy. Please read all the information regarding the side effects.

Patient: Well, I hope this medicine does the trick. I don't want to get another ulcer.

Pharmacist: Well there are things you can do to take care of yourself. I'm sure your doctor mentioned that smoking can increase stomach acid, and that excessive drinking can also irritate the lining of your stomach and possibly cause bleeding. And it's a good idea to avoid taking pain relievers such Motrin and Aleve. If you need to take a pain reliever, take Tylenol.

Patient: Well, I am trying to quit smoking and I'm not a big drinker, but I'll watch myself. You have some good advice.

Pharmacist: OK, then. If you have problems with the medication, call your doctor.

CHAPTER 8

Pharmacist/Patient Dialogues

Dialogue #1

Pharmacist: Hello, are you Rachel Lipton?

Patient: Yes, I am.

Pharmacist: Good morning, I'm Walter Cronin, the pharmacist. You can call me Walt. How would you prefer to be called, Rachel or Mrs. Lipton?

Patient: I've been called Mrs. Lipton for so long, why stop now? Walt, you can call me Mrs. Lipton.

Pharmacist: OK, Mrs. Lipton. I see that you are here today to get your prescription for sulfasalazine to help treat your rheumatoid arthritis.

Patient: Is that what Dr. Solomon ordered?

Pharmacist: Yes.

Patient: I hope it helps me. My rheumatoid is really getting bad. The pain and swelling has gotten worse, especially on my fingers. My fingers are curling up and becoming deformed. My hips, knees, and feet are stiff. My muscles hurt. I hurt all over. It's so painful, but I try to keep a stiff upper lip.

Pharmacist: I'm sorry to hear that it's getting worse. I have reviewed your chart, and I see that you've had arthritis for quite a while, and you've taken other medications. I guess they haven't worked for you.

Patient: No. Not really. The Aleve didn't help, and the prednisone didn't help but it made me gain weight. I was even on Vioxx, and it killed some people and it was taken off the market. So now the doctor wants me to try this new drug. What did you say the name of the drug is?

Pharmacist: It's sulfasalazine. It will help to reduce the joint pain, swelling, and stiffness you've been having. Hopefully it will help to slow down the progression of the disease and prevent further joint damage. Your doctor also wants you to continue with Aleve. Sulfasalazine is an antiarthritic drug that is used with a nonsteroidal anti-inflammatory drug such as Aleve. Hopefully, you'll start to notice a difference after taking the Aleve with the sulfasalazine.

Patient: I hope so. How often do I take it, and what does it look like? Pills come in so many different colors I get confused sometimes.

Pharmacist: I know what you mean. Well, it's a gold-color, 500-mg tablet. It looks like this. It's a delayed-released tablet...

Patient: What does that mean?

Pharmacist: It means the drug doesn't take effect as soon as you take it. You take one tablet with breakfast in the morning and make sure to drink a glass of water, too. And make sure that you swallow it whole. Don't chew, crush it, or break it. And take the Aleve, too, which as you know is yellow.

Patient: Yeah, but it won't make it easier to swallow.

Pharmacist: That may be so, but you don't want to increase the chance of getting an upset stomach if you crush, chew, or break it.

Patient: The prednisone made me gain weight. What's this new medicine going to do to me?

Pharmacist: Well, first, it's intended to help reduce the pain you're having. However, as with all medicines, patients will experience some side effects. You may experience nausea, vomiting, and headaches along with some other effects that are listed on the drug information sheet I will give you. However, call your doctor if you have ringing in the ear, painful urination, or blood in your urine or have difficulty breathing.

Patient: Is this one of those medicines that won't let you out in the sun?

Pharmacist: Yeah. It may make you sensitive to the sun, so avoid being out in the sun too long and, as always, wear sunscreen. Have you had any problems with the Aleve, like stomach bleeding?

Patient: No, nothing like that. So if I take this new pill without chewing, crushing, or breaking it and drink lots of water with it and take it every day, I won't be feeling all this pain? Sometimes I just want to yell at the top of my lungs, it hurts so bad.

Pharmacist: I understand. But you need to know that it may take 1 to 3 months before you feel any improvement.

Patient: That long? I'll be tearing my hair out.

Pharmacist: I understand, but along with the medications, it's important to exercise. You can ask your doctor to refer you to a physical therapist who can teach you how to exercise your fingers. And exercise is good for the entire body. Of course, it's important to control weight. Too much weight can add stress to the joints on your back, hips, knees, and feet.

Patient: If weight is bad for arthritis, then why do doctors give patients like me prednisone, which makes you gain weight?

Pharmacist: That's a good question. But you found that prednisone is not good for you. Is there anything that you do to help reduce the pain?

Patient: Sometimes, especially at night, I put hot pads around my fingers and on my knees and feet and my muscles. I heat the hot pads in the microwave and they do feel good on my joints. And of course, Mr. Lipton massages my feet and knees almost every night.

Pharmacist: Well, you're very lucky to have Mr. Lipton. You can also try to use a cold pack. It can help to dull the sensation of the pain. Do you have any other questions about the sulfasalazine?

Patient: No, you've been very helpful, Walt. Is that it?

Pharmacist: Almost. I just need to confirm some information in your chart about your age, allergies, and medical history before I send you home.

Patient: Sure.

Dialogue #2

Pharmacist: Good morning, Mr. Brady. How are you today? Do you remember me? I know it's been a while.

Patient: Not really. The last time I was here was over 2 months ago.

Pharmacist: That's right. I'm Henrietta Washington.

Patient: Henrietta. Now I remember. How are you?

Pharmacist: I'm fine. How are you doing? How are you feeling?

Patient: Well, not so good.

Pharmacist: I remember that you started to see us after you were diagnosed with COPD and chronic bronchitis. Are you using your Atrovent inhaler?

Patient: Yes. But I'm not here for that. I now have arthritis in my spine. The name of the arthritis is hard to pronounce and remember so I just call it AS.

Pharmacist: Is it ankylosing spondylitis?

Patient: Yeah. I think that's it. Here's the prescription. I can't really read the doctor's handwriting.

Pharmacist: Thank you. Okay, I see Dr. Anderson has prescribed Rheumatrex. He's also indicated that if we don't have Rheumatrex, which is the brand-name drug, we can give you methotrexate.

Patient: Give me whatever is easier to pronounce, even if it costs more. I have a good drug prescription plan.

Pharmacist: Sure. But, Mr. Brady, first I'd like to ask you some questions and review your medical and drug history.

Patient: Sure, Henrietta. And you can call me Steven.

Pharmacist: Sure, Steven. First thing's first. You mentioned earlier that you're using your Atrovent inhaler?

Patient: Yes.

Pharmacist: How many inhalations do you take a day?

Patient: I take two to four inhalations every day two times a day.

Pharmacist: Is it working for you? Has it made breathing easier for you?

Patient: Yes, very much.

Pharmacist: Have you experienced any side effects that you weren't having before using the inhaler?

Patient: No, none really, except in the beginning I did have a sore throat, but then it went away and my throat has just been fine. And now I have AS.

Pharmacist: Can you tell more about that and what took you to see Dr. Anderson?

Patient: I was having soreness in my lower back and pain and a tender feeling down my spine, and then it spread to my ribs and my shoulders. I thought it was related to my COPD so I went to see my lung doctor, Dr. Posner. He gave me some blood tests and an MRI and then he told me I had AS. I really got hit between the eyes. He sent me to Dr. Anderson. He's an arthritis doctor.

Pharmacist: Well, thank you for sharing that with me. I'm sure both of your doctors will monitor you carefully. They may have explained to you that AS can also cause the rib cage to stiffen and restrict lung capacity and function.

Patient: Yeah, I know. Dr. Anderson also told me that I will have difficulty walking and standing, and that I'll be hunched and stooped over when the joints begin to fuse.

Pharmacist: Did he mention that you may experience breathing difficulty as a result of the bones in your rib cage fusing together?

Patient: So I'll have more breathing problems in addition to my COPD.

Pharmacist: Have you noticed increased breathing difficulty?

Patient: No, not really. But my doctor says I could have more breathing problems.

Pharmacist: Well, it would be a good idea to get physical therapy. It will help relieve pain and give you physical strength and flexibility. And as the disease progresses, you'll develop a stooped posture, but with physical therapy you can work on standing upright as much as you can. And of course, not smoking will help. You're not smoking, are you?

Patient: No, I gave that up when I was told I had COPD.

Pharmacist: Good. Now, let me tell you about your new medication, Rheumatrex. Rheumatrex is a very potent medication. You need to take one pill a week. You can take it with food, but you don't have to. But you should drink plenty of fluid when you take the pill. And keep an eye out for any possible side effects such as mouth sores, a persistent cough, and black stools. I'll give you a patient information sheet with detailed side effects. Read it carefully. Also, it's important to avoid alcohol and limit your time in the sun. You may become more sensitive to the sun.

Patient: I hope I get relief right away.

Pharmacist: Well, it will take up to several months before you feel relief. But of course, if you're having difficulty breathing and moving and you feel you're getting worse, please call both of your doctors. And of course, you can always call me or any of our other pharmacists.

Patient: Thank you so much, Henrietta.

Pharmacist: Sure, Steven. Now, before you leave with your Rheumatrex, I just want to double-check some personal and medical history. Are you still at the same address, do you have any new allergies, and are you taking any other new medications that I don't know about?

Patient: I'm still at the same address, no new allergies, and I'm taking Atrovent and now I'll be taking Rheumatrex, too.

Mini Dialogue Listening Exercises

Mini Dialogue #1

Person A: You know Patty is really mad at you.

Person B: Yeah, I know. Her nose is all out of joint because I didn't invite her to my graduation party.

Mini Dialogue #2

Person A: I don't know how much longer I can take working here. All Teresa does is criticize and nag me all day.

Person B: You need to tell her to get off your back.

Mini Dialogue #3

Person A: What did you think of Dr. Smith's lecture on arthritis treatments?
Person B: I'm just glad it's over. I was bored stiff.

Mini Dialogue #4

Person A: Did you hear what happened last night at the dance club?
Person B: Yeah, I heard that some students became angry after they couldn't get in because it was crowded with so many people, so they decided to muscle their way in, but security came and took them away.

Mini Dialogue #5

Person A: How did you do on your research paper?
Person B: I can't believe I broke my back writing that stupid paper just to get a C+.

Mini Dialogue #6

Person A: Don't worry. I'll work for you this weekend.
Person B: Are you sure? You always work your fingers to the bone. Thank you so much for switching weekends with me.

Mini Dialogue #7

Person A: I'm never going to lend Jack money again. He still hasn't given me back the $20 he borrowed a month ago.
Person B: Forget about it. Last year, he stiffed me out of $25.

Mini Dialogue #8

Person A: I can't believe I almost got a perfect score on my pharmacy licensing exam.
Person B: Are you kidding me? You just send chills up my spine! Wow!

Mini Dialogue #9

Person A: Are you speaking to Eric and Debbie?
Person B: Are you kidding me? How can I? As soon as we broke up, he stabbed me in the back and began dating her, my own roommate. They both stabbed me in the back.

Mini Dialogue #10

Person A: She's never going to enjoy working here if she doesn't learn to adjust to our rules.
Person B: It's too bad she's so stiff-necked, because she's actually a very good worker.

Chapter 8 Post-Assessment

Dialogue #1

Pharmacist: Good morning. Are you Mr. Eric Gallagher?
Patient: Yes, I am. Good morning.
Pharmacist: I'm the clinic pharmacist, Elizabeth New. How are you feeling this morning?
Patient: Well, I have felt better, but it's been hard for me to walk. My right toe has been hurting a lot. It's real inflamed and burning.
Pharmacist: Have you had problems with your big toe for a while?
Patient: Yeah. I have gout, and I'm having a real big flare-up.
Pharmacist: How long have you had gout?
Patient: Oh, I guess about 10 years. You know, it comes and goes. I went to the emergency room 3 nights ago. It was really bad. My toe was so swollen and real tender. I couldn't even wear my shoes. I wore my sandals.
Pharmacist: Are you currently taking any medication?

Patient: No, but the last time I had a real bad flare-up about a year ago, and my doctor gave me a cortisone shot and he also gave me a medicine called probene. I think that's what it's called.

Pharmacist: I think you mean probenecid. What did the ER doctor give you?

Patient: He gave me a prescription. Here it is.

Pharmacist: OK, I see she has also written a prescription for probenecid and over-the-counter Aleve. OK, Mr. Gallagher, since this is your first time in the clinic, I need to ask you a few questions about your medical history, and then I'll go over your prescription with you and tell you a bit more about how to treat your gout.

Patient: Sure.

Pharmacist: OK. How old are you?

Patient: I'm 53.

Pharmacist: Are you currently taking any other medications?

Patient: Well, I just finished taking an antibiotic for my swimmer's ear. I had a bad ear infection in my right ear.

Pharmacist: Do you remember the name of the antibiotic?

Patient: I think it was Cort- something. Yeah, it was Cortisporin, I think.

Pharmacist: Did it clear up your ear infection?

Patient: Yeah. It really worked fast.

Pharmacist: Any other medications?

Patient: No, but I take my multivitamins. And I take Metamucil every day just so I don't get constipated.

Pharmacist: Have you had any surgery?

Patient: Yeah. I had my appendix taken out about 10 years ago. And about 15 years ago, I had surgery on my left knee.

Pharmacist: Do you have a family history of gout?

Patient: Yeah, my dad. He passed away about 4 years ago.

Pharmacist: Do you smoke?

Patient: Not anymore. I used to be a two-pack-a-week smoker, but I quit about 3 years ago, after my best buddy died of lung cancer. He was a chain smoker.

Pharmacist: Quitting was the wise thing to do. Do you have any allergies?

Patient: Yeah, I'm allergic to CAT scan dye.

Pharmacist: You're allergic to iodine. OK, Mr. Gallagher, now let's talk about how to treat your gout. The doctor has prescribed probenecid. Probenecid is used to help lower the high levels of uric acid in your body. When your body produces too much uric acid, crystals form in the joints and cause gout. Hopefully the medication will reduce the chance and severity of a future gout attack. The doctor also wants you to take Aleve, which will help to reduce the inflammation. Have you taken Aleve before?

Patient: Yeah.

Pharmacist: Any problems with it?

Patient: No, should I watch for any problems?

Pharmacist: Well, in some patients it can cause stomach bleeding and ulcers. So just keep an eye out.

Patient: How often do I take the gout medicine?

Pharmacist: Take the probenecid twice daily. And make sure you take it with food to reduce stomach upset. It's important to also drink a glass of water with the tablets. And drink at least eight 8-ounce glasses of water a day to prevent kidney stones.

Patient: I hope this gets rid of my gout.

Pharmacist: Well, I need to warn you. It's possible that you may experience more gout attacks in the next month while the medication helps the body remove the extra uric acid in your body, so don't stop taking probenecid if you get another gout attack.

Patient: But isn't the probenecid going to take the pain away?

Pharmacist: No, it's not a pain reliever. That's why you need to take Aleve for pain relief. Also, keep in mind that in some patients probenecid can cause dizziness, loss of appetite, sore gums, and frequent urination. I'll give you a complete list of the side effects. Please read them very carefully.

Patient: These gout attacks are really difficult to stomach.

Pharmacist: I know. But it's important to know that there are also other ways to help relieve symptoms. First, avoid or limit alcohol. Alcohol prevents the excretion of uric acid. Second, always maintain a healthy weight, and drink plenty of fluids.

Patient: No beer with my buddies?

Pharmacist: Try not to have more than two drinks a day. But right now I would advise against drinking. Do you have any other questions, Mr. Gallagher?

Patient: No. You have really educated me.

Pharmacist: OK, now I just need to ask some personal information questions, and then I'll get the prescription for you.

Dialogue #2

Pharmacist: Good afternoon, Mrs. Vo. How are you today?

Patient: OK, and you? Please, you can call me Vicky.

Pharmacist: Sure, Vicky. I'm Anthony Gonzalez and I'm fine today. I'm the clinic pharmacist and I'm here to see how you're doing and to review your prescriptions with you. And you are here today because you have a prescription for osteoporosis.

Patient: Yeah, osteoporosis. I have weak bones, and my doctor said I have brittle bones.

Pharmacist: I also see from your chart that you have had two cataracts removed, one on each eye.

Patient: And now I can see better and more clearly.

Pharmacist: When did you have the cataracts removed?

Patient: I remember very well. It was October 6, 2005.

Pharmacist: Did the doctor give a medication for any reason?

Patient: Yes, Dr. Wu, W-U, not Dr. Woo—W-O-O. He gave me Lotemax—L-O-T-E-M-A-X.

Pharmacist: Thank you for spelling both the name of the medication and the doctor's name. You make my job easier.

Patient: Sure. No problem.

Pharmacist: Can you tell me why Dr. Wu gave you Lotemax?

Patient: He told me to help with eye inflammation.

Pharmacist: Did it help?

Patient: Yes, very much. I can see good again.

Pharmacist: Mrs. Vo, I mean Vicky, are you taking any other medication?

Patient: No. I am healthy but now Dr. Jones told me I have os-te-o-po-ro-sis. Not easy to pronounce.

Pharmacist: I know what you mean. Were you feeling pain in your body before you went to see Dr. Jones?

Patient: Yeah. Sometimes I have a little pain in my back and I don't walk with my back straight.

Pharmacist: Yes, people with osteoporosis will experience back pain, and very strong pain if they have a fracture. A fracture is a break in the bone. And people with osteoporosis will begin walking with a stooped posture, which means the back is no longer as straight as it used to be. Some people will get shorter.

Patient: Yeah. I'm starting to walk like an old lady.

Pharmacist: How old are you, Mrs. Vo?

Patient: 68, but I feel strong, but now I have osteoporosis.

Pharmacist: Did Dr. Jones give you a prescription?

Patient: Yeah, she told me it's FO-SA-MAX.

Pharmacist: OK. That's Fosamax. Did Dr. Jones explain how to take this medicine?

Patient: She said take one pill a day and I will feel better. If any problems, I'm to call her.

Pharmacist: OK, I will give you some more important information.

Patient: Good.

Pharmacist: It's very important that you take the pill every day. Are you taking any other medications?

Patient: No.

Pharmacist: OK. Now, it's important to take the tablet with a full glass of water and that you swallow the tablet whole. Don't chew it or suck it. Do you understand me?

Patient: Yeah, just take quickly with water.

Pharmacist: Yes. Then make sure you do not lie down. Your body must be upright. Sit on a chair, stand, or walk, but do so for 30 minutes. After 30 minutes, then you can eat your meal and have your tea or coffee or juice. Do not drink water.

Patient: I must be very careful. This is serious medicine. This helps my osteoporosis?

Pharmacist: Yes. Fosamax will help to stop osteoporosis and help you from losing bone. Stopping osteoporosis or bone loss will help you to keep your bones healthy and help your bones from breaking, or from getting fractures.

Patient: Good. I will take my medicine every day as you say.

Pharmacist: Also, pay attention to some problems you may have. Some medicines have side effects. For example, some people who take Fosamax have stomach pain. I will give you the patient information leaflet that explains all the side effects. Read it carefully.

Patient: I will read it with my son, and I have Vietnamese and English dictionary. I will read carefully.

Pharmacist: That's a very good idea. Vicky, do you have any allergies?

Patient: Yes, bees!

Pharmacist: Now, it's important to remember that you cannot eat certain foods with this medicine. For example, you should not eat foods such as citrus fruit, like oranges. Don't eat tomatoes or tomato sauce. And try not to drink coffee, chocolate, soda, peppermint, or pepper.

Patient: No problem. I don't eat those foods.

Pharmacist: OK. Do you have any questions?

Patient: No, not now. You are very helpful. I can call you, if I have question?

Pharmacist: Sure, you can call me. Here's my card with my name and phone number on it. And of course, you can also call Dr. Jones.

Patient: OK. I have an appointment with her in 1 month for a checkup.

CHAPTER 9

Pharmacist/Patient Dialogues

Dialogue #1

Pharmacist: Good morning. I'm Richard Mendez and I'm the pharmacist working with your doctor, Dr. Gabby Lucas. Are you Ariana Snow?

Patient: Yes.

Pharmacist: How are you today?

Patient: I'm OK. Can I go home now?

Pharmacist: Well, you are being discharged from the hospital today, but first I need to go over your new medication with you and your mom. Are you Mrs. Snow?

Patient's mother: Yes, I am.

Pharmacist: It's very nice to meet you both. Like I said, I just want to review the new medication and answer any questions you have. I see from your chart that you have been diagnosed with epilepsy after having two seizures, and that this is the first time you'll be taking medication to control your seizures.

Patient: Yeah.

Patient's mother: Out of nowhere she had a terrible seizure. We didn't know what was wrong so we raced her to the emergency room and she was admitted overnight.

Pharmacist: Did you lose consciousness, Ariana?

Patient: Yeah, I guess so. I don't remember any of it. But my mom told me that my legs and arms were jerking out of control and that my body got real stiff.

Pharmacist: Well, hopefully your new medication will leave you free of seizures or at least control your seizures. Dr. Lucas has prescribed Tegretol. That's the brand name. It's also known as carbamazepine. That's the generic name. This is what the Tegretol looks like. It's a red-speckled, pink chewable tablet. How old are you, Ariana?

Patient: I'm 16.

Pharmacist: Tegretol is known as an antiepileptic drug and anticonvulsant drug that helps to treat your type of seizures, which are called grand mal seizures.

Patient's mother: Yes, that's what the doctor said. How often does she take it?

Pharmacist: Dr. Lucas has prescribed that you take one tablet twice daily. Ariana, take the pill with or without food, and make sure you take it the same time each day. But you shouldn't have grapefruit or grapefruit juice with this medication, unless your doctor says it's okay.

Patient's mother: Ariana has always been very healthy. When she was younger, she used to get a lot of ear infections. And she was allergic to Ceclor, the antibiotic to stop the infection. It made her body break out in a rash and she'd get very watery diarrhea.

Pharmacist: Well, it could cause unsteadiness as she adjusts to the medicine. Keep your eye out for nausea, dizziness, and vomiting. And it's not uncommon to feel fatigued. I'll give you a complete list of possible side effects, including serious, but rare, side effects.

Patient: What kind of serious side effects?

Pharmacist: Well, though unlikely, pay attention to your chest and ankles. For example, if you get chest pains or if your ankles swell up, call your doctor immediately. And if you notice problems with speech or coordination, call your doctor. Ariana, do you have any other allergies?

Patient: I'm allergic to cats and latex.

Pharmacist: Mom, does Ariana have any other medical conditions?

Patient's mother: No, just ear infections in the past. She hasn't had one since she was 5. She did develop an eye infection when she first got her contacts, but she's fine now. And she's had stitches three times.

Patient: Yeah, on my head. I got hit with a hockey stick. I got six stitches. I also got five stitches on my chin. I got hit with a tennis racket. And I broke my right arm when I was 12 on a water slide.

Pharmacist: Wow. Are you playing any sports now?

Patient: Yeah, I play softball. I'm a pitcher. I can still play, even though I have epilepsy, right?

Pharmacist: Talk to Dr. Lucas, but I'm sure you can continue to be physically active and participate in sports, as long as you take your medication and follow up with your doctor. But Dr. Lucas might want to talk to you about wearing a helmet when you participate in certain sports or recreational activities with a high risk of head injury. Also, it's very important that you wear a medical alert bracelet. And don't swim alone.

Patient's mother: What should we do when she has another seizure?

Pharmacist: Well, roll Ariana to one side and put a soft pillow under her head. And don't put your fingers in her mouth. She will not swallow her tongue. And don't try to restrain her or yell or shake her when she's having a seizure.

Patient: Am I going to have seizures forever?

Pharmacist: Well, everyone is different, but the good news is that most people with epilepsy do become seizure free as long as they take medication. And we know that more than half of children with epilepsy eventually stop taking their medication and become seizure free. And if you feel that the Tegretol is not working for you, call your doctor.

Patient: Good. I can still play sports.

Pharmacist: That's right. As long you take your medication as prescribed. And never stop taking your medication unless directed by your doctor. Any other questions?

Patient: No.

Pharmacist: Mom?

Patient's mother: No, not right now. You've been very helpful. Ariana is tough as nails. She'll be fine.

Dialogue #2

Pharmacist: Hi. Are you Susan Wilson?

Patient: Yes, I am.

Pharmacist: How are you today? My name is Lucas Page and I'm the pharmacist on duty in the clinic today. I'm here to talk to you about the medication Dr. Lena Kasporova has prescribed. She has prescribed Betaseron. Do you know why you need to take Betaseron?

Patient: Well, I've been diagnosed with MS. Dr. Kasporova said I have relapsing multiple sclerosis and that I'm in the early stages of MS.

Pharmacist: That's right. Betaseron will not cure your MS, but it will help to reduce the number of flare-ups and the attacks that make you weak. The medication will slow down the disease.

Patient: My doctor said that it's interferon.

Pharmacist: Yes, it's the same as interferon, which is a protein that your body produces naturally. This protein helps the body's immune system. If you have MS, adding more interferon may help your body to fight the effects of MS. Did your doctor tell you that you need to inject the interferon?

Patient: Yes.

Pharmacist: Okay, now, before we go on I just need to ask you a few questions. Is your birth date May 21, 1964, and are you 44?

Patient: Yes.

Pharmacist: Do you have any allergies?

Patient: I can't eat shrimp or shellfish; I'm so allergic.

Pharmacist: Do you have any questions?

Patient: I have to wait 3 to 6 months before I can urinate normal again? That's a long time.

Pharmacist: I know, but there are a few things that you can do in the meantime to help control your symptoms. You say you feel like you need to urinate frequently at night. To prevent that, try not to drink water or other drinks, especially drinks that contain caffeine, after seven at night. Caffeine can produce more urine and irritate your bladder. And try to limit alcohol. Also try sitting on the toilet seat, rather than standing, to empty your bladder. And believe it or not, exercise can help your difficulty urinating. Lack of exercise helps us to keep our urine in.

Patient: I'll try to do what you tell me. I hope it works.

Pharmacist: Sometimes simple lifestyle changes can really help. And of course, if your symptoms get worse and you are very uncomfortable, please tell your doctor.

Patient: I will.

Pharmacist: OK, now the prescription is for 1 month, but you have five refills, so come back to see me or another pharmacist on duty when you need a refill. In the meantime, if you have any questions about the medication, call us or your doctor. Our phone number is on the medication label.

Patient: OK, thank you very much.

Chapter 10 Post-Assessment

Dialogue #1

Pharmacist: Good morning.

Patient: Good morning.

Pharmacist: I'm the clinic pharmacist, Jude Berger. How can I help you?

Patient: Yes, my name is Joan Brown and I need a prescription filled. I'm having problems with my bladder. The doctor says I have an overactive bladder and she gave me this prescription. I think it's for Detrol. Here it is.

Pharmacist: You're right. Have you had Detrol before?

Patient: No. This is the first time. I've been having problems losing my urine every time I have the urge to urinate. It's so embarrassing. My doctor told me I have urge incontinence.

Pharmacist: I see that Dr. Susan Hoffman is your doctor.

Patient: Yeah. She said the Detrol should help stop my urge to urinate and the leakage. I've even started to wear absorbent pads, you know, Depends. Can you hurry up? I'm afraid I'm going to need to go to the bathroom soon.

Pharmacist: Sure, I'll try, but first I need to ask you a few questions. Are you currently taking any medication?

Patient: Yes. I'm on Amaryl. I have type II diabetes.

Pharmacist: Do you have any allergies?

Patient: Latex and Ceclor.

Pharmacist: When were you taking Ceclor?

Patient: Oh, a long time ago, years ago when I had an ear infection. I haven't had an ear infection since and I know not to take Ceclor.

Pharmacist: OK. How old are you?

Patient: I'm 48.

Pharmacist: Do you have any other medical conditions?

Patient: Well, I have three fibroids and I have had two breast biopsies that were benign, thank God. But now I have this overactive bladder.

Pharmacist: Did the doctor explain to you how Detrol works and how to take it?

Patient: She just told me to take it twice a day and to see her in 6 weeks.

Pharmacist: OK, then, let me explain how Detrol works. Detrol will help to treat your overactive bladder by relaxing the muscles in your bladder and helping you to control your urination. And yes, you'll take the 2-mg, round, white tablet twice a day.

Patient: Do I take it with food?

Pharmacist: You can take it with or without food.

Patient: Will it have any side effects?

Pharmacist: It's not uncommon for some people to get dry mouth and dry eyes, constipated, dizzy, or headaches. To prevent constipation, make sure you have a diet rich in fiber and drink enough water.

Patient: But won't drinking water make me want to urinate even more?

Pharmacist: Yes, that's true. If you get constipated, tell your doctor and she'll recommend an appropriate laxative and stool softener. Also, keep in mind that this medication may cause you to feel dizzy and drowsy and have blurred vision, so be careful when driving. Also, Detrol can cause decreased sweating, so be careful not to overheat if you exercise or do strenuous activities.

Patient: Are you certain this medication is going to stop my overactive bladder? So far it doesn't sound so good. Now I need to worry about constipation, blurred vision, and overheating. Isn't there something else that I can take or do?

Pharmacist: Well, your doctor has prescribed Detrol because it will be beneficial to you. But in the meantime, there are things that you can do to take care of yourself and to reduce the number of times you have the urge to urinate and the number of leakages. Control the amount of fluids you take and when you take them during the day. You'll also need to learn how to control your bladder.

Patient: Oh, yeah. My doctor told me how to delay urinating every time I have the urge. She said I should begin delaying the urge for 10 minutes, then go, and continue to increase the time delay until I can delay it for up to 2 hours. I hope I can do it.

Pharmacist: Training your bladder is important. You should also try to double void, meaning when you urinate, wait a few minutes and try to go again until your bladder is completely empty. You should also learn how to do Kegel exercises to help strengthen your pelvic floor muscles. A physical therapist can teach you how to do these exercises.

Patient: I'll try to remember everything that you've told me.

Pharmacist: I strongly suggest you take a look at the National Association for Continence. You can find them on the web. It has great information on support groups for people with overactive bladders and great tips on how to stay motivated using the strategies I've just told you. You'll find that you're not alone and that there are others who can help you.

Patient: Thank you so much. You've been great, but can you tell me where the bathroom is? I need to go now!

Dialogue #2

Patient: Hi, are you the pharmacist?

Pharmacist: Yes, I am. I'm Leonard Chase. How can I help you?

Patient: I need to get a prescription for Ma...cro...dantin. I think that's how it's pronounced.

Pharmacist: Do you have the prescription from your doctor?

Patient: Yeah, here it is.

Pharmacist: What is your name?

Patient: Jacklyn Cho.

Pharmacist: How do you spell your first name?

Patient: J-A-C-K-L-Y-N.

Pharmacist: And your last name?

Patient: C-H-O.

Pharmacist: Have you been here before?

Patient: No.

Pharmacist: Jacklyn, what's your date of birth?

Patient: February 12, 1989. I'm 18.

Pharmacist: OK. I just need to get your address and your phone number.

Patient: I live on 27 Sunset Terrace in Watertown, and my phone number is 467-4485.

Pharmacist: What type of insurance do you have?

Patient: I'm covered by my father's insurance. It's Health Choice Medical and Drug Plan. I have the card. Do you need it?

Pharmacist: Sure. I need to enter the insurance information in our computer. Jacklyn, who is your doctor?

Patient: Dr. Varsha Patel.

Pharmacist: Do you have any allergies?

Patient: I don't have allergies to medicines, I don't think, but I get hay fever in the spring and I'm lactose intolerant and allergic to tomatoes.

Pharmacist: Are you currently on any medications?

Patient: Just birth control pills.

Pharmacist: Have you been taking anything to treat your urinary tract infection?

Patient: Just cranberry juice. My friend told me it's supposed to help.

Pharmacist: Well, cranberry juice can help to prevent the bacteria from spreading, but you need an antibiotic and that's why Dr. Patel has prescribed Macrodantin. Have you ever taken an antibiotic?

Patient: No, I don't think so.

Pharmacist: OK, well I'll explain to you how Macrodantin works and how to use it. Macrodantin is an antibiotic that helps to stop the bacteria from growing in your bladder.

Patient: I hope it gets rid of the burning sensation I get when I urinate.

Pharmacist: It should, as long as you take your medication until the full prescribed amount is finished. Don't stop taking it if you start to feel better. Finish the entire prescription. However, if the condition gets worse, tell your doctor. Dr. Patel wants you to take a capsule four times a day, so try to take one every 6 hours. Make sure you swallow the capsule whole.

Patient: OK.

Pharmacist: Also, since you've never taken an antibiotic, keep your eye out for some side effects. You might notice that your urine might look dark yellow or a little brown. Don't worry about this. This is quite normal. You might also feel nauseous, lose your appetite, get a headache, or feel dizzy. If you feel nauseous, take the medication with food. I'll give you a pamphlet with more details about the medication.

Patient: OK. Should I stop drinking cranberry juice?

Pharmacist: You can continue to drink cranberry juice. And make sure you drink plenty of water. Water helps to dilute the bacteria and to flush it out.

Patient: Can I still drink alcohol like beer and wine?

Pharmacist: Well, I wouldn't recommend it. Avoid alcohol, caffeine, and citrus drinks until your infection has cleared. These tend to irritate the bladder.

Patient: I hope I don't get another infection. I'm so uncomfortable.

Pharmacist: Well, there are things you can do to prevent future infections. It's important to empty your bladder and not to hold in your urine. Also, after urinating it's important to wipe from front to back, and very important to empty your bladder and to drink plenty of water to flush out any bacteria after sexual intercourse. If you take your medication as prescribed, your symptoms should start clearing up.

Patient: OK, thanks.

CHAPTER 11

Pharmacist/Patient Dialogues

Dialogue #1

Pharmacist: Hello, I'm Justine Barry, the hospital pharmacist on duty. Are you Jonathan Libster?

Patient: Yeah.

Pharmacist: How are you doing this morning?

Patient: Well, I'm happy to be leaving the hospital and going home.

Pharmacist: Well, before you can go home, I need to talk to you about the medication that Dr. Sorenson has prescribed. He has prescribed Aldactone. Do you know why?

Patient: Because I have cirrhosis. I have a bad liver. I guess the medicine will make my liver better.

Pharmacist: Well, it won't make your liver better. Cirrhosis of the liver causes irreversible scarring of the liver. But what the medication will help you with is the removal of the excess fluid in your body caused by cirrhosis. Aldactone is a diuretic.

Patient: Yeah. I still have a lot of water in my abdomen and my legs are swollen even though I don't drink as much as I used to and I don't eat as much salt as I used to.

Pharmacist: It's really important that you stop drinking alcohol all together. Alcohol is a toxin that is filtered through your liver, but in the process the alcohol damages the liver. It's crucial that you stop drinking alcohol.

Patient: I know. That's how I got cirrhosis in the first place. I have a drinking problem. But I also don't want to have to get a new liver or die. And I want to get rid of this water in my abdomen and legs. It's hard to move and walk. How many times do I take this pill?

Pharmacist: Well, your doctor has prescribed that you take two 25-mg tablets, one in the morning and one in evening, but not too late, or you might be getting up in the middle of the night to urinate.

Patient: I'm also taking rifampin to help me with my itching. I itch a lot with this cirrhosis. Can I take both medications at the same time?

Pharmacist: Yes. Have you had any side effects with the rifampin?

Patient: No. I'm getting some relief.

Pharmacist: Aldactone has some side effects that you may or may not experience. You may notice that your breasts may become enlarged. Other rare side effects include diarrhea, drowsiness, and impotence. If you notice any of these side effects, call your doctor. I'll give you a pamphlet to take with you that tells you all the side effects.

Patient: Can I take it with food?

Pharmacist: You can take it with or without food. While I have your chart here, I just want to confirm a few things. According to your chart, you're allergic to bees, wasps, shellfish, iodine, and sulfa?

Patient: That's right.

Pharmacist: Well, I'm glad you don't eat shellfish. It's one of the foods that people with cirrhosis need to avoid altogether.

Patient: Really? Why?

Pharmacist: Well, uncooked shellfish, including oysters and clams, is not always free from bacteria, and bacteria are extremely dangerous to people with cirrhosis.

Patient: I didn't know that.

Pharmacist: According to your chart, you're still drinking about two cans of beer a week?

Patient: I think that's good. I've cut back a lot, and I'm not drinking hard liquor.

Pharmacist: Mr. Libster, I can't emphasize this enough. You need to stop drinking alcohol entirely. You have a damaged liver that can lead to liver failure, a liver transplant, or death. I'm sure your doctor has told you this.

Patient: Well, I don't smoke.

Pharmacist: That's good. Do you use drugs?

Patient: When I was much younger I smoked pot, but it's been years.

Pharmacist: I'm sure your doctor has told you that there are things you can do to reduce liver damage as a result of your cirrhosis. But just in case, let me give you important advice. First...

Patient: I know. Don't drink alcohol.

Pharmacist: Second, eat healthy—fruits and vegetables. Restrict salt because salt causes your body to retain water. Be careful not to take aspirin or Aleve or Motrin. And stay away from sick people because your body is not able to fight off infections like you would if you were healthy.

Patient: Yeah, I know about staying away from sick people. My doctor vaccinated me against hepatitis A and B and the flu and pneumonia.

Pharmacist: Good. I see that in your chart. One more thing, I just want to confirm your age and date of birth.

Patient: I'm 43. I was born June 28, 1964.

Dialogue #2

Pharmacist: Good morning. How are you today?

Patient: Not so good.

Pharmacist: Are you Samantha Duffy?

Patient: Yes. Are you a doctor?

Pharmacist: No, I'm the clinic pharmacist, Mustafa Pasdar. I'm going to take care of your medication needs today. Do you have a prescription with you?

Patient: Yeah. Here it is. The doctor is giving me medicine for my hepatitis. I have hepatitis B.

Pharmacist: Samantha, how old are you?

Patient: I'm 25, and you can call me Sam.

Pharmacist: Sam, what's your date of birth?

Patient: May 14, 1982.

Pharmacist: OK, your doctor...is your doctor Ben Whitman?

Patient: Yeah.

Pharmacist: Dr. Whitman has prescribed Hepsera. Do you know why you've been prescribed Hepsera?

Patient: Because I got hepatitis B. I got infected after having unprotected sex with a person who's infected. I started to get sick and had pain around my abdomen. I had dark urine and I noticed my skin was turning yellow, and my eyes too. That's when I went to Dr. Whitman, and he gave me tests and then told me I had hepatitis B.

Pharmacist: I'm sorry to hear that you have hepatitis B. It's a very serious liver infection. I can tell you Hepsera will help to slow down the virus, but it will not cure your hepatitis. And this is very important: It will not prevent you from spreading the virus to others, so you need to be careful. I'll explain more about how to do this, but first let me tell you how to use Hepsera.

Patient: OK.

Pharmacist: Dr. Whitman has prescribed that you take Hepsera, which is spelled H-E-P-S-E-R-A, once a day. You can take it with or without food.

Patient: How long will I have to take it?

Pharmacist: Well, your doctor will decide that and will monitor how you're doing on the medication. It's possible that your hepatitis could worsen if you discontinue the medication. It's very important that you keep all your blood work appointments. You'll be getting your blood tested on a regular basis to monitor your liver and kidney function.

Patient: What else can happen to me on this drug?

Pharmacist: Well, there are side effects you'll need to pay attention to. You might experience headaches, fever, weakness, and diarrhea. Serious side effects include rash, swelling, and a change in your urine amount. If you experience any of these, contact your doctor. I'll give you a leaflet for you to read carefully.

Patient: OK. I can't believe I'm going to have hepatitis forever.

Pharmacist: Well, if you have the virus in your system for less than 6 months, you should be able to recover. Your immune system may be able to clear up the virus. However, if you have had the virus for more than 6 months, you have chronic hepatitis B and it may be lifelong because your body has not been able to fight the infection. Like I said earlier, it's important to see your doctor and keep all your appointments so that he can monitor your condition.

Patient: This just boggles the mind. I can't believe it.

Pharmacist: Did Dr. Whitman explain to you the other ways hepatitis B is transmitted?

Patient: Yeah. He told me through sharing contaminated needles. Even people like you, healthcare workers can accidentally get it if they come in contact with contaminated human blood. And even infected pregnant mothers can pass it on to their babies. And of course, having unprotected sex with an infected person. I've learned my lesson.

Pharmacist: Sam, since you are infected, it's very important to protect your partners from the virus and to protect them from exposure to blood, saliva, and vaginal secretions. It's important that your partner wear a condom for vaginal and anal sex and that you both wear dental condoms for oral sex. And of course, let your partner know that you have the virus. Of course, don't share intravenous needles and syringes and don't share razors and toothbrushes. I know this is a lot of information to digest.

Patient: Can I still drink?

Pharmacist: I would not advise drinking alcohol. Alcohol can speed up the progression of the disease. But eat a healthy diet of fruits, vegetables, whole grains, and protein. Exercise and get enough sleep. These lifestyle changes are important.

Patient: I'll try.

Pharmacist: Remember, Sam, not taking your medicine and not making important lifestyle changes can lead to other serious complications such as cirrhosis of the liver, which is permanent scarring of the liver, liver cancer, and liver damage. Talk to your doctor if you have any questions and concerns.

Patient: I will. Thanks so much.

Chapter 11 Post-Assessment

Dialogue #1

Pharmacist: Good morning.

Patient: Good morning.

Pharmacist: I'm the clinic pharmacist, Felicia Arroyo. How can I help you?

Patient: Well, I need a prescription filled. The doctor says I have hepatitis C and he gave me this prescription. I think it's a prescription for two things. She said I need to get injections and take capsules, too. I think it's called Rebetron.

Pharmacist: You're right. Rebetron is a combination drug of interferon alpha-2b solution and ribavirin capsules.

Patient: That sounds confusing.

Pharmacist: I know. I'll explain it to you and you can ask me any questions you have, but first I need to get your name.

Patient: Right. My name is James Richter. That's R-I-C-H-T-E-R. This is my first time in this clinic.

Pharmacist: James, what is your date of birth?

Patient: September 21, 1975. I'm 32.

Pharmacist: Your home address?

Patient: 701 Julia Lane in Willamstown.

Pharmacist: Phone number?

Patient: 876-5321.

Pharmacist: James, do you have any allergies?

Patient: No, I don't think so, but I can't eat onions. I'm allergic to those.

Pharmacist: And your doctor's name?

Patient: Charles Borden.

Pharmacist: Did your doctor talk to you about hepatitis C?

Patient: Yeah, he told me that it looks like I got it from a contaminated needle when I got my last tattoo. I have five tattoos and I never had any problems before. And I noticed that after I got my last tattoo, I started to feel sick, like I had the flu. I went to the clinic doctor in the hospital and after a few blood tests he told me I had hepatitis C. I don't use drugs or inject drugs, and I haven't gotten a blood transfusion ever, so it looks like it was the tattoo.

Pharmacist: Did Dr. Borden explain to you how to take the medication?

Patient: He told me I need to inject myself and I need to take a pill. The nurse showed me how to inject, and I almost fainted. I don't like needles. They make me feel queasy.

Pharmacist: If you feel queasy, make sure someone is with you when you inject. You will inject the interferon alpha-2b, which comes in the form of prepared solution in vials called Intron A. You will inject subcutaneously, or in your skin. And then you will take the ribavirin 200-mg capsule. Ribavirin is an antiviral medication. You'll do this once a day, but make sure you do it the same time every day. I would recommend you do this at bedtime.

Patient: That's it?

Pharmacist: Well, it's important that you drink a full glass of water with the capsule. Ribavirin can cause dehydration, so it's very important that you drink fluids every day. And you can take the capsules with or without food, but make sure that you do the same thing every day. Also, it's important to keep both medicines in the refrigerator and don't shake the vials.

Patient: So this medication should take care of my hepatitis, right?

Pharmacist: Well, it's not known if Rebetron cures hepatitis C or if it prevents the transmission of the virus to others or if it prevents cirrhosis of the liver, which is permanent scarring of the liver, or if it prevents liver cancer.

Patient: Are you kidding me? Is this medicine going to make me sicker?

Pharmacist: Well, there are side effects. This medication can cause some patients to have flu-like symptoms and to become anemic, become dehydrated, feel dizzy, feel nauseous, and even experience hair loss and hair thinning.

Patient: You mean I could become bald?

Pharmacist: Like I said, in some patients it can cause hair loss and hair thinning.

Patient: Any more bad side effects?

Pharmacist: Well, this medication has caused some serious side effects in some patients, such as depression, mood and behavior changes, and thoughts of suicide.

Patient: Are you serious?

Pharmacist: I will give you the complete patient pamphlet describing this medication, its benefits, and its side effects. Your doctor has prescribed this medication to treat your hepatitis C because he has determined that the benefits to you are greater than the risks of the side effects, which can also include allergic reactions such as a rash, swelling of the lips and mouth, and difficulty breathing. Call your doctor immediately or get medical attention immediately if this happens.

Patient: Can I at least have sex?

Pharmacist: Good question. It's very important for your partner not to get pregnant while taking this drug, so it's very important to avoid pregnancy. Interferon is known to cause birth defects in unborn children, so it's very important that women and partners taking this medication avoid getting pregnant while on the medication and for 6 months after the treatment is over. So please make sure you use reliable birth control and don't engage in unprotected sex.

Patient: Wow. I'm not married or planning to get any woman pregnant, but thanks for the warning. Looks like my life is over.

Pharmacist: No, not at all. You just need to make a few adjustments to prevent spreading the virus to others, and to take measures to protect your health and the health of others. There are a few things you can do and you can begin by avoiding alcohol, which speeds the progression of liver diseases. Eat a healthy diet of fruits, vegetables, and whole grains, and make sure that others don't come in contact with your blood, so avoid sharing razors and toothbrushes, and cover and protect any wounds you may get. Of course, you can't donate blood, semen, or organs and it's always a good idea to let other health workers you come in contact with know that you have the virus.

Patient: I can't believe this. All because I got a tattoo.

Dialogue #2

Patient: Hi, are you the pharmacist?

Pharmacist: Yes, I am. I'm Victor Watson. How can I help you?

Patient: I need to get a prescription for pred-ni-sone.

Pharmacist: Do you have the prescription from your doctor?

Patient: Yeah, here it is.

Pharmacist: What is your name?

Patient: Sonia Sanchez.

Pharmacist: How do you spell your first name? Do you spell it S-O-N-Y-A or S-O-N-I-A?

Patient: S-O-N-I-A.

Pharmacist: And your last name?

Patient: Sanchez. S-A-N-C-H-E-Z.

Pharmacist: Have you been here before?

Patient: No.

Pharmacist: What's your date of birth?

Patient: 1/5/49.

Pharmacist: OK. And your address and your phone number?

Patient: My address is 6 Moonlight Terrace in Ivytown, and my phone number is 367-7644.

Pharmacist: What type of insurance do you have?

Patient: It's Personal Health. I have the card. Do you need it?

Pharmacist: Sure. I need to enter the insurance information in our computer. Who's your doctor?

Patient: Dr. Michelle Drake.

Pharmacist: Do you have any allergies?

Patient: I'm allergic to penicillin and eggs.

Pharmacist: Are you currently on any medications?

Patient: Just Fosamax for my bones. I'm in menopause.

Pharmacist: Did the doctor tell you why you need prednisone?

Patient: I have autoimmune hepatitis. Same thing my mother had. She died a few years ago after several other health complications.

Pharmacist: I'm sorry to hear that your mother died. Heredity is one cause of autoimmune hepatitis, but if it's discovered early and treated early, it can be controlled with medication such as prednisone to suppress the immune system and to slow the progression of the disease. But it's important to be careful with the medication.

Patient: How much prednisone do I take?

Pharmacist: Your doctor has prescribed one 40-mg tablet per day. This prescription comes in 20-mg tablets, so you will take two at the same time, once a day. And it's recommended that you take it with food.

Patient: I hope it helps me. My doctor said the good news is that I don't have cirrhosis of the liver. My liver biopsy was negative, thank God.

Pharmacist: Well, that's good. The prednisone should help to inhibit the disease, as long as you take your medication as directed by your doctor. It will not cure your condition. And I'm sure your doctor has told you that you need to get more frequent blood tests to monitor your liver.

Patient: Yeah, she did. I've never been on prednisone, but I have a friend whose dog is on prednisone to shrink her cancer tumors. She seems to be doing fine. My liver should be getting better soon, right?

Pharmacist: Well, you might not see immediate improvement, and it may take some time. However, there are side effects that you should be aware of. Prednisone can cause fluid and salt retention; weight gain; puffiness in the face, or what we call moon face and high blood pressure.

Patient: Weight gain and moon face?

Pharmacist: It can also cause osteoporosis, and patients will also take Fosamax, but since you're already taking Fosamax, that's good. I would also recommend a calcium supplement of 600 mg and vitamin D, both twice daily. This will help treat your osteoporosis and prevent further erosion while taking prednisone.

Patient: Well, I do exercise regularly. I go to the gym and lift weights and jog and walk around the indoor track. But I'll take your suggestion and get calcium and vitamin D, too.

Pharmacist: I'm glad you exercise. I would continue doing that as long as you're feeling good and strong.

Patient: Am I going to need to take prednisone for the rest of my life?

Pharmacist: Well, your doctor will determine that. As soon as your symptoms—

Patient: You mean like my fatigue, discomfort around my abdomen, and my jaundice?

Pharmacist: Yes, those symptoms and other symptoms you have may improve, and your doctor may want to reduce the dose of the medication while still controlling the disease. Every individual is different. Some will be on prednisone for life, others for a few years. Some will go into remission, but usually the disease will return if the medication is discontinued. The good news is that because you were diagnosed early and because you're getting treatment, you don't run the risk of developing cirrhosis of the liver and liver failure.

Patient: I guess I should consider myself pretty lucky.

CHAPTER 12

Pharmacist/Patient Dialogues

Dialogue #1

Pharmacist: Hello. My name is Frank Walker, and I'm the clinic pharmacist for today. Are you Emily Lynch?

Patient: Yeah.

Pharmacist: How are you today?

Patient: Well, I could be doing better. I guess you know why I'm here. Dr. Alexander said you would talk to me about my medication for my vaginal yeast infection.

Pharmacist: That's right. Dr. Alexander prescribed a nonprescription medication called Monistat. You can buy it over the counter in any pharmacy or supermarket. I'm going to give you a sample to take home with you, but you'll need to go to your local pharmacy to buy some more. Do you know what Monistat is?

Patient: Well, I've seen commercials for it on TV. I've never had this problem before, you know, yeast infection. This is so embarrassing.

Pharmacist: Well, it's quite common. It fact, three out of four women will experience vaginal yeast infection, and there's no reason to be embarrassed. Dr. Alexander wants you to take Monistat-7 suppositories.

Patient: I don't take a pill?

Pharmacist: No. You will insert a suppository using the applicator into your vagina as if you were inserting a tampon. It's a 100-mg suppository.

Patient: How often do I insert it?

Pharmacist: You need to insert a suppository using the applicator once nightly for 7 nights. This medication will help to treat your yeast infection.

Patient: Is the medicine going to hurt?

Pharmacist: No, the medicine should not hurt you, but you might feel some irritation or burning after inserting the suppository. These are the only potential side effects. And I would recommend wearing a light panty liner as discharge from the suppositories can occur.

Patient: Is it going to get rid of the itch and the thick discharge that looks like cottage cheese?

Pharmacist: Yes, it should. Those are typical symptoms of a vaginal yeast infection.

Patient: I've never had a yeast infection. Is this considered a sexually transmitted disease?

Pharmacist: No, it's not a sexually transmitted disease. You can relax.

Patient: Then how did I get it?

Pharmacist: Well, certain changes in your environment can trigger an overgrowth of a naturally occurring fungus called *Candida*.

Patient: Fungus?

Pharmacist: Relax. A lot of factors can trigger a yeast infection, like certain antibiotics, pregnancy, birth control pills, and menopause.

Patient: Well, I'm not pregnant or menopausal. I'm only 21. But I am on birth control pills. But I've been on the pill for 3 years and I've never had a yeast infection.

Pharmacist: Sometimes bubble baths, vaginal contraceptives, and tight clothes can trigger the growth of the fungus.

Patient: Really? Bubble bath? I got a new bottle of bubble bath recently. Maybe that's how I got it.

Pharmacist: It could be. The good news is that you saw your doctor soon, and now you can start treating it.

Patient: OK. Thanks for the info. Now I know to stay away from bubble bath. If I stop using the bubble bath, I'll be OK and not get another yeast infection?

Pharmacist: Well, it's a good idea to stop using the bubble bath. And there are other things that women in general should do to prevent vaginitis and yeast infections. Try to avoid whirlpools and hot tubs. It's a good idea to avoid scented pads and tampons. They can irritate the vagina.

Patient: Can I still douche? I douche once in a while.

Pharmacist: I wouldn't douche. Douching can actually cause vaginal infections. It certainly doesn't clear up infections.

Patient: Really? I didn't know that. I'll have to tell all my girlfriends.

Pharmacist: I would recommend eating yogurt that contains active *Lactobacillus* cultures. *Lactobacillus* is a good bacterium that is common in the vagina.

Patient: Are you serious? I had no idea. Wow, I've really learned a lot. Dr. Alexander didn't tell me any of this. He just said "take Monistat."

Pharmacist: Well, I'm glad you've learned a lot. And don't forget to take the entire dosage. Finish the entire course of treatment even if you start to feel better...

Patient: You mean, finish all seven suppositories?

Pharmacist: That's right.

Patient: Will do. Thanks a lot.

Dialogue #2

Pharmacist: Good morning. How are you today?

Patient: OK. I need a prescription filled.

Pharmacist: Sure. What's the prescription for?

Patient: I have ED. You know.

Pharmacist: Sure. I understand.

Patient: Here it is. I've been here before.

Pharmacist: OK. Let me look you up in our computer. What is your name?

Patient: Lester Greenwald II.

Pharmacist: Lester Greenwald the second. Is your date of birth July 16, 1951?

Patient: Yes. All the information is the same. Same address. Same insurance.

Pharmacist: 22 Ardmore Road in Westmont, and you have Healthy Life Insurance?

Patient: Yeah.

Pharmacist: I want you to know that your insurance plan does not cover Viagra.

Patient: Are you serious? You gotta be kidding me. This is ridiculous. I pay part of the cost of my insurance. Those lousy insurance companies get you all the time.

Pharmacist: Mr. Greenwald, I can understand your frustration. I would suggest calling your insurance company.

Patient: Oh, you bet I will. I'm sorry. You can call me Les.

Pharmacist: That's OK, Les. Like I said, your prescription is for Viagra. Did Dr. Ahmet talk to you about Viagra?

Patient: Well, he told me it will probably take a while before I improve. You know, I was having a lot of pressure and stress at work. And I was depressed. I was taking Zoloft for a while. The doctor told me that what's causing my ED. It's psychological. I'm not physically abnormal, you know.

Pharmacist: Are you still taking Zoloft?

Patient: No, I started to feel better so I don't take it anymore, but I think maybe the Zoloft could be a reason why I've been having this ED problem. It's never been a problem in the past. I've had ED for more than 2 months. That's when I went to see Dr. Ahmet, our family doctor. My wife has been patient and understanding, but, well, you know.

Pharmacist: I understand. There are several reasons for erectile dysfunction, or as you say, ED. Your doctor is prescribing Viagra because he feels it will treat your situation. You're not alone. Many men experience ED. And you're lucky you have a patient and understanding wife. Would you like to know how Viagra works?

Patient: I guess.

Pharmacist: Viagra will help to relax the smooth muscles in your penis. What this will do is increase the amount of blood in the penis to cause an erection during sexual stimulation. Viagra will help an erection to occur.

Patient: Is it a pill or a liquid?

Pharmacist: It's a blue, diamond-shaped tablet. Your doctor has ordered 50-mg tablets. You take one tablet only before sexual activity.

Patient: How soon before my wife and I can get intimate? You know.

Pharmacist: Well, you can take it between 4 hours and 30 minutes before, but taking one tablet about an hour before sexual intimacy is most effective. And it's very important to remember that Viagra can be taken only once in a 24-hour period.

Patient: How soon will the Viagra start working, and how long will it last?

Pharmacist: Well, the Viagra should start to work 30 minutes after taking it. The medication should last for 4 hours, but after 2 hours it works less effectively.

Patient: How about side effects? Is there anything I should worry about?

Pharmacist: Well, there are some common side effects to look out for. You can become dizzy, become flushed, get back pain, or get diarrhea. Viagra is also known to cause blue vision, which is sensitivity to light. I'll give you a complete patient leaflet for you to read very carefully.

Patient: Do I eat when I take the tablet?

Pharmacist: No. You don't have to, but if you do, don't eat a high-fat meal. A high-fat meal may delay the onset of Viagra.

Patient: Well, Dr. Ahmet thinks Viagra will help me. I'm not taking any medications right now that would be a problem. I don't have any medical problems except this problem.

Pharmacist: That's good to know. You should also know that men on Viagra should not take heart medications that contain nitrates. Do you have any other questions?

Patient: Yeah. When will this problem go away?

Pharmacist: Well, you're not going to see changes immediately. Every patient is different. If you see that your situation is not improving, please see your doctor again. He may need to adjust the dosage.

Patient: OK. Thanks so much.

Chapter 12 Post-Assessment

Dialogue #1

Pharmacist: Good morning.

Patient: Good morning.

Pharmacist: I'm the clinic pharmacist, Rosa Mendez. Do you need help?

Patient: Yeah. I gotta get a medication. I have the clap. Doctor said I have gonorrhea.

Pharmacist: What is your name?

Patient: David Cunningham.

Pharmacist: Did your doctor give you a prescription?

Patient: Yeah. It's right here.

Pharmacist: Your doctor, Dr. Sanderson, has prescribed two antibiotics, doxycycline and azithromycin.

Patient: He did? Two? Why two?

Pharmacist: Doxycycline is used to treat gonorrhea and azithromycin is used to treat chlamydia.

Patient: Chlamydia? I have gonorrhea and chlamydia?

Pharmacist: According to your doctor, yes. Let me explain to you how both antibiotics work.

Patient: As long as it stops this burning sensation when I piss, you know, urinate. And I also have some kind of discharge coming from my penis. My doctor told me my urethra is infected.

Pharmacist: Gonorrhea and chlamydia are both bacterial infections spread through sexual contact. The antibiotics will help to treat the infection.

Patient: How long will I have to take both antibiotics?

Pharmacist: You're going to take both antibiotics for 7 days. You're going to take the light yellow doxycycline tablet, which is 100 mg, twice a day for 7 days. Take one tablet in the morning and one tablet in the evening. And you're also going to take the red azithromycin capsule once a day for 7 days.

Patient: Can I take them together?

Pharmacist: Yes, but don't eat food with them. Doxycycline should not be taken with food. And you don't need to eat food with azithromycin. Take both medications at least 1 hour before or 2 hours after meals.

Patient: OK. That's it, huh?

Pharmacist: Well, you need to be aware of possible side effects.

Patient: Like what?

Pharmacist: Well, with doxycycline you could experience nausea, upset stomach, dizziness, trouble sleeping, and lightheadedness. And try to avoid sun exposure as it may cause photosensitivity. And with azithromycin you could experience diarrhea, loose stools, vomiting, and abdominal pain. I'll give you a complete computer printout of the side effects for you to take with you and read carefully.

Patient: Sure. Is that it?

Pharmacist: It's really important that you finish the entire prescription. If you stop taking your medication too early, the infection could return.

Patient: Oh, I'll finish it. I don't want this stuff to return. It's no way to live. I guess sex is out of the question.

Pharmacist: Avoid sexual intercourse until after your infections are completely gone. See your doctor after you finish the prescribed antibiotics. And use latex condoms when you're ready to resume sexual intercourse and avoid oral intercourse. Gonorrhea and chlamydia are contagious. You can get both infections again if you don't take measures to prevent getting and spreading both. And it's critical to let your partner...

Patient: Or partners know. I know. I hear you. I just hope these antibiotics do the trick.

Pharmacist: It's important to practice safe sex. If you have any concerns, please call your doctor or call the clinic pharmacy. The phone number is on the medication bottle label. Now, David, I need to confirm some information that appears in your chart.

Patient: Sure.

Pharmacist: Your date of birth?

Patient: May 18, 1983. I'm 24.

Pharmacist: Address?

Patient: 643 Millbrook Road, Apartment 4C, in Morton.

Pharmacist: Phone?

Patient: 543-0090.

Pharmacist: According to your doctor and your patient records in your chart, you have no allergies and you're not taking any medications?

Patient: That's right.

Pharmacist: And do you have insurance?

Patient: No, I'll be paying cash.

Dialogue #2

Patient: Hi, are you the pharmacist?

Pharmacist: Yes, I am. I'm Stuart Robertson. How can I help you?

Patient: I have a prescription for two medicines I can't pronounce.

Pharmacist: Do you have the prescription with you?

Patient: Yeah, here it is.

Pharmacist: OK, your doctor, Dr. Gerber, has prescribed levofloxacin and metronidazole. Do you know why she has prescribed these medications?

Patient: Yeah. I have PID, short for pelvic inflammatory disease.

Pharmacist: OK. What is your name?

Patient: Roberta Livingston.

Pharmacist: OK, Roberta. Have you been to this pharmacy before?

Patient: No.

Pharmacist: What's your date of birth?

Patient: June 19, 1985. I'm 22.

Pharmacist: Home address?

Patient: 65 Springdale Road in Cherryville.

Pharmacist: How do you spell Springdale?

Patient: S-P-R-I-N-G-D-A-L-E.

Pharmacist: You doctor is Dr. Francesca Gerber?

Patient: Yes.

Pharmacist: Roberta, do you have any allergies?

Patient: Just iodine. I can't have CAT scan dye or shellfish.

Pharmacist: Are you currently on any medications?

Patient: No. I just take Tylenol when I have a headache. I take vitamins, too.

Pharmacist: Are you on birth control?

Patient: Not now. I had an IUD but my doctor removed it, and now that I have PID.

Pharmacist: Have you taken levofloxacin or metronidazole before?

Patient: No. How often should I take them?

Pharmacist: Your doctor has prescribed that you take levofloxacin once a day. It's a terra cotta pink, 250-mg tablet. You need to take metronidazole twice daily. It's a white, round, 250-mg tablet. You can take them together. You can take one levofloxacin and one metronidazole in the morning, and one metronidazole in evening. They will stop the growth of the bacteria that is causing your PID.

Patient: Can I take them with food?

Pharmacist: You need to take both of them with a glass of water or with milk to prevent an upset stomach. Both medications can cause an upset stomach.

Patient: How long do I take both medications?

Pharmacist: You doctor has prescribed they be taken for 14 days.

Patient: Besides maybe an upset stomach, are there any other side effects? Can I still drink alcohol?

Pharmacist: No, you can't drink alcohol when you take metronidazole. And you should also know that because you take vitamins, you need to take the levofloxacin either 2 hours before or 2 hours after you take your vitamins. Vitamins and antacids bind with the medication to prevent the medication from being fully absorbed. Now, as for the other side effects, both can cause an upset stomach, diarrhea, drowsiness, nausea, headache, and loss of appetite. In addition, metronidazole can cause constipation and dry mouth, and levofloxacin can cause trouble sleeping.

Patient: OK. You mentioned that they help the bacteria in my body. Is it going to stop the pain in my pelvis and my lower abdomen, and in my back and in the heavy vaginal discharge I have?

Pharmacist: Those are typical symptoms of PID. The medications will help, but it's important to take the fully prescribed dosage. Don't stop taking the tablets even if you start feeling better. PID is a serious disease that needs to be treated. It can lead to complications such as chronic pelvic pain, ectopic pregnancy, and infertility. I'm sure your doctor has discussed this with you.

Patient: She has.

Pharmacist: And of course it's important to tell one's partner and to abstain from sexual intercourse until the infection has cleared up, and to...

Patient: Practice safe sex and to use a condom.

Pharmacist: Good. If you have any problems with the medications, call Dr. Gerber or call us. Roberta, do you have any other questions?

Patient: Can I use my credit card to pay for these? I don't have insurance.

Pharmacist: Sure.

Pharmacotherapy Workup Notes

Pharmacotherapy Workup© **NOTES**	**ASSESSMENT**

CONTACT INFORMATION

Name				
Address	City		State	Postal Code
Telephone (h)	(w)	(cell)	e-mail	
Pharmacy Name		Clinic Name		
(tel)		(tel)		

DEMOGRAPHICS

Age	Date of Birth		Gender: M/F
Weight	Height	Lean Body Weight	
Pregnancy status: Y/N	Breast Feeding: Y/N	Due Date	
Occupation			
Living Arrangements/Family			
Health Insurance (coverage issues):			

REASON FOR THE ENCOUNTER

MEDICATION EXPERIENCE

	Needs attention in care plan	
	Y	N
What is the patient's general attitude toward taking medication?		
What does the patient want/expect from his/her drug therapy?		
What concerns does the patient have with his/her medications?		
To what extent does the patient understand his/her medications?		
Are there cultural, religious, or ethical issues that influence the patient's willingness to take medications?		
Describe the patient's medication taking behavior		

		Birth	1 mo	2 mos	4 mos	6 mos	12 mos	15 mos	18 mos	24 mos	4–6 yrs	11–12 yrs	13–18 yrs
CHILDHOOD IMMUNIZATIONS*	Hepatitis B	Dose 1		Dose 2				Dose 3					
	Diphtheria, Tetanus, Pertussis			1	2	3		4					
	Haemonphilus influenzae Type b			1	2	3	4						
	Polio-inactivated			1	2		3				4		
	Measles, Mumps, Rubella						1				2		
	Varicella (chicken pox)												
	Pneumococcal			1	2	3	4						
	Hepatitis A(children in high risk regions)										Hepatitis A Series		
	Influenza (Children ≥6 with asthma, diabetes, HIV, sickle cell, cardiac disease)							Yearly					

☐ Current on all childhood immunizations

		19–49 YEARS	50–64 YEARS	65 YEARS & OLDER
ADULT IMMUNIZATIONS*	Tetanus, Diphtheria (Td)	1 booster every ten years	1 booster every ten years	1 booster every ten years
	Influenza	1 dose annually for persons with medical or occupational indications or household contacts of persons with indications	1 annual dose	1 annual dose
	Pneumococcal (polysaccharide)	1 dose for persons with medical or other indications. (1 dose revaccination for immunosuppressive conditions)	1 dose for person with medical or other indications. (1 dose revaccination for immunosuppressive conditions)	1 dose for unvaccinated persons 1 dose revaccination

☐ Current on all adult immunizations
*see http:///www.cdc.gov/nip for more information

	Substance	History of Use	Substance	History of Use
SOCIAL DRUG USE	Tobacco ☐ No tobacco use	☐ 0–1 packs per day ☐ >1 packs per day ☐ previous history of smoking ☐ attempts to quit	Alcohol ☐ No alcohol use	☐ < 2 drinks per week ☐ 2–6 drinks per week ☐ > 6 drinks per week ☐ history of alcohol dependence
	Caffeine ☐ No caffeine use	☐ < 2 cups per day ☐ 2–6 cups per day ☐ > 6 cups per day ☐ history of caffeine dependence	Other recreational drug use	

ALLERGIES & ALERTS

Medication Allergies (drug, timing, reaction—rash, shock, asthma, nausea, anemia)

Adverse reactions to drugs in the past

Other Alerts/Health Aids/Special Needs (sight, hearing, mobility, literacy, disability)

CURRENT MEDICAL CONDITIONS AND MEDICATIONS

INDICATION	DRUG PRODUCT	DOSAGE REGIMEN dose, route, frequency, duration	START DATE	RESPONSE effectiveness/safety

PAST DRUG THERAPIES

INDICATION	DRUG THERAPY	RESPONSE	DATE

PAST MEDICAL HISTORY (RELEVANT ILLNESSES, HOSPITALIZATIONS, SURGICAL PROCEDURES, INJURIES, PREGNANCIES, DELIVERIES)

NUTRITIONAL STATUS (NOTE DAILY INTAKE OF CALORIES, CALCIUM, SODIUM, CHOLESTEROL, FIBER, POTASSIUM, VITAMIN K)

calories	K$^+$	cholesterol	Vitamin K
calcium	Na$^+$	fiber	

OTHER FOOD OR DIETARY RESTRICTIONS/NEEDS

Vital signs: BP _____/_____   HR _____bpm   Resp Rate _____   Temp____

		y/n				y/n
REVIEW OF SYSTEMS	General Systems	Poor appetite		GU/Reproductive	Dysmenorrhea/menstrual bleeding	
		Weight change			Incontinence	
		Pain			Impotence	
		Headache			Decreased sexual drive	
		Dizziness (vertigo)			Vaginal discharge or itching	
	EENT	Change in vision			Hot flashes	
		Loss of hearing		Kidney/Urinary	Urinary frequency	
		Ringing in the ears (tinnitus)			Bloody urine (hematuria)	
		Bloody nose (epistaxis)			Renal dysfunction	
		Allergic rhinitis		Hematopoietic Symptoms	Excessive bruising	
		Glaucoma			Bleeding	
		Bloody sputum (hemoptysis)			Anemia	
	Cardiovascular	Chest pain		Musculoskeletal	Back pain	
		Hyperlipidemia			Arthritis pain (osteo/rheumatoid)	
		Hypertension			Tendonitis	
		Myocardial Infarction			Painful muscles	
		Orthostatic hypotension		Neuropsychiatric	Numb, tingling sensation in extremities (parasthesia)	
	Pulmonary	Asthma			Tremor	
		Shortness of breath			Loss of balance	
		Wheezing			Depression	
	Gastrointestinal	Heartburn			Suicidal	
		Abdominal pain			Anxiety, nervousness	
		Nausea			Inability to concentrate	
		Vomiting			Seizure	
		Diarrhea			Stroke/TIA	
		Constipation			Memor loss	
	Skin	Eczema/Psoriasis		Infectious Disease	HIV/AIDS	
		Itching (pruritis)			Malaria	
		Rash			Syphilis	
	Endocrine Systems	Diabetes			Gonorrhea	
		Hypothyroidism			Herpes	
		Menopausal Symptoms			Chlamydia	
	Hepatic	Cirrhosis			Tuberculosis	
		Hepatitis				
	Nutrition/Fluid/Electrolytes	Dehydration				
		Edema				
		Potassium deficiency				

DRUG THERAPY PROBLEMS TO BE RESOLVED

MEDICAL CONDITION AND DRUG THERAPY INVOLVED	INDICATION
	Unnecessary Drug Therapy __No medical indication __Duplicate therapy __Nondrug therapy indicated __Treating avoidable ADR __Addictive/recreational ***Needs Additional Drug Therapy*** __Untreated condition __Preventive/prophylactic __Synergistic/potentiating

MEDICAL CONDITION AND DRUG THERAPY INVOLVED	EFFECTIVENESS
	Needs Different Drug Product __More effective drug available __Condition refractory to drug __Dosage form inappropriate __Not effective for condition ***Dosage Too Low*** __Wrong dose __Frequency inappropriate __Drug interaction __Duration inappropriate

MEDICAL CONDITION AND DRUG THERAPY INVOLVED	SAFETY
	Adverse Drug Reaction __Undesirable effect __Unsafe drug for patient __Drug interaction __Dosage administered or changed too rapidly __Allergic reaction __Contraindications present ***Dosage Too High*** __Wrong dose __Frequency inappropriate __Duration inappropriate __Drug interaction __Incorrect administration

MEDICAL CONDITION AND DRUG THERAPY INVOLVED	COMPLIANCE
	Noncompliance __Directions not understood __Patient prefers not to take __Patient forgets to take __Patient cannot afford __Cannot swallow/administer __Drug product not available

(Left vertical label: DRUG THERAPY PROBLEMS)

___**No Drug Therapy Problem(s) at this time**

Pharmacotherapy Workup © NOTES   **CARE PLAN**

INDICATION_____
(Description and history of the present illness or medical condition including previous approaches to treatment and responses)

GOALS OF THERAPY (improvement or normalization of signs/symptoms/laboratory tests or reduction of risk)

1.

2.

DRUG THERAPY PROBLEMS to be resolved

☐ None at this time

Therapeutic Alternatives (to resolve the drug therapy problem)

1.

2.

PHARMACOTHERAPY PLAN (Includes current drug therapies and changes)

MEDICATIONS (DRUG PRODUCTS)	DOSAGE INSTRUCTIONS (DOSE, ROUTE, FREQUENCY, DURATION)	NOTES CHANGES

Other interventions to optimize drug therapy

SCHEDULE FOR NEXT FOLLOW-UP EVALUATION:

Pharmacotherapy Workup© **NOTES**	**EVALUATION**

Medical Condition:_____

	Outcome Parameter	Date: / / Pretreatment/ Baseline	/ / First Evaluation	/ / Second Evaluation
EFFECTIVENESS	Sign/symptom			
	Sign/symptom			
	Laboratory value			
	Laboratory value			
SAFETY	Sign/symptoms			
	Signs/symptoms			
	Laboratory value			
	Laboratory value			
	Other			
OUTCOME STATUS	**Initial:** goals being established, initiate new therapy **Resolved:** goals achieved, therapy completed **Stable:** goals achieved, continue same therapy **Improved:** adequate progress being made, continue same therapy **Partial Improvement:** progress being made, adjustments in therapy required **Unimproved:** no progress yet, continue same therapy **Worsened:** decline in health, adjust therapy **Failure:** goals not achieved, discontinue current therapy and replace with different therapy			
	New Drug Therapy Problems Identified		○ none at this time ○ documented	○ none at this time ○ documented

Date	Schedule for next follow-up	Comments

Signature_____Date _____

PARAMETERS COMMONLY USED TO EVALUATE EFFECTIVENESS AND/OR SAFETY OF DRUG THERAPY		
PARAMETER	**GOALS OF THERAPY (NORMAL VALUES)**	**CLINICAL USE**
Blood pressure	Goals of therapy include: systolic blood pressure of 110–140 mmHg diastolic blood pressure of 75–85 mmHg <130/80 with diabetes or kidney disease	Used to evaluate effectiveness and safety of antihypertensive drug therapies such as diuretics, beta blockers, ACE inhibitors, angiotensin II receptors blockers, aldosterone antagonists, calcium blockers.
Total Cholesterol	Goal of therapy < 200 mg/dl (SI < 5.17 mmol/L)	Represents all of the different kinds of cholesterol in the blood and includes high-density lipids (HDL), low-density lipids (LDL), and triglycerides (TG).
LDL Low-density lipoprotein	Goal of therapy varies depending on other risk factors including cigarette smoking, hypertension, HDL<40mg/dl, family history of CHD and male>45 or female>55. • without other risk factors <160 mg/dl (SI <4.1 mmol/L) • with 2 risk factors <130 mg/dl (SI <3.4 mmol/L) • with CHD and ≥2 risk factors <100 mg/dl (SI <2.6 mmol/L) Optional high risk <70 mg/dl	Used to evaluate the effectiveness of lipid lowering drug therapies including atorvastatin (Lipitor®), fluvastatin (Lescol®), lovastatin (Mevacor®), pravastatin (Pravachol®), rosuvastatin (Crestor®), simvastatin (Zocor®) ezetimibe/simvastatin (Vytorin®) nicotinic acid (Niacin®) gemfibrozil (Lopid®), clofibrate (Atromid-S®) colestipol (Colestid®), cholestyramine (Questran®)
HDL High-density lipoprotein	Goals of therapy > 40 mg/dl (SI >1.04 mmol/L)	HDL removes excess cholesterol from peripheral tissues and is considered "good" cholesterol. Elevated HDL levels are associated with decreased risk for coronary heart disease.
Triglycerides	<160 mg/dl <1.8 mmol/L	Elevated triglycerides considered an independent risk factor for coronary heart disease.
Glucose	Goal of therapy includes: preprandial blood glucose of 80–120 mg/dL bedtime blood glucose of 100–140 mg/dL Fasting plasma glucose of > 126 mg/dL on two occasions is consistent with the diagnosis of diabetes mellitus	Used to evaluate drug therapy to manage hyperglycemia associated with diabetes mellitus including insulin (Humulin®) (Novolin®), glipizide (Glutcotrol®), glyburide (Diabeta®) (Mircronase®), pioglitazone (Actos®), rosiglitazone (Avandia®)
HbA$_{1c}$ Hemoglobin A$_{1c}$	Goal of therapy < 7% Normal range 4–6%	Used to evaluate the effectiveness of glucose control in patients with diabetes. Reflects the blood glucose control over the past 2 to 3 months.
TSH Thyroid Stimulating Hormone	Goals of therapy include the reduction of TSH levels to the normal range of 0.3–5 μU/ml (SI 0.3–5 mU/L)	Used to evaluate the effectiveness of thyroid replacement therapy to manage hypothyroidism, levothyroxine (Synthroid®). Elevated TSH levels are indicative of hypothyroidism.
INR International Normalized Ratio	Goal of therapy varies with the indication. INR 2.0–3.0 for atrial fibrillation, deep vein thrombosis, pulmonary emboli INR 2.5–3.5 for mechanical prosthetic values	Used to evaluate the effectives and safety of anticoagulant therapy. Used to determine dosage adjustments for warfarin (Coumadin®) therapy.
K$^+$ Serum Potassium	Goal of therapy is to maintain serum potassium within the normal range of 3.5–5.0 mEq/L (SI 3.5–5.0 mmol/L)	Used to evaluate and prevent cardiac toxicity associated with hypokalemia caused by diuretics, diarrhea/vomiting. Can aggravate digoxin (Lanoxin®) toxicity. Hyperkalemia associated with renal dysfunction, ACE inhibitors including captopril (Capoten®), enalapril (Vasotec®), lisinopril (Prinivil®) (Zestril®), ramipril (Altace®)
Creatinine serum creatinine (SCr) creatinine clearance (CrCl)	Creatinine normal range 0.6–1.3 mg/dL (SI 53–115 μmol/L) Creatinine Clearance normal range 80–100 ml/min Drug dosage adjustments often required when CrCl is <30 ml/min	Used as a guideline to determine appropriate dosage of medications which are dependent on renal function for elimination. Used to determine if drug therapy is causing nephrotoxicity or if drugs are accumulating to unsafe levels due to decreasing renal function.
ALT Alanine aminotransferase AST Aspartate aminotrasnferase	Normal values Males 10–40 Units/ml Females 8–35 Units/ml Males 20–40 Units/ml Females15–30 Units/ml	Used to evaluate liver damage caused by medications such as simvastatin (Zocor®), pravastatin, lovastatin (Mevacor®), atorvastatin (Lipitor®) (Pravachol®), fluvastatin (Lescol®), rosuvastatin (Crestor®), carbamazepine, phenytoin, acetaminophen If elevated 2–3 times, drug-induced hepatic damage suspected

Index

A

Abbreviations, 303–318, 329
Abdomen, 79, 83, 86, 157
  Chinese pronunciations, 167
  dialogues, 360–365
  dictation, 167–168
  Gujarati pronunciations, 166
  idiomatic expressions using, 174
  Korean pronunciations, 167
  medical conditions and patient
    complaints, 160–161
  multiple choice questions, 155–156,
    176–177
  parts of speech, 157–164
  pharmacist/patient dialogues,
    168–173, 177–180
  pronunciation exercise, 164–166
  Russian pronunciations, 167
  Spanish pronunciations, 166
  true/false questions, 155, 175–176
  Vietnamese pronunciations, 166
  vocabulary, 156–157, 161–164
  word forms, 157–161
Abdominal, 98, 164
Abdominal pain, 156
Abscess, 10
Absorbency, 233
Absorbent, 240, 247
Absorption, 157, 164
Ache, 79, 81, 86, 183
Aching, 190
Acne, 6, 10
Acute, 112
Acute pyelonephritis, 235
Acuteness, 105
Adam's apple, 82
Addison's disease, 86
Adenoids, 59
Adenomyosis, 281, 284–285, 295
Adrenaline, 138
"After one's blood," 95
Agitated, 77
Agitation, 79, 86, 207
Airplane ear, 28, 30–31, 33
Airway, 112
Alcoholic cirrhosis, 253, 256
Alcoholism, 255, 261
"All ears," 25, 44

Allergens, 53, 55, 107–108
Allergic, 54, 71
Allergy, 53
Alopecia, 6–7, 10
Alzheimer's disease, 207, 210,
  212–213, 216
Amenorrhea, 275, 277, 279, 283–285, 293
Amyotrophic lateral sclerosis,
  211–214, 216
Anemia, 81, 86
Aneurysm, 129, 131, 134, 138
Angina, 129–131, 133, 136, 138, 150
Angioplasty, 138
Ankylosing spondylitis, 185, 188, 190
Antihistamines, 55, 58–59
Anus, 157, 164
Anxiety, 131, 138, 149
Aorta, 131, 138
Aortic aneurysm, 134
Appendicitis, 155, 159
Appendix, 157, 164
Appetite, 81, 86
Armpit, 86
Arrhythmia, 138
Arteriosclerosis, 132, 134–135
Artery, 131, 134, 138
Arthritis, 181, 183, 186, 190
Ascites, 255, 261
Aspirate, 216
Aspiration, 209
Asthma, 103, 105, 107, 110, 112, 122
Asthmatic, 105
Astigmatism, 33
Atherosclerosis, 131, 133–134, 138
Athlete's foot, 1, 20
Atonic, 216
Atonicity, 209
Atrial fibrillation, 135, 138
Atrophic vaginitis, 281, 284–285, 295
Autoimmune, 82, 183, 190
Autoimmune hepatitis, 253, 256–260,
  268–270

B

Backwash, 164
Bacteria, 277
Bacterial vaginosis, 285
"Bad mouth," 67

Balance, 209, 216
Barking cough, 107
Barrett's esophagus, 155, 159
"Bated breath," 120
"Beat one's brains," 224
Bed wetting, 240
"Behind one's back," 199
Belch, 158, 160, 163–164
Belly button, 164
Bellyache, 158, 164
"Bend someone's ear," 42
Benign, 86
Benign prostatic hyperplasia, 232
Bile, 164
Bile duct, 261
Bipolar disorder, 211, 216
Birth control, 285
Birthmark, 10
"Bite someone's head off," 224, 226
Black nail, 10
Black toe, 7, 10
Bladder, 240
Bladder training, 240
Bleed, 53
Blink, 27–28
Blinking, 33
Blister, 1, 4, 10, 21, 56
Bloating, 158–159, 163–164, 176–177
Block, 53
Blocked nose, 56, 59
Blood, 79, 86, 95
"Blood boil," 95–97
"Blood from a stone," 95
"Blood is thicker than water," 95–96
Blood pressure, 130
"Blood run cold," 95–96
Bloodshot, 30, 33
Blood-streaked, 112
Blood-tinged, 112
Blow, 53
Bluish color, 112
Blur, 27, 33
Blurred vision, 26
"Boggles the mind," 224
Boil, 4, 10
Bone marrow, 82, 86
"Bone of contention," 199
"Bone to pick," 199

Bony lump, 190
Booger, 55, 59
"Bored stiff," 199
Bout, 164
Bowel, 164
Bowel movement, 86
Bradycardia, 131, 138
"Break one's back," 199, 201
Breakout, 10
Breast lump, 285
Breath, 78
"Breath of fresh air," 120, 123
"Breathe down someone's neck," 120
"Breathe easy," 120
Brittle, 4, 6, 10
Brittleness, 183, 190
Bronchial, 106
Bronchial tubes, 110
Bronchitis, 103, 105, 107–109, 112, 123
Bronchodilator, 105, 107–109
Bruise, 4, 10, 20
Bruising, 56, 81
Bulge, 27, 44
Bulginess, 27
Bulging eye, 33
Bump, 4, 7, 10, 44, 54
Bumpy, 29
Burning, 232
Burp, 164
Bursitis, 181, 190
"Butterflies in one's stomach," 174, 176
Buzzing, 34

C
Canker sore, 51–52, 54, 57, 59
"Can't stomach someone or something,"
    174, 176
Cardiac catheterization, 138
Cardiomyopathy, 138
Cardiovascular system
    Chinese pronunciations, 141
    dialogues, 354–360
    dictation, 141–142
    Gujarati pronunciations, 140–141
    idiomatic expressions using, 147–148
    Korean pronunciations, 141
    medical conditions and patient
        complaints, 134–135
    multiple choice questions, 129–130,
        135–137, 149–151
    parts of speech, 131–138
    pharmacist/patient dialogues,
        142–147, 151–154
    pronunciation exercise, 138–140
    Russian pronunciations, 141
    Spanish pronunciations, 140
    true/false questions, 129, 137, 149
    Vietnamese pronunciations, 140
    vocabulary, 130–131, 135–138
    word forms, 131–133

Carpal tunnel syndrome, 190
Cartilage, 190
Cataract, 25, 29, 33–34
"Catch one's breath," 120
Catheter, 237, 240
Cauliflower ear, 34
Celiac disease, 161–162, 164
Cerebral hemorrhage, 138
Cerebrovascular accident, 138
Cervical cancer, 280
Cervicitis, 281, 283
Cervix, 277, 285
Chapped lips, 51, 59, 71
Cheek, 59
Chest
    Chinese pronunciations, 114
    dialogues, 349–354
    dictation, 114–115
    Gujarati pronunciations, 113–114
    idiomatic expressions using, 120
    Korean pronunciations, 114
    medical conditions and patient
        complaints, 107–109
    multiple choice questions, 103–104,
        122–123
    parts of speech, 105–111
    pharmacist/patient dialogues,
        115–119, 123–127
    pronunciation exercise, 86–87
    Russian pronunciations, 114
    Spanish pronunciations, 113
    true/false questions, 103, 122
    Vietnamese pronunciations, 113
    vocabulary, 104–105
    word forms, 105–109
Chiggers, 10
Chills, 105, 112
"Chills up/down one's spine," 199
Chinese pronunciations, 13, 36, 62, 89,
    114, 141, 167, 193, 218, 242,
    262, 288
Chipped tooth, 60
Chlamydia, 293–294
Cholesterol, 129, 131, 138
"Chopped liver," 254
Chronic bronchitis, 109
Chronic infection, 110
Chronic obstructive pulmonary disease,
    103, 108–110, 112
Chronicity, 105
Cigarettes, 107
Circulation, 131
Cirrhosis, 253–256, 258–261, 268, 270
Clammy, 112
Claudication, 134
Clear, 55
Clog, 27, 34, 54
Clogged nose, 60
Clogging, 134
Clot, 131, 138

Cloud, 53
Cloudiness, 53
Cloudy discharge, 60
Coagulability, 132
Coagulation, 132, 138
Coarse, 10, 81
Cold intolerance, 81–82, 86
Cold sore, 51, 60
Collagen, 183, 190
Collapse, 105
Collapsed lung, 109, 112
Collapsibility, 105
Colon, 158, 164
Colon cancer, 163
Colostomy, 164
Community-acquired bladder infection,
    236–237
Compulsion, 209
Concentration, 81
Condoms, 280, 285, 294
Congenital, 139
Congenital heart disease, 130
Congested, 51–52
Congestion, 53, 60, 129
Congestive heart failure, 130, 134, 149
Conjunctivitis, 25, 34
Connective tissue, 190
Constipation, 77, 79, 81, 86, 96, 156,
    158–159, 163–164, 176
Contact lens, 34
Contagion, 53, 253, 255
Contagious, 56, 109, 269
Contaminant, 270
Contamination, 255, 261
Contents, 240
Contraception, 278, 280
Contraceptive, 278, 285
Contract, 240
Contraction, 158, 164
Controllability, 278
Coordination, 79, 86
COPD, 103, 108–110, 112
Cornea, 34
Cough, 53, 107
Cough up, 107
Coughing, 53, 55, 60
Crack, 4, 53
Cracked, 10
Cracked lips, 60
Crackles, 112
Cramp, 132, 139, 158, 165, 278, 285
Creak, 105
Creaking, 112
Crohn's disease, 156, 159, 161–162, 268
Cross-eyed, 34
Croup, 105, 107–108, 110, 112
Crushing sensation, 139, 150
Crust, 4, 31
Crusty, 10, 29
Crusty eyelid, 34, 45

Cushing's disease, 86
Cuticle, 10
Cyst, 6, 10, 285
Cystic fibrosis, 107–109, 112
Cystitis, 231, 234–236, 238–240

D
"Dance one's heart out," 148
Dandruff, 1, 6–7, 10
Deaf, 34
Deafness, 27
Debilitation, 183, 191, 202
Decongestants, 55, 60
Deformity, 183, 191
Degeneration, 183
Degenerative, 191, 226
Delirious, 77
Delirium, 77, 79, 83, 86, 96
Demented, 209
Dementia, 207, 213–214, 216
Dentures, 60
Depression, 207–209, 211–214, 216, 227
Dermatitis, 10
Deterioration, 201
Deviated septum, 51, 56, 60
Dexterity, 207, 210, 216
Diabetes, 77, 79, 81–83, 85–86, 97, 133, 136, 236
Diagnosed, 81
Diaper rash, 10
Diaphragm, 158, 165, 285
Diarrhea, 81, 156, 158, 165
"Difficult to stomach," 174, 176
Digestion, 158, 165, 176
Diphtheria, 105, 112
Discharge, 26, 30
Disorder, 81
Disorientation, 207, 210, 216
Distorted, 34
Distortion, 27
Distracted, 216
Distraction, 210
Diuretic, 132, 139
Diverticula, 159, 161, 165
Diverticular disease, 155
Diverticulitis, 155, 165
Diverticulosis, 159, 165
Dizziness, 27
Dizzy, 34, 83
"Don't hold your breath," 120
Double vision, 30, 34
Double voiding, 240
Douche, 285
Drain, 34, 240
Drainage, 28, 44, 55, 233
Dribble, 233, 240, 248
Drip, 54
Drool, 54, 56, 60
Droop, 28
Droopy eye, 25

Drowsiness, 54, 80–81
Drowsy, 55, 86
Dry cough, 60
Dry eye, 30, 32–34, 44
Dry mouth, 51, 56, 60
Dryness, 4
Duct, 255
Dysfunction, 278
Dysmenorrhea, 278, 280, 284–285
Dyspareunia, 285
Dysphagia, 158, 161, 165
Dyspnea, 104–105, 110, 112

E
Ear(s)
    Chinese pronunciations, 36
    dialogues, 336–338
    dictation, 36–37
    Gujarati pronunciations, 36
    idiomatic expressions using, 41–42
    Korean pronunciations, 36
    medical conditions and patient
        complaints, 29–30
    multiple choice questions, 25–26,
        43–45
    parts of speech, 27–33
    pharmacist/patient dialogues, 37–41,
        45–49
    pronunciation exercise, 33–35
    Spanish pronunciations, 35
    true/false questions, 25, 43
    Vietnamese pronunciations, 35
    vocabulary, 26–27, 31–33
    word forms, 27–30
Ear infection, 25, 29, 31
Ear lobe, 34
Ear plugs, 30
Ear popping, 25
Ear wax, 25
Earache, 25, 34
Eardrum, 28, 31
Echocardiogram, 139
Ectopic, 278
Ectopic pregnancy, 279, 285, 294
Eczema, 4, 10
Edema, 105, 112, 132, 139
Ejaculation, 278, 285
Electric shock, 216
Electrocardiogram, 139
Embolism, 105, 132, 139
Emergency contraception, 280, 284
Emphysema, 103–104, 106–107,
    109–110
Emphysemic, 122
Emptiness, 233
Encephalopathy, 255
Endocrine system
    Chinese pronunciations, 89
    dialogues, 345–349
    dictation, 89–90

Gujarati pronunciations, 88
idiomatic expressions using, 94–95
Korean pronunciations, 88
medical conditions and patient
    complaints, 82–83
multiple choice questions, 77–78, 96–98
parts of speech, 79–85
pharmacist/patient dialogues, 90–96,
    98–101
pronunciation exercise, 86–87
Russian pronunciations, 89
Spanish pronunciations, 88
true/false questions, 77, 96
Vietnamese pronunciations, 88
vocabulary, 78–79
word forms, 79–83
Endometrial cancer, 282, 294
Endometriosis, 278, 281, 284–285,
    294–295
Enlarged prostate, 237, 239–240
Enlarged spleen, 77
Enlargement, 80–81, 86, 233
Epigastric area, 160, 165
Epigastrium, 158
Epilepsy, 207, 210–212, 215, 217, 227
Epinephrine, 139
Episode, 106
Episodic, 112
Erectile dysfunction, 275, 279, 283–284,
    286, 293–294
Erection, 278
Erode, 165
Erodibility, 158
Erythrocyte sedimentation rate, 191
Esophagus, 155, 158, 165
Exacerbation, 132, 139, 150, 217
Excessive, 54, 70
Excessiveness, 54
Excrete, 10
Excretion, 4
Exertion, 106, 112
Exhalation, 106
Exhale, 112
Exhaustion, 80, 86, 106
Expectorant, 106, 108, 123
Expectorate, 107, 110, 112, 122
Expectoration, 106
Eye(s)
    Chinese pronunciations, 36
    dialogues, 336–338
    dictation, 36–37
    Gujarati pronunciations, 36
    idiomatic expressions using, 41
    Korean pronunciations, 36
    medical conditions and patient
        complaints, 29–30
    multiple choice questions, 25–26, 43–45
    parts of speech, 27–33
    pharmacist/patient dialogues, 37–41,
        45–49

Eye(s) (*Cont.*)
  pronunciation exercise, 33–35
  Russian pronunciations, 36
  Spanish pronunciations, 35
  true/false questions, 25, 43
  Vietnamese pronunciations, 35
  vocabulary, 27, 31–33
  word forms, 27–30
Eye herpes, 34
Eye pressure, 34
Eye strain, 30, 34
"Eye to eye," 26
Eyeball, 34
Eyelid, 29
"Eyes are bigger than one's stomach,"
  174–175
"Eyes in the back of one's head," 41, 43
"Eyes like a hawk," 41, 43–44
"Eyes were glued," 41–42

F
Faintness, 132, 139
Fallopian tube, 286
Farsighted, 30–31, 34
Farsightedness, 33
Fatigue, 80–81, 86, 108, 123, 135
Febrile, 112
Fecal impaction, 155, 159, 162, 176
Fecal incontinence, 161
Feces, 158–159, 165
"Feel it in my bones," 182
"Feel something in one's bones," 199
Fertile, 286
Fertility, 275, 278
Fever, 106
Fever blisters, 52, 56–57, 59–60, 71
Fibrillation, 135
Fibrocystic breasts, 286
Fibroid, 278, 286
Fibromyalgia, 182, 185–187,
  190–191, 203
Fibrosis, 106
Fine, 10
Flakes, 4, 30
Flakiness, 4
Flaky, 1, 10
Flare, 165
Flatulence, 165
Flexibility, 183, 191
Floaters, 29, 34
Flow, 233, 240, 247
Fluid, 28–30, 34
Fluidity, 28
Flushness, 132, 139
Flutter, 130, 139
"Foam at the mouth," 67, 70
Focus, 28–29, 34, 45
Foreign body, 25, 34
Foreign objects, 29
Forgetfulness, 210, 217

Fracture, 183, 186, 191
"From the bottom of one's heart," 147
Froth, 106, 112
Frothiness, 278
Frothy discharge, 286
Functional incontinence, 236, 239
Fungal infection, 10
Fungus, 56
Fusion, 183, 191
Fuzz, 28
Fuzziness, 28
Fuzzy, 34

G
Gag, 54
Gag reflex, 60
Gait, 217
Gallbladder, 165
Gangrene, 78, 80, 86, 133
Gargle, 54–55, 60
Gas, 159, 165
Gash, 7, 10
Gasping, 139
Gastric, 177
Gastric ulcers, 161, 165
Gastritis, 161, 164–165
Gastroenteritis, 160, 162, 164–165
Gastroesophageal reflux disease, 155,
  159–160, 162–163
Gastrointestinal system
  Chinese pronunciations, 167
  dialogues, 360–365
  dictation, 167–168
  Gujarati pronunciations, 166
  idiomatic expressions using, 174
  Korean pronunciations, 167
  medical conditions and patient
    complaints, 160–161
  multiple choice questions, 155–156,
    176–177
  parts of speech, 157–164
  pharmacist/patient dialogues,
    168–173, 177–180
  pronunciation exercise, 164–166
  Russian pronunciations, 167
  Spanish pronunciations, 166
  true/false questions, 155, 175–176
  Vietnamese pronunciations, 166
  vocabulary, 156–157, 161–164
  word forms, 157–161
Generalized anxiety disorder, 207, 211,
  214–216
Generalized seizures, 208
Genital herpes, 275, 282–283, 285
"Get in my hair," 18–19
"Get off one's back," 199
"Get something off your chest,"
  103, 120
"Get under my skin," 17, 19
Gingivitis, 60

Gland, 86
Glare, 28–29, 34
Glaucoma, 25, 34
Glucose, 77, 81–82, 86
Gluten, 159
Goiter, 81, 84, 86
Gonorrhea, 275, 278–279, 281,
  284–286, 294
"Good eye," 41
"Good head on one's shoulders," 208
Gout, 181, 183, 185–186, 188,
  190–191, 202
Gouty arthritis, 184
Grade, 83
Grand mal seizure, 207
Graves disease, 78, 85–86
"Green behind the ears," 43
"Grin from ear to ear," 42
Grit, 28
Grittiness, 28
Gritty, 34
Gujarati pronunciations, 12, 36, 62, 88,
  113–114, 140–141, 166, 192, 218,
  241, 262, 287
Gums, 60

H
Hacking cough, 104, 112
Hair
  Chinese pronunciations, 13
  dialogues, 333–336
  Gujarati pronunciations, 12
  idiomatic expressions using, 18
  Korean pronunciations, 12–13
  loss of, 10
  medical conditions and patient
    complaints, 5–7
  multiple-choice questions for, 1–2,
    20–21
  parts of speech, 3–9
  pharmacist/patient dialogues
    involving, 14–17, 21–23
  pronunciations, 10–11
  Russian pronunciations, 13
  Spanish pronunciations, 12
  true/false questions regarding,
    1, 19–20
  Vietnamese pronunciations, 12
  vocabulary for, 3, 7–9
  word forms, 3–7
"Hair stand on end," 18–19
Hairy tongue, 60
Halitosis, 51, 56, 58, 60, 70
Halos, 29, 34
"Hang one's head," 224, 227
Hard, 149
"Hard as nails," 18
"Hard nosed," 67, 70
"Hard to stomach," 174
Hardening, 132, 139

"Hardly have time to breathe," 120
Hashimoto's disease, 84–86
"Have a heart," 147
Hay fever, 60
Head lice, 6, 10, 20
Hearing loss, 29, 34
Heart
    Chinese pronunciations, 141
    dialogues, 354–360
    dictation, 141–142
    Gujarati pronunciations, 140–141
    idiomatic expressions using, 147–148
    Korean pronunciations, 141
    medical conditions and patient
        complaints, 134–135
    multiple choice questions, 129–130,
        135–137, 149–151
    parts of speech, 131–138
    pharmacist/patient dialogues,
        142–147, 151–154
    pronunciation exercise, 138–140
    Russian pronunciations, 141
    Spanish pronunciations, 140
    true/false questions, 129, 137, 149
    Vietnamese pronunciations, 140
    vocabulary, 130–131, 135–138
    word forms, 131–133
Heart attack, 129, 133–134, 138
Heart failure, 129, 133–136, 138–139
"Heart of gold," 147, 149
"Heart of stone," 147, 149
"Heart sank," 148
"Heart skips a beat," 147, 149
"Heart was in the right place," 147
Heartburn, 139, 155, 159–160, 165
"Heart-to-heart," 147
Heat intolerance, 86
"Heavy heart," 147, 149
Hematuria, 233, 240
Hemochromatosis, 259, 261
Hemolysis, 255
Hemolytic anemia, 261
Hemorrhage, 134
Hemorrhoids, 158, 160, 162, 165
Hepatic encephalopathy, 258–259,
    261, 269
Hepatic system
    Chinese pronunciations, 262
    dialogues, 381–386
    dictation, 263–264
    Gujarati pronunciations, 262
    idiomatic expressions using, 268
    Korean pronunciations, 262
    medical conditions and patient
        complaints, 257–258
    multiple choice questions, 253–254,
        269–270
    parts of speech, 255–260
    pharmacist/patient dialogues,
        264–268, 270–274

pronunciation exercise, 261–262
Russian pronunciations, 263
Spanish pronunciations, 262
true/false questions, 253, 268–269
Vietnamese pronunciations, 262
vocabulary, 254–255, 258–260
word forms, 255–258
Hepatitis A, 253, 256–257, 259–260,
    268, 270
Hepatitis B, 253–254, 256, 259–260,
    268–269
Hepatitis C, 253, 256, 259–260, 268
Hiatal hernia, 155, 159–160, 165
High blood pressure, 139
"Hit between the eyes," 41, 197
Hives, 10
Hoarse voice, 60
Hoarseness, 54
Hodgkin's lymphoma, 85–86
"Hold your tongue," 68
Hormone, 80–82, 86, 278, 286
Hot flashes, 275, 279, 286, 293
Human papillomavirus, 281–283, 285
Hyperglycemia, 83–84
Hypertension, 132, 139
Hyperthyroidism, 77, 85–86
Hypoglycemia, 77, 80
Hypothyroidism, 77, 82, 85–86, 97
Hysterectomy, 278, 281, 284, 286, 295

I
Idiomatic expressions
    back, 198–199
    blood, 95
    bone, 198–199
    brain, 224
    chest, 120
    ears, 41–42
    endocrine system, 94–95
    eyes, 41
    hair, 18
    head, 224
    heart, 147–148
    hepatic system, 268
    joint, 198–199
    lung, 120
    lymphatic system, 94–95
    mind, 224
    mouth, 67–68
    muscle, 198–199
    musculoskeletal system, 198–199
    nails, 18
    nose, 67
    reproductive system, 293
    respiratory system, 120
    skin, 17–18
    spine, 198–199
    stiff, 198–199
    stomach, 174
    urinary system, 247

Immune, 191
Immune globulin, 258, 261
Immune system, 86
Immunization, 183, 255, 261
Impaction, 156
Impairment, 210
Impede, 240
Impediment, 233
Incontinence, 80, 86, 158–159, 161,
    165, 231, 233, 239–240
Indigestion, 86, 158, 160–161,
    164–165
Infected, 29
Infection, 25, 51
Infertility, 275, 278, 280, 286, 295
Inflamed sinuses, 55
Inflammation, 4, 10, 29–30, 56, 81
Inflexible, 202
Influenza, 106, 112
Ingrown nail, 10
Inhalant, 106
Inhalation, 103, 106
Inhale, 112
Inhaler, 103, 106
Inoperability, 255, 261
Inseminate, 286
Insemination, 278
Insomnia, 80–81, 87
Insomniac, 80
Insulin, 81–82, 87
Intercourse, 286
Intermittence, 132
Intermittent claudication, 139
Interstitial cystitis, 231, 234–235,
    239–240, 248
Intestine, 158
Intolerable, 97
Intolerance, 77, 80
Intolerant, 97
Intrauterine device, 286
Involuntariness, 233
Involuntary contraction, 240
Irregular heartbeat, 139
Irreversibility, 210, 217
Irritable, 56
Irritable bowel syndrome, 155, 159–160,
    163–164
Irritant, 4
Irritation, 4, 10, 54
Ischemia, 132–133, 136, 139, 149
Isolation, 210, 217
Itch, 4, 10
Itchiness, 4
Itching, 55
Itchy, 21, 25, 29
Itchy throat, 60

J
Jaundice, 28, 34, 256, 258, 261
Joint, 184, 191

K

"Keep an eye out," 41, 198
"Keep me abreast," 276
"Keep one's head," 224
"Keep your hair on," 18
"Keep your head above water," 224
"Keep your nose clean," 67
Kegel exercises, 240, 247
Keloid, 2, 6, 11
Kidney infection, 231, 236–237, 239–240
Knife-like pain, 112
Knuckle, 184, 191
Korean pronunciations, 12–13, 36, 62, 88, 114, 141, 167, 192, 218, 241, 262, 288

L

Labored, 107
Labored breathing, 112, 123
Laceration, 2, 4, 11
Lactation, 278–279, 286
Lapse, 210, 217
Lazy eye, 29, 34
Leak, 231, 233, 240
"Lend an ear," 41
Lesion, 11
"Let my hair down," 18
Lethargy, 77, 80, 87
Leukemia, 77, 84–85
Lice, 6
Ligament, 184, 191
Light therapy, 217
Lightheaded, 83–84, 87
Lightheadedness, 80
Limp, 134
Lips, 68
Liver cancer, 254
Liver transplant, 261
"Lose one's head," 224, 226
Lou Gehrig's disease, 212
Lower esophageal sphincter, 165
Low-grade, 108
Lump, 28
Lung
    Chinese pronunciations, 114
    dialogues, 349–354
    dictation, 114–115
    Gujarati pronunciations, 113–114
    idiomatic expressions using, 120
    Korean pronunciations, 114
    medical conditions and patient complaints, 107–109
    multiple choice questions, 103–104, 122–123
    parts of speech, 105–111
    pharmacist/patient dialogues, 115–119, 123–127
    pronunciation exercise, 86–87
    Russian pronunciations, 114

Spanish pronunciations, 113
true/false questions, 103, 122
Vietnamese pronunciations, 113
vocabulary, 104–105
word forms, 105–109
Lupus, 182, 184–185, 187, 190–191
Lymph nodes, 77–78, 87
Lymphatic system
    Chinese pronunciations, 89
    dialogues, 345–349
    dictation, 89–90
    Gujarati pronunciations, 88
    idiomatic expressions using, 94–95
    Korean pronunciations, 88
    medical conditions and patient complaints, 82–83
    multiple choice questions, 77–78, 96–98
    parts of speech, 79–85
    pharmacist/patient dialogues, 90–96, 98–101
    pronunciation exercise, 86–87
    Russian pronunciations, 89
    Spanish pronunciations, 88
    true/false questions, 77, 96
    vocabulary, 78–79
    word forms, 79–83
Lymphoma, 77, 82, 85

M

Macular degeneration, 34
"Make my mouth water," 67
"Make my skin crawl," 18
"Make one's blood boil," 95–97
Malaise, 87
Malignant, 87
Manic-depressive disorder, 211, 227
Marfan syndrome, 181
Mask, 80, 87
Mastectomy, 286
Mastitis, 275, 278, 286, 293
Measles, 87
Medical conditions
    cardiovascular system, 134–135
    chest, 107–109
    ears, 29–30
    endocrine system, 82–83
    eyes, 29–30
    hair, 5–7
    heart, 134–135
    hepatic system, 257–258
    lung, 107–109
    lymphatic system, 82–83
    mental health, 212–213
    mouth, 55–56
    musculoskeletal system, 185–187
    nails, 5–7
    neurologic system, 212–213
    nose, 55–56

reproductive system, 280–282
respiratory system, 107–109
skin, 5–7
urinary system, 235–236
"Melt in your mouth," 67
Menarche, 278
Menopause, 278–279, 281, 285–286
Menorrhagia, 275, 278, 282–284, 286
Menses, 286
Menstruation, 275, 278, 286, 295
Mental health
    Chinese pronunciations, 218
    dialogues, 371–378
    dictation, 219–220
    Gujarati pronunciations, 218
    idiomatic expressions using, 223–224
    Korean pronunciations, 218
    medical conditions and patient complaints, 212–213
    multiple choice questions, 207–208, 226–227
    parts of speech, 209–216
    pharmacist/patient dialogues, 220–223, 227–230
    pronunciation exercise, 216–217
    Russian pronunciations, 218
    Spanish pronunciations, 218
    true/false questions, 207, 226
    Vietnamese pronunciations, 218
    vocabulary, 213–214
    word forms, 209–213
Mental impairment, 217
Metabolism, 80, 82, 87, 97
Middle ear infection, 34
"Mind goes blank," 224
"Mind-numbing," 224
Mini-stroke, 136
Miscarry, 276, 278, 286
Mitral valve prolapse, 135, 139
Mittelschmerz, 276, 286
Mobility, 182, 184, 191, 203
Mobilization, 203
Moderation, 158, 165
Moist, 11
Moistness, 4
Mole, 11
Mononucleosis, 87
Mood swing, 87
Morning after pill, 280, 284
Mouth
    Chinese pronunciations, 62
    dialogues, 341–345
    dictation, 62–63
    Gujarati pronunciations, 62
    idiomatic expressions using, 67–68
    Korean pronunciations, 62
    medical conditions and patient complaints, 55–56
    multiple choice questions, 51–52, 70–71

parts of speech, 53–59
pharmacist/patient dialogues, 63–66, 71–75
pronunciation exercise, 59–61
Russian pronunciations, 62
Spanish pronunciations, 61
true/false questions, 51, 69–70
Vietnamese pronunciations, 61
vocabulary, 52–53, 57–59
word forms, 53–55
Mouth sore, 54, 60
Mucous discharge, 51
Mucus, 51, 54–56, 59–60
Multiple sclerosis, 207, 211–215, 217
Mumbler, 210
Mumbling speech, 217
Mumps, 87
Muscle cramp, 87
"Muscle one's way in," 199
Muscle wasting, 214
Musculoskeletal system
    Chinese pronunciations, 193
    dialogues, 365–371
    dictation, 193–194
    Gujarati pronunciations, 192
    idiomatic expressions using, 198–199
    Korean pronunciations, 192
    medical conditions and patient complaints, 185–187
    multiple choice questions, 181–182, 202–203
    parts of speech, 183–190
    pharmacist/patient dialogues, 194–198, 203–206
    pronunciation exercise, 190–192
    Russian pronunciations, 193
    Spanish pronunciations, 192
    true/false questions, 181, 201–202
    Vietnamese pronunciations, 192
    vocabulary, 182–183, 187–190
    word forms, 183–185
"My heart goes out to you," 130
Myelin sheath, 217
Myocardial infarction, 139
Myoclonic, 217

N
Nail(s)
    Chinese pronunciations, 13
    dialogues, 333–316
    Gujarati pronunciations, 12
    idiomatic expressions using, 18
    Korean pronunciations, 12–13
    medical conditions and patient complaints, 5–7
    multiple-choice questions for, 1–2, 20–21
    parts of speech, 3–9
    pharmacist/patient dialogues involving, 14–17, 21–23

pronunciations, 10–11
Russian pronunciations, 13
Spanish pronunciations, 12
true/false questions regarding, 1, 19–20
Vietnamese pronunciations, 12
vocabulary for, 3, 7–9
word forms, 3–7
"Nail biting," 18
Nasal, 54
Nasal aspirator, 57
Nasal congestion, 51
Nasal discharge, 55, 60
Nasal flaring, 109, 112
Nasal passages, 56, 58
Nausea, 80, 87
Nauseation, 80
Navel, 165
Nearsighted, 34
Nearsightedness, 33
"Need to take a piss," 232, 247
Nervous, 87
Nervousness, 80
Neurologic system
    Chinese pronunciations, 218
    dialogues, 371–378
    dictation, 219–220
    Gujarati pronunciations, 218
    idiomatic expressions using, 223–224
    Korean pronunciations, 218
    medical conditions and patient complaints, 212–213
    multiple choice questions, 207–208, 226–227
    parts of speech, 209–216
    pharmacist/patient dialogues, 220–223, 227–230
    pronunciation exercise, 216–217
    Russian pronunciations, 218
    Spanish pronunciations, 218
    true/false questions, 207, 226
    Vietnamese pronunciations, 218
    vocabulary, 213–214
    word forms, 209–213
Neurology, 210, 217
Night sweats, 81
Night vision, 34
Nipple, 286
Nitroglycerin, 139
"No bones about something," 199
Nocturia, 240
Nocturnal enuresis, 232, 237, 239–240
Node, 191
Nodule, 87
Non-Hodgkin's lymphoma, 85, 87
Nose
    Chinese pronunciations, 62
    dialogues, 341–345
    dictation, 62–63
    Gujarati pronunciations, 62

idiomatic expressions using, 67
Korean pronunciations, 62
medical conditions and patient complaints, 55–56
multiple choice questions, 51–52, 70–71
parts of speech, 53–59
pharmacist/patient dialogues, 63–66, 71–75
pronunciation exercise, 59–61
Russian pronunciations, 62
Spanish pronunciations, 61
true/false questions, 51, 69–70
Vietnamese pronunciations, 61
vocabulary, 52–53, 57–59
word forms, 53–55
"Nose around," 67
Nose job, 60
"Nose out of joint," 198, 201
Nose spray, 57
"Nose to the grindstone," 67
Nosebleed, 51, 56, 59–60
Nostril, 51, 54, 60
"Not breathe a word," 120
"Not have the heart to do something," 147
"Not have the stomach for," 174
Numbness, 80, 87

O
Obesity, 129
Obsession, 210
Obsessive-compulsive disorder, 217
Obstruction, 106, 158, 165
Obstructiveness, 106
Obstructor, 106
Occult blood, 165
Oil, 4
Oiliness, 4
Oily, 11
Onset, 217
Ooze, 4, 11, 21
Optic nerve, 34
Oral herpes, 60
Oral thrush, 56, 58, 60
Osteoarthritis, 184–187, 189, 191, 203
Osteomyelitis, 181
Osteoporosis, 181–182, 184, 187–189, 191
"Out of breath," 122
Outbreaks, 261
Ovarian cancer, 282
Ovarian cyst, 276, 282
Ovary, 278, 286
Overactive, 77, 87
Overactive bladder, 231, 234–236, 238–240, 248
Overactivity, 80, 233
Overflow, 240
Overflow incontinence, 239

Overproduction, 87
Ovulation, 278, 286

P
Pacemaker, 130
Paget's disease, 181
"Paid through the nose," 51
Pain, 134
Painful, 55
Palate, 58, 60
Paleness, 80–81
Pallor, 80, 87
Palpitations, 129, 132, 139
Pancreas, 158, 165
Panic, 210, 226
Panic attack, 217
Pap smear, 286
Paralysis, 130, 132, 139, 150
Parkinson's disease, 207, 211–212, 214,
    216, 232
Partial seizures, 208
"Pat on the back," 199, 201
Patch, 4, 11
Patient complaints
    cardiovascular system, 134–135
    chest, 107–109
    ears, 29–30
    endocrine system, 82–83
    eyes, 29–30
    hair, 5–7
    heart, 134–135
    hepatic system, 257–258
    lung, 107–109
    lymphatic system, 82–83
    mental health, 212–213
    mouth, 55–56
    musculoskeletal system, 185–187
    nails, 5–7
    neurologic system, 212–213
    nose, 55–56
    reproductive system, 280–282
    respiratory system, 107–109
    skin, 5–7
    urinary system, 235–236
Patient history and physical database
    form, 322–329
"Peace of mind," 224
Peeling, 11
Pelvic inflammatory disease, 275,
    279–280, 284, 286
Pelvis, 240, 278, 286
Penis, 278, 286, 293
Peptic ulcers, 159–160, 162, 165
Perforated eardrum, 28, 34, 44
Pericarditis, 135–136
Perimenopause, 280, 283, 285–286, 294
Peripheral artery disease, 133, 137, 139
Peripheral vascular disease, 136, 139
Peripheral vision, 34
Pernicious anemia, 261, 269

Persistence, 106
Persistent cough, 112, 123
Perspiration, 106, 112
Perspiring, 103
Pertussis, 104, 106, 108, 110, 112
Pessary, 240
Pharmacist/patient dialogues
    answers to, 413–471
    cardiovascular system, 142–147,
        151–154
    chest, 115–119, 123–127
    ears, 37–41, 45–49
    endocrine system, 90–96, 98–101
    eyes, 37–41, 45–49
    hair, 14–17, 21–23
    heart, 142–147, 151–154
    hepatic system, 264–268, 270–274
    lung, 115–119, 123–127
    lymphatic system, 90–96, 98–101
    mental health, 220–223, 227–230
    mouth, 63–66, 71–75
    musculoskeletal system, 194–198,
        203–206
    nails, 14–17, 21–23
    neurologic system, 220–223, 227–230
    nose, 63–66, 71–75
    reproductive system, 289–293,
        295–299
    respiratory system, 115–119, 123–127
    skin, 14–17, 21–23
    urinary system, 243–247, 249–252
Pharmacotherapy workup notes,
    473–480
Pharmacy documentation, 301–332
Phlegm, 55–57, 59–60
Phobia, 210, 217
Photophobia, 33–34
Photosensitivity, 184, 191
"Pick someone's brain," 224, 226
Pick the nose, 60
"Piece of one's mind," 224, 226
Pill rolling, 217
Pimples, 4, 7, 11, 29
Pink eye, 25–26, 31, 33–34
Pins and needles, 11
Pituitary gland, 87
Plaque, 60, 139
Platelet, 261
Pleurisy, 103, 106, 108, 112
Pneumonia, 103, 106–109
Pneumothorax, 103, 107
"Poke your nose into something," 67
Polycystic ovary syndrome, 280, 286
Portal hypertension, 261
Postnasal drip, 51, 55, 57, 60
Postpartum, 286
Posture, 184
Postvoid residual urine, 240
Pouch, 165
Pregnancy, 278

Premature ovarian failure, 282, 284
Premenstrual syndrome, 276, 281, 286,
    293, 295
Presbyopia, 28–29, 32, 34
Pressure, 28, 30, 81
Prickly heat, 11
Progesterone, 286
Progress, 210
Progressive, 217
Prolapse, 135
Pronunciations
    abdomen, 164–166
    cardiovascular system, 138–140
    chest, 86–87
    Chinese variations, 13, 36, 62, 89,
        114, 141, 167, 193, 218, 242,
        262, 288
    ears, 33–35
    endocrine system, 86–87
    eyes, 33–35
    gastrointestinal system, 164–166
    Gujarati variations, 12, 36, 62, 88,
        113–114, 140–141, 166, 192, 218,
        241, 287
    hair, 10–11
    heart, 138–140
    hepatic system, 261–262
    Korean variations, 12–13, 36, 62, 88,
        114, 141, 167, 192, 218, 241,
        262, 288
    lung, 86–87
    lymphatic system, 86–87
    mental health, 216–217
    mouth, 59–61
    musculoskeletal system, 190–192
    nails, 10–11
    neurologic system, 216–217
    nose, 59–61
    reproductive system, 285–287
    respiratory system, 86–87
    Russian variations, 13, 36, 62, 89,
        114, 141, 167, 193, 218, 242,
        263, 288
    skin, 10–11
    Spanish variations, 12, 35, 61, 88,
        113, 140, 166, 192, 218, 241, 262,
        287
    urinary system, 240–241
    Vietnamese variations, 12, 35, 61, 88,
        113, 140, 166, 192, 218, 241,
        262, 287
Prostate cancer, 231, 234
Protruding, 77, 81, 87
Protrusion, 80
Psoriasis, 4, 11
Puff, 80, 112
Puffiness, 80–81, 84, 97
Puffy, 87
Pulmonary embolism, 103, 108, 112
Pulse, 132, 139

Pump, 139
Pupil, 34
Pus, 1–2, 4, 11

R
"Rack one's brains," 224
Radioactive iodine therapy, 84
Ragweed, 60
Range of motion, 191
Rapid breathing, 112
Rash, 11, 81
Rectal, 177
Rectum, 158, 165
Recurrence, 54
Reflux, 165
Regulate, 87
Regulation, 80
Regurgitation, 158, 165
Relapse, 80, 87, 191
Relief, 54–55
Relieve, 70
Remission, 191
Reproductive system
    Chinese pronunciations, 288
    dialogues, 386–391
    dictation, 288–289
    Gujarati pronunciations, 287
    idiomatic expressions using, 293
    Korean pronunciations, 288
    medical conditions and patient
        complaints, 280–282
    multiple choice questions, 275–276,
        294–295
    parts of speech, 277–285
    pharmacist/patient dialogues,
        289–293, 295–299
    pronunciation exercise, 285–287
    Russian pronunciations, 288
    Spanish pronunciations, 287
    true/false questions, 275, 293–294
    Vietnamese pronunciations, 287
    vocabulary, 276–277, 282–285
    word forms, 277–282
Residue, 233
Respiratory system
    Chinese pronunciations, 114
    dialogues, 349–354
    dictation, 114–115
    Gujarati pronunciations, 113–114
    idiomatic expressions using, 120
    Korean pronunciations, 114
    medical conditions and patient
        complaints, 107–109
    multiple choice questions, 103–104,
        122–123
    parts of speech, 105–111
    pharmacist/patient dialogues,
        115–119, 123–127
    pronunciation exercise, 86–87
    Russian pronunciations, 114

Spanish pronunciations, 113
    true/false questions, 103, 122
    Vietnamese pronunciations, 113
    vocabulary, 104–105
    word forms, 105–109
Rest, 150
Retention, 80
Retentiveness, 80
Retina, 34
Rheumatism, 184, 191
Rheumatoid arthritis, 181, 184, 186,
    188–189
Rhinoplasty, 51, 60
Rigidity, 210, 217, 227
Ring, 28
Ringing, 34
Rouse, 217
"Run in one's blood," 95
Runny nose, 51, 55, 59–60
Rupture, 4, 11, 29–30
Ruptured cyst, 8
Ruptured eardrum, 31, 33
Russian pronunciations, 13, 36, 62, 89,
    114, 141, 167, 193, 218, 242,
    263, 288

S
Saliva, 56, 60
"Save your breath," 120
"Say something under one's breath," 120
Scab, 4, 6–7, 11
Scabies, 11, 286
Scales, 11
Scar, 1, 4, 8, 11
"Scared stiff," 199, 202
Scarred, 21
Scarring, 30, 261
Schatzki's ring, 161–162, 165
Scleroderma, 181, 185–188,
    190–191, 202
Scrape, 4, 6, 8, 11
Scratch, 11, 20
Scratchiness, 55–56
"Scratching one's head," 207
Scratchy throat, 60
"Scream at the top of one's lungs," 120
"Sealed lips," 68
Seasonal affective disorder, 207–208,
    211–216, 227
Secrete, 34
Seizures, 207–208, 210, 217
Semen, 278, 286, 294
Seminal fluid, 286
Sensitivity, 184
Septicemia, 233, 240
Sex, 279
Sexually transmitted disease, 286
Sexually transmitted infection, 286
Shakiness, 106
Shaking chills, 112

Shallow breathing, 104, 112
Shallowness, 106
Sharp pain, 112
Sharpness, 106
Shingles, 7–8, 11
Shiver, 106
Shivering, 112
"Shivers up/down one's spine," 199
"Shoots his or her mouth off," 52
Shortness of breath, 103–104, 108, 112,
    123, 135
"Shouting at the top of one's lungs," 103
Shuffling walk, 217
Silk, 11
"Sing one's heart out," 148
Sinus infection, 55–56, 60
Sinus passages, 60
Sinusitis, 51
Sjögren's syndrome, 181, 184–185,
    190–191
Skin
    Chinese pronunciations, 13
    dialogues, 333–336
    Gujarati pronunciations, 12
    idiomatic expressions using, 17–18
    Korean pronunciations, 12–13
    medical conditions and patient
        complaints, 5–7
    multiple-choice questions for, 1–2,
        20–21
    parts of speech, 3–9
    pharmacist/patient dialogues
        involving, 14–17, 21–23
    pronunciations, 10–11
    Russian pronunciations, 13
    Spanish pronunciations, 12
    true/false questions regarding, 1, 19–20
    Vietnamese pronunciations, 12
    vocabulary for, 3, 7–9
    word forms, 3–7
"Skin deep," 18
"Skin of my teeth," 17
"Skin off one's nose," 67
Skipping heart beat, 139
Sleepiness, 82
"Slip of the tongue," 68
Slur, 210
Slurred speech, 217
"Smile from ear to ear," 42
Smoking, 107–108, 187
Sneeze, 54
Sneezing, 60
Snores, 52, 56
Snoring, 60
SOAP notes, 318–322
Sore, 4, 11
Sore throat, 59–60
Spanish pronunciations, 12, 35, 61, 88,
    113, 140, 166, 192, 218, 241,
    262, 287

Spasm, 132, 139
Sperm, 282, 286, 294
Spermicide, 286
Spider angioma, 261
Spinal tap, 217
Spine, 184, 191
Spit, 60, 106, 112
Sputum, 55–56, 59–60
Squeezing, 132, 139, 151
Squint, 28, 34
Squinter, 28
"Stab someone in the back," 199
Stage, 83
Stare, 210
Staring spells, 217
"Stick your nose into something," 67
Stiff, 87, 181, 191
"Stiff," 199
"Stiff upper lip," 68, 195
"Stiff-necked," 199, 202
Stiffness, 80, 97, 184
Stomach acid, 165
Stool, 81, 165
Stooped posture, 191, 202, 226
Strain, 165
Strep throat, 55, 59–60
Stress, 184, 191
Stress incontinence, 231, 234–235,
    239, 247
Stretchability, 184, 191
Stroke, 129, 133, 135, 139
Stuffiness, 54
Stuffy nose, 52, 54, 57, 59
Stye, 25, 29–31, 33
Subside, 191
Substance abuse, 281
Sufferer, 54–55
Suffering, 54
Suicide, 210, 217
Sunscreen, 11
Superficial, 11
Superficial wound, 8, 21
Susceptible, 191
Susceptibleness, 184
Swallow, 54, 80, 87, 158, 165
Swallowing, 56, 156
Sweat, 4, 11, 20
Swell, 4, 21, 25, 44, 51
Swelling, 30, 56, 81, 83
Swimmer's ear, 30, 32–34
Swollen, 11, 54
Syncope, 132, 139
Syndrome, 279
Synovitis, 184, 191, 201
Syphilis, 279

T
Tachycardia, 132, 139
"Take someone's words out of his or her
    mouth," 68

Taste buds, 56, 61
Tear, 28–30, 34
"Tear my hair out," 18–20, 196
Tearfulness, 28
Tearing, 30
Teething, 56–57, 70–71
Temporomandibular joint, 191
Tender, 87
Tenderness, 54, 80, 158, 165
Tendonitis, 181, 191
Testicle, 279, 286
Testicular cancer, 280, 284, 294
Testosterone, 286
Therapy, 210
"Thick skinned," 17
Thickening, 132, 139
Thirst, 80, 87
Throb, 132, 139
Thrombosis, 133, 139
Thrush, 51, 56, 58
Thyroid, 77, 80
Thyroid cancer, 82
Thyroid nodule, 78
Thyroiditis, 80
TIA, 129, 134
Tick bite, 11
Tightness, 104, 106, 112, 123
Tingle, 54, 61
Tingling, 70
Tinnitus, 30, 34
Toilet, 240
Tolerance, 80
Tolerated, 98
Tongue, 68
Tonsils, 61
Tooth, 54, 61
Total incontinence, 232
"Tough as nails," 18–20
Toxic, 255
Toxic shock syndrome, 275, 286
Toxicity, 269
Toxin, 253, 261
Trachea, 82
Transient ischemic attack,
    129, 134
Transmission, 279
Transplant, 255, 268
Transplantation, 135
Tremble, 80, 87, 96
Trembler, 80
Tremor, 80–81, 217
Tuberculosis, 103, 109
Tug, 28, 35
Tugged, 45
Tugging, 29
Tunnel vision, 26, 33
"Turn a deaf ear," 42
"Turn one's stomach," 174–175
"Turn your stomach," 156
Twitch, 28, 35, 210, 217

U
Ulcer, 4, 11
Ulcerates, 54
Ulceration, 4
Ulcerative colitis, 156, 159–160,
    162, 164
"Under one's nose," 67
Underactive, 87
Underarm, 87
Underproduction, 87
Unquenchable, 87
Unsteadiness, 210, 217
"Up to your ears," 42
Urethra, 233, 240
Urethritis, 231, 235–236, 240, 247
Urge incontinence, 238–239
Urgency, 155
Urinalysis, 233, 240
Urinary incontinence, 231–232, 234
Urinary sphincter, 240
Urinary system
    Chinese pronunciations, 242
    dialogues, 377–381
    dictation, 242–243
    Gujarati pronunciations, 241
    idiomatic expressions using, 247
    Korean pronunciations, 241
    medical conditions and patient
        complaints, 235–236
    multiple choice questions, 231–232,
        248–249
    parts of speech, 233–239
    pharmacist/patient dialogues,
        243–247, 249–252
    pronunciation exercise, 240–241
    Russian pronunciations, 242
    Spanish pronunciations, 241
    true/false questions, 231, 247
    Vietnamese pronunciations, 241
    vocabulary, 232–233, 237–239
    word forms, 233–236
Urinary tract infection, 231–232, 234,
    238–240
Urinate, 87, 240
Urination, 80, 247
Urine, 80–81, 233, 240
Uterine fibroids, 275, 286
Uterus, 279

V
Vaccination, 261
Vaccine, 255
Vagina, 279
Vaginitis, 275, 279, 281, 286
Varices, 268
Vein, 132, 139
Venereal disease, 287
Vertebrae, 191
Vertigo, 29, 35
Vessel, 132

Vietnamese pronunciations, 12, 35, 61, 88, 113, 140, 166, 192, 218, 241, 262, 287
Viral hepatitis, 261
Virus, 255
Vocabulary
    abdomen, 156–157, 161–164
    cardiovascular system, 130–131, 135–138
    chest, 104–105
    ears, 26–27, 31–33
    endocrine system, 78–79
    eyes, 27, 31–33
    gastrointestinal system, 156–157, 161–164
    hair, 3, 7–9
    heart, 130–131, 135–138
    hepatic system, 254–255, 258–260
    lung, 104–105
    lymphatic system, 78–79
    mental health, 213–214
    mouth, 52–53, 57–59
    musculoskeletal system, 182–183, 187–190
    nails, 3, 7–9
    neurologic system, 213–214
    nose, 52–53, 57–59
    pharmacy documentation, 302–318
    reproductive system, 276–277, 282–285
    respiratory system, 104–105
    skin, 3, 7–9
    urinary system, 232–233, 237–239
Void, 231, 240
Voluntary muscles, 217
Volunteer, 210
Vomit, 132, 139

W
"Wait with bated breath," 120
Walking pneumonia, 107, 113
Wanderer, 210
Wandering, 217
Wart, 7–8, 11
"Waste one's breath," 120

Water, 54
Water retention, 87
Wax, 28, 30, 35
Wear and tear, 191
"Wear one's heart on one's sleeve," 148
Weight loss, 81
"Wet behind the ears," 42
Wheezer, 106
Wheezing, 103, 109, 113
Whooping cough, 108, 113, 122
Windpipe, 77, 82, 84, 87, 96
"Work one's fingers to the bone," 199
Workup notes, 473–480
Wound, 4, 11, 21, 71
Wrinkles, 11

Y
Yeast, 279
Yeast infection, 275, 284, 287, 293
"Yell at the top of one's lungs," 120, 196

Z
Zit, 11